Jeanett

COGNITIVE THERAPY OF SUBSTANCE ABUSE

Cognitive Therapy of Substance Abuse

Aaron T. Beck, M.D.
Fred D. Wright, Ed.D.
Cory F. Newman, Ph.D.
Bruce S. Liese, Ph.D.

THE GUILFORD PRESS
New York   London

© 1993 The Guilford Press
A Division of Guilford Publications, Inc.
72 Spring Street, New York, NY 10012

Printed in the United States of America

This book is printed on acid-free paper.

Last digit is print number: 9 8 7 6 5 4 3 2

Library of Congress Cataloging-in-Publication Data

Cognitive therapy of substance abuse / Aaron T. Beck . . . [et al.].
    p. cm.
  Includes bibliographical references and index.
  ISBN 0-89862-115-1
  1. Substance abuse—Treatment. 2. Cognitive therapy. I. Beck,
Aaron T.
  [DNLM: 1. Cognitive Therapy—methods. 2. Substance Abuse—
therapy. WM 270 C6765 1993]
RC564.C623 1993
616.86'0651—dc20
DNLM/DLC
for Library of Congress   93-5208
                                      CIP

To Phyllis, Gwen, Jane, and Ziana

Preface

Substance abuse is widely recognized as a serious social and legal problem. In fact, the use of illegal drugs may be responsible for more than 25% of property crimes and 15% of violent crimes. Financial losses related to these crimes have been estimated at $1.7 billion per year. Homicides are also strongly linked to drug dealing. Approximately 14% of homicides per year are causally related to drugs. The costs for criminal justice activities directed against drug trafficking on the federal level were approximately $2.5 billion in 1988, compared to $1.76 billion spent in 1986.

There are also many health problems caused by these drugs. Alcohol can damage almost every body organ, including the heart, brain, liver, and stomach. Illegal drugs such as cocaine can have a serious effect on the neurological, cardiovascular, and respiratory systems. Cigarettes can cause cancer, heart disease, and more. The most widely used and abused drug in the world is alcohol. In the United States, two-thirds of the population drink alcohol. About ten out of a hundred people have problems with alcohol so serious that they can be considered "alcoholic" or "alcohol-dependent." (Interestingly, this 10% of Americans buys and drinks more than half of the alcoholic beverages!)

At least 14 million Americans take illegal drugs every month. During "peak months" this number climbs to more than 25 million users. Some experts have estimated that approximately 2.3% of Americans over 12 years of age have a problem with illegal drugs serious enough to warrant drug treatment.

To a large degree, we have tried to put a halt to drug abuse by making drugs illegal. For example, heroin and cocaine are presently illegal in the United States. Cigarette smoking is becoming increasingly proscribed. At one time we tried to stop alcoholism by legal mechanisms (i.e., prohibition). Obviously, these methods will never make substances completely unavailable.

Not all people who use drugs become addicted to them, although many people have asked themselves, "Am I [or is someone else] an alcoholic [or a substance abuser]?" The American Psychiatric Association has defined the addictions very specifically. In fact, the official term for an addiction is "substance dependence." There are some specific signs of substance dependence, including (1) heavy use of the substance, (2) continued use even though it may cause problems to the person, (3) tolerance, and (4) withdrawal symptoms.

Cultural and historical factors are implicated in substance use and abuse. The patterns and consequences of drug use have been influenced by historical developments, which have had positive and negative effects. Two centuries ago, the extraction of pure chemicals from plant materials created more powerful medicinal agents. The invention of the hypodermic needle in the middle of the nineteenth century was also a medical boon, which, on the other hand, allowed drug users to circumvent the body's natural biological controls consisting of bitter taste and slow absorption through the digestive tract. Many synthetic drugs developed in the twentieth century had medical application but created further opportunities for abuse and addiction. In short, any activity that affects the reward mechanisms of the brain may lead to compulsive, self-defeating behavior.

Social, environmental, and personality factors have affected substance use and abuse in ways that go far beyond the simple pharmacological properties of these agents. Alcoholism, for example, is prevalent among certain ethnic groups and practically absent among others, such as the Mormons, who require abstinence for group acceptance. On the other hand, other social subgroups may condition group acceptance on using or drinking. The social milieu may influence using. Soldiers used illegal drugs extensively in Vietnam but, for the most part, relinquished heavy drug use after returning home. Impoverished environments have been shown in both animal experiments and human studies to lead to addiction. As pointed out by Peele, the common denominator is the lack of other opportunities for satisfaction. Finally, our clinical experiences have indicated that addicted individuals have certain clusters of addictive attitudes that make them abusers rather than users.

Successful treatment depends on clinicians' effectiveness in dealing with these addictive potentials. And what form will this care take? As pointed out by Marc Galanter, president of the American Academy of Psychiatrists in Alcoholism and Addiction, the long-term efficacy of new pharmacological treatments is open to question. "Tricyclics, dopaminergic agents, and carbamazapine for cocaine abusers have yet to be substantiated as a vehicle for continuing care. For opiates, naltrexone and buprenorphine offer only a modest niche in the domain that was traditionally occupied by methadone maintenance. Intervention in GABAergic transmission may hold promise for alcoholism, but that promise is far from clinical application" (Galanter, 1993, pp. 1–2).

We have written this book in response to the ever-growing need to formulate and test cost-effective treatments for substance abuse disorders, problems that seem to be multiplying in the population in spite of society's best efforts at international interdiction and domestic control and education. We believe that cognitive therapy, a well-documented and demonstrably efficacious treatment model, can be a major boon to meeting this pressing need.

At one time, "drug abuse rehabilitation counseling" was regarded as a specialty area in the field of psychotherapy—now it is apparent that almost all who engage in clinical practice will encounter patients who use and abuse drugs. Therefore, it would be desirable for all mental health professionals to receive some sort of routine training and education in the social and psychological phenomena that comprise the addiction disorders. Our volume is intended to provide a thorough, detailed set of methods that can be of immediate use to therapists and counselors—regardless of the amount of experience they might have had with cognitive therapy, or in the field of addictions. Toward this end, we have strived to make our model and our procedures as specific and complete as possible. We certainly recommend that those who read this book also read the many valuable sources we have cited in the text. Nevertheless, our intention in writing *Cognitive Therapy of Substance Abuse* has been to provide a convenient, centralized source that is comprehensive, teachable, and testable.

Although advances in the field have been made in the form of pharmacological interventions (e.g., antabuse, methadone, and naltrexone), 12-step support groups (e.g., Alcoholics Anonymous, Narcotics Anonymous, and Cocaine Anonymous), and social-learning models and programs (relapse prevention, rational recovery, etc.), each of these approaches has posed problems that limit its respective potential efficacy. For example, pharmacological interventions have produced promising short-term data but are fraught with compliance and long-term maintenance difficulties—patients may not take their chemical agonists and antagonists, and they are prone to relapse when the medications are discontinued. Twelve-step programs provide valuable social support and consistent guidance principles for individuals who voluntarily join and faithfully attend the program meetings, but cannot address the needs of those who will not enter the programs or who drop out. Social-learning approaches provide sophisticated models of substance abuse and relapse, and hold promise to produce and accumulate empirical data, but thus far the resultant treatments (with very few exceptions) have been less well described than the theories that gave rise to them.

Although the cognitive approach that we have explicated is most closely related to the social-learning theories of substance abuse, we want to emphasize that we find value in all of the aforementioned treatment modalities. Cognitive therapy is not in "opposition" to 12-step or psychobiological models of substance abuse. We have found that these alternative treatment systems may be *complementary* to our procedures. Many of the substance abuse patients that we treat at the Center for Cognitive Therapy concurrently attend Narcotics Anonymous and similar 12-step groups. Other patients take the full spectrum of pharmacologic agents, from antidepressants to antabuse, under strict medical guidance. The individualized conceptualization of patients' belief systems and the long-term coping skills (to deal with everyday life concerns, as well as to manage cravings and urges specific to drug use) that cognitive therapy provides for patients can mesh well with medication and 12-step meetings. The main variable that seems to influence whether or not patients avail themselves of all of these treatment opportunities (once they have been presented to the patients in a feasible manner) is *not* the practical compatibility of the treatments, but rather *the attitudes of the treatment providers*!

At present, an earlier draft of this book is serving as a treatment manual in a National Institute on Drug Abuse collaborative, multisite study on the respective efficacy of cognitive therapy, supportive–expressive therapy, and general drug counseling. Data obtained from this project will help us to answer two important questions: (1) Does *Cognitive Therapy of Substance Abuse* succeed as a manual for the training of competent cognitive therapists for patients with addictions? and (2) Do patients who receive the treatment outlined in the text make demonstrable and lasting gains? In order to answer these questions, therapists are provided with intensive supervision (note: the authors of this text serve in that role), complete with competency and adherence ratings on a regular basis; treatment is *not* confounded with adjunct medications, urinalyses are routinely conducted, and a host of measures *other* than drug monitoring per se are being administered and evaluated (to examine changes in mood and global adaptational functioning).

Drug abuse is a sociological problem as well as a psychological issue. Factors such as poverty and lack of adequate educational and vocational opportunities play a role in the epidemic. However, we believe that it is harmful to assume that low socioeconomic status patients cannot be treated as effectively as those of higher socioeconomic status. While social change is desirable, individual change is not necessarily dependent on it. We are optimistic that cognitive therapy can serve as an important individual-focused treatment in today's society, and that the data will support this.

Acknowledgments

We would like to offer our thanks to our highly esteemed colleagues in the field of substance abuse treatment and research, Drs. Dan Baker, Lino Covi, Tom Horvath, Jerome Platt, Hal Urschel, David Wilson, and Emmett Velten, for their extremely helpful insights and suggestions on earlier versions of this manuscript. Special thanks are due Dr. Kevin Kuehlwein, an important member of our own cognitive therapy team in Philadelphia, for his thorough evaluations and editorial work on many of the chapters in this book. The input of all of the above has been invaluable during the course of this project. We would also like to offer our thanks and appreciation to Tina Inforzato, who did yeoman work in typing this volume, and its many revisions. Without her tireless efforts, this volume would still be "on the drawing board."

Contents

CHAPTER 1

Overview of Substance Abuse

The fabric of America is profoundly affected by problems of substance abuse. They are problems that directly affect those millions of Americans who suffer from substance abuse and indirectly touch the lives of millions more in the larger social and vocational networks around them. One in every ten adults in this country has a serious alcohol problem (Institute of Medicine [IOM], 1987) and at least one in four is addicted to nicotine (Centers for Disease Control [CDC], 1991a). Approximately 1 in 35 Americans over the age of 12 abuses illicit drugs (IOM, 1990a). This level of substance abuse has profound social, medical, and psychological ramifications on both the individual and the larger societal levels. The CDC (1991b), for example, estimate that approximately 434,000 people in this country die each year as a result of cigarette smoking, and many thousands also die as a result of alcoholism (IOM, 1987) and/or illicit drug abuse (IOM, 1990a). It must be emphasized, however, that substance abuse spans many more areas and the toll taken is far greater than these simple mortality figures convey.

In this introductory chapter we set the stage for the cognitive therapy of substance abuse. We begin with an overview of psychoactive substances and substance abuse, we briefly review the history of psychoactive substance use, we describe the most commonly used and abused psychoactive substances, we discuss cognitive models for understanding substance abuse and relapse, and we scan traditional methods for treating substance abuse.

BACKGROUND: PSYCHOACTIVE
SUBSTANCES AND SUBSTANCE ABUSE

Psychoactive substances are chemicals that affect the central nervous system, altering the user's thoughts, moods, and/or behaviors. The revised third edition of the *Diagnostic and Statistical Manual of Mental Disorders* (DSM-III-R; American Psychiatric Association [APA], 1987) categorizes psychoactive substances into 10 classes: alcohol; amphetamines or similarly acting sympathomimetics; cannabis; cocaine; hallucinogens; inhalants; nicotine; opioids; phencyclidine (PCP) or similarly acting arylcyclohexylamines; and sedatives, hypnotics, or anxiolytics. Each of these substances has unique properties and effects. Some substances that are abused have low addictive potential (e.g., hallucinogens), while others have high addictive potential (e.g., crack cocaine). Some are typically smoked (e.g., nicotine, cannabis, and crack cocaine); others are ingested orally (e.g., hallucinogens and sedatives); while still others are taken intranasally (e.g., powdered cocaine and inhalants). Some drugs lead the user to feel "up" or energized (e.g., amphetamines and cocaine); some cause the user to feel "down" or relaxed (e.g., sedatives, hypnotics, and anxiolytics); while others (e.g, alcohol and nicotine) simultaneously have both effects on the user.

DSM-III-R distinguishes between substance abuse and dependence. *Abuse* is defined as a maladaptive pattern of psychoactive substance use while *dependence* (considered more serious than abuse) is defined as "impaired control of use" (i.e., physiological addiction). In this volume, we do not go to great lengths to emphasize this distinction. Instead, we view any pattern of psychoactive substance use as problematic and requiring intervention if it results in adverse social, vocational, legal, medical, or interpersonal consequences, regardless of whether the abuser experiences physiological tolerance or withdrawal. Further, although we caution against an all-or-none view of addiction and recovery, and although we acknowledge that some patients seem to be more successful at engaging in controlled, moderate substance use than are others, we advocate a program of treatment that strives for abstinence. In this manner we maximize the patients' chances of maintaining an able and responsible lifestyle, reduce the risk of relapse, and avoid giving patients the false impression that we view a mere *reduction* in drug use as the optimal outcome.

History of Psychoactive Substance Use

Psychoactive substances have been used by most cultures since prehistoric times (Westermeyer, 1991). In fact, for centuries psychoactive substances have served many individual and social functions. On an individual level, they have provided stimulation, relief from adverse emotional states and uncomfortable physical symptoms, and altered states of consciousness. On a social level, psychoactive substances have facilitated religious rituals, ceremonies, and medical functions. Egyptian and Chinese opiate use was evident from the earliest writings of these people (Westermeyer, 1991). Marijuana was referenced in India "as far back as the second millennium B.C." (Brecher, 1972, p. 397). Evidence of Mayan, Aztec, and Incan medicinal and ritual drug use was evident from their statues and from drawings on their buildings and pottery (Karan, Haller, & Schnoll, 1991; Westermeyer, 1991). Alcohol use goes back to paleolithic times (Goodwin, 1981) and Mesopotamian civilization gave one of the earliest clinical descriptions of intoxication and hangover cures.

In modern times the World Health Organization (WHO) has been concerned about drug and alcohol abuse problems on a worldwide scale (Grant, 1986). As early as 1968 the WHO conducted an international study of drug use in youth (Cameron, 1968), and in a more recent study (Smart, Murray, & Arif, 1988) drug abuse and prevention programs in 29 countries were reviewed. However, Smart and his colleagues concluded from their review that "the seriousness of the drug problem is well recognized in some countries but not in others" (p. 16). Presently the WHO is addressing the issue of alcohol-related problems by developing an international secondary prevention protocol (Babor, Korner, Wilber, & Good, 1987).

Drug policies in the United States have been profoundly affected by historical and sociocultural attitudes regarding psychoactive drugs on a spectrum from less restrictive (e.g., libertarian) to more restrictive (i.e., criminal). Between the late 1700s and the late 1800s, for example, psychoactive drugs (especially narcotics) were widely used in the United States. In fact, Musto (1991) reported that opium and cocaine were legally available during this time from "the local druggist." A Consumers Union report (Brecher, 1972) described the nineteenth century as "a dope fiend's paradise" due to such minimal restrictions. In the late 1800s and the early 1900s, medical conceptualizations of addiction began to develop, however, influenced to some extent by Dr. Benjamin Rush's (1790) earlier interest in the course of addictions. Magnus Huss, a Swedish physician, first used the term "alcoholism" in 1849 (IOM, 1990b). At the same time (late 1800s and early 1900s), criminalization of drug use was increasingly becoming U.S. policy. In the 1960s and 1970s, however, attitudes about drugs became less restrictive as U.S. sociopolitical attitudes generally became more liberal. Simultaneously, the disease model of addictions was gaining widespread acceptance, partly due to the work of Jellinek (1960).

Since the 1980s, the United States has again become less tolerant and more restrictive about drugs. At least two explanations can account for this phenomenon: (1) The negative effects of drugs on individuals, families, and society have become more apparent with increased use, and (2) sociopolitical attitudes in the United States generally have become more conservative. At the same time, however, there is increasing controversy about the disease model of addiction ("Current Disease model," 1992; Fingarette, 1988; Peele & Brodsky, with Arnold, 1991) and the criminalization of psychoactive substances (R. L. Miller, 1991).

The Most Commonly Used Drugs

Alcohol

Alcohol is simultaneously a chemical, a beverage, and a drug that "powerfully modifies the functioning of the nervous system" (Levin, 1990, p. 1). Approximately 10% of Americans in the United States have a serious drinking problem; 60% are light to moderate drinkers; and the remaining 30% of adults in the United States do not consume any alcohol. Alcohol abuse, however, accounts for approximately 81% of hospitalizations for substance abuse disorders (IOM, 1987). Remarkably, half the alcohol consumed in this country is consumed by the 10% who are heavy drinkers. A larger percentage of men than women drink and a greater percentage of men than women are heavy drinkers.

Alcohol initially acts as a general anesthetic, interfering with subtle functions of thought, reason, and judgment (Miller & Munoz, 1976). As blood alcohol concentration (BAC) increases, however, the effects become more intense until gross motor functioning is also affected. At still higher BAC levels, sleep is induced, and ultimately death may occur as a result of respiratory depression.

"Alcohol affects almost every organ system in the body either directly or indirectly" (National Institute of Alcohol Abuse and Alcoholism [NIAAA], 1990, p. 107). Thus with chronic use, alcohol can cause serious multiple medical problems, including damage to the liver, pancreas, gastrointestinal tract, cardiovascular system, immune system, endocrine system, and nervous system. Alcohol has also been strongly linked to the leading causes of accidental death in the United States: motor vehicle accident, falls, and fire-related injuries. Furthermore, approximately 30% of suicides and half of all homicides are alcohol related (IOM, 1987), and estimates of annual deaths related to alcohol use range between 69,000 and 200,000 per year (IOM,

1987). In addition, a significant percentage of both violent and non-violent crimes are committed under the influence of alcohol (cf. McCord, 1992). Chronic alcohol use can also have other profound negative social consequences, including loss of career, friends, and family. A great deal of physical and sexual abuse, for example, is related to the intoxicated state of the offender (Clayton, 1992; Frances & Miller, 1991; Harstone & Hansen, 1984), and general family dysfunction often is associated with the alcoholism of one or more adult members (Heath & Stanton, 1991). Medical complications can even reach insidiously into the next generation, in that maternal drinking during pregnancy can cause fetal alcohol syndrome and other serious birth defects. In fact, "prenatal alcohol exposure is one of the leading known causes of mental retardation in the western world" (NIAAA, 1990, p. 139).

Illicit Drugs

According to the IOM (1990a), at least 14 million persons consume illicit drugs monthly. During peak months this figures climbs to more than 25 million users. It is estimated that approximately 2.3% of the U.S. population over 12 years old has an illicit drug problem sufficiently serious to warrant treatment. This statistic is substantially higher, however, for individuals who are incarcerated (33%) or on parole or probation (25%). When these people are included in the epidemiologic data, the estimate of illicit drug use problems in the overall population increases to 2.7%.

Regarding the social costs of illicit drug abuse, it is estimated that more than 25% of property crimes and 15% of violent crimes are related to illicit drug use by the criminal. Financial losses related to these crimes have been estimated at $1.7 billion per year. Homicides are also strongly linked to activities surrounding drug dealing. Approximately 14% of homicides per year are causally related to drugs. The costs for criminal justice activities directed against drug trafficking on the federal level were approximately $2.5 billion in 1988, compared to $1.76 billion spent in 1986. In the following sections we present brief descriptions of the three most commonly used illicit drugs: marijuana, cocaine, and the opioids.

In 1972, a Consumers Union report identified marijuana as the fourth most popular psychoactive drug in the world, after caffeine, nicotine, and alcohol (Brecher, 1972, p. 402). Although marijuana's use has declined since its peak in 1979, it still remains the most widely used illicit drug in Western society (APA, 1987; Weiss & Millman, 1991).

Marijuana is typically smoked, although it can also be ingested. According to Weiss and Millman (1991), in spite of its generally sedating effects, marijuana's psychoactive effects in the user are quite varied, "profoundly dependent upon the personality of the user, his or her expectation, and the setting" (p. 160).

The health effects of marijuana have been widely debated and remain quite controversial, probably due to the inconsistent effects of the drug on the individual user and across different users. For some time marijuana was considered relatively safe and nonaddictive (Brecher, 1972). Presently, however, it is associated with multiple adverse physical and psychological effects, including labile affect and depression, amotivational syndrome, impaired short-term memory, and pulmonary disease (Weiss & Millman, 1991). According to DSM-III-R, marijuana dependence is characterized by heavy use of the drug (e.g., daily) with substantial impairment. Marijuana dependence also puts one at risk for other psychological problems, as those who are dependent on cannabis are also likely polysubstance abusers or afflicted with other psychiatric disorders (APA, 1987; Weiss & Millman, 1991).

Cocaine is a major central nervous system stimulant that produces euphoria, alertness, and a sense of well-being. It may also lower anxiety and social inhibitions while increasing energy, self-esteem, and sexuality. Presently cocaine is among the most widely used illicit drugs. In fact, cocaine use increased in 1991, "despite the Bush administration's three-year war against drugs" (Mental Health Report, 1992, p. 5). Clearly, for many people the positive short-term physiological and psychological effects of cocaine maladaptively supersede the dangers associated with acquiring and using the drug. According to Gawin and Ellinwood (1988), "The pursuit of this direct, pharmacologically based euphoria becomes so dominant that the user is apt to ignore signs of mounting personal disaster" (p. 1174).

Cocaine is an alkaloid (as are caffeine and nicotine) which is extracted from the coca leaf. In its pure form, raw coca leaves can be chewed, although this practice is generally limited to native populations in the cocaine-producing countries (APA, 1987).

In the United States, cocaine is most commonly taken intranasally (i.e., snorted or "tooted") in the powder form of cocaine hydrochloride. In this form, the user pours the powder on a hard surface and then arranges it into "lines," one of which is snorted into each nostril (Karan et al., 1991). In powdered form, cocaine hydrochloride can also be mixed with water and administered by intravenous injection. This process is known as "shooting" or "mainlining" (Karan et al., 1991). Intravenous injection of cocaine results in intense subjective and physiologic effects within 30 seconds (Jones, 1987).

Cocaine can also be smoked as a paste or in alkaloid form (i.e., "freebased"). In this form it also produces its effects within seconds. Crack cocaine (named for the sound made by the cocaine as it is freebased) is the currently popular form of freebase which is sold in relatively inexpensive, prepackaged, and ready-to-use small doses (Karan et al., 1991). According to Karan et al. (1991), low-cost crack, approximately $2–$10 per vial, "has been widely available on the streets in many American cities since 1985" (p. 125), making it easily within the financial grasp of most teenagers and even the impoverished. Adding to this high availability is the especially troublesome fact that crack cocaine produces an enormously intense and almost instant high. Crack cocaine is, therefore, extremely addictive, leading to significant impairment in life functioning after only a few weeks' use on average (Gawin & Ellinwood, 1988; Smart, 1991), much faster than, for example, intranasal usage of cocaine. These characteristics of crack cocaine make it especially prone to rapid increase in the prevalence of its abuse.

Indeed, many observers suggest that cocaine use has already reached epidemic levels (Weinstein, Gottheil, & Sterling, 1992). In the popular press, for example, a graphic biographical *Reader's Digest* article describes cocaine as "the devil within" (Ola & D'Aulaire, 1991). This contrasts starkly with the glorification of cocaine in movies and songs of the 1970s and early 1980s, when cocaine was seen as the drug of choice of the affluent and powerful. In the scientific literature, Gawin and Ellinwood (1988) explain that "believing that the drug was safe, millions of people tried cocaine, and cocaine abuse exploded" (p. 1173). These authors report that 15% of Americans have tried cocaine, and 3 million people had abused cocaine regularly by 1986, resulting in "more than five times the number addicted to heroin" (p. 1173). Smart and Adlaf (1990) report also that an increasing number of cocaine abusers have sought treatment since the 1980s. Cohen (1991) attributes the "cocaine outbreak" to supply factors (e.g., low cost, availability, and high profitability), external factors (e.g., peer pressure and media portrayals of drug usage), internal factors (e.g., hedonism, sociopathy, depression, and life stress), and intrinsic drug factors (e.g., "the pharmacologic imperative"). Strikingly, cocaine abuse occurs and persists in spite of dramatic medical problems that are associated with its use: central nervous system damage, cardiac arrest, stroke, respiratory collapse, severe hypertension, exacerbation of chronic diseases, infection, and psychiatric complications (Estroff, 1987). Because cocaine abuse research has produced fewer pharmacological treatment alternatives than has research on some other illicit drugs such as heroin (Alterman, O'Brien, & McLellan, 1991; Covi, Baker, & Hess, 1990; Stine, 1992), and because of the extent and severity of cocaine-related problems, we have placed proportionately greater emphasis on cocaine and crack cocaine than on other drugs in this treatment manual.

The opioids, including heroin, methadone, and codeine, are drugs that pharmacologically resemble morphine. Drugs in this class produce feelings of euphoria, relaxation, and mood elevation. They also have the potential for reducing pain, anxiety, aggression, and sexual drives (IOM, 1990a), and are considered highly addictive. According to Thomason and Dilts (1991):

> Opioids have the capacity to commandeer all of an individual's attention, resources, and energy, and to focus these exclusively on obtaining the next dose at any cost. This vicious cycle repeats itself every few hours, 24 hours a day, 365 days a year, for years on end. Comprehending the implications of opioid abuse shocks and staggers the inquiring mind. (p. 103)

Although the use of pharmacologic agonists such as methadone (and antagonists such as naltrexone) traditionally has represented an important component of treatment in the heroin abuser, methadone itself is unfortunately subject to various forms of abuse (e.g., black market dealings or use with other drugs). Further, many heroin abusers find methadone to be inferior to the "real stuff," leading to high noncompliance and dropout (Grabowski, Stitzer, & Henningfield, 1984) rates with these programs. Therefore, we posit that pharmacologic approaches (even for heroin) represent an incomplete treatment strategy unless utilized in combination with psychosocial approaches such as support groups and cognitive therapy.

Nicotine

Cigarette smoking is by far the single most preventable cause of death in the United States. In fact, it has been estimated that 434,000 people died in 1988 due to cigarette smoking (CDC, 1991b). This figure includes those who died of cancer, lung disease, heart disease, house fires caused by careless smoking, and renal and pancreatic disease. Approximately 49.4 million Americans (28.1%) are regular cigarette smokers (CDC, 1991a), despite the fact that cigarette smoking is known to be a leading cause of morbidity and mortality in this country.

Since the mid-1970s, however, the number of smokers has admittedly decreased steadily. Historically, more men than women have smoked; however, a higher proportion of men than women have also *quit* smoking. It has thus been projected that by the year 1995, more women than men will be smokers. Ironically, in spite of cigarettes' historical and advertising linkage with status, wealth, and desirability, it is increasingly the case that the socially disadvantaged are over-represented as smokers. The number of minorities, poor, and less educated people who smoke, for example, has been disproportionately higher than those who do not smoke, and this trend is expected to continue (Pierce, Fiore, & Novotny, 1989).

Nicotine is the psychopharmacologically addictive ingredient in cigarettes. As mentioned earlier, nicotine dependence is included in DSM-III-R, along with the dependence on other psychoactive substances (alcohol, opiates, cocaine, etc.). Not surprisingly, we have found the addictive process in cigarette smoking to be analogous to the addictive process involved in the other psychoactive substances. Therefore, although nicotine addiction is not associated with the same degree of social, vocational, and legal consequences as is addiction to illicit drugs, its medical hazards and the fact that early-life regular smoking often leads to addiction to "harder" substances (Henning-field, Clayton, & Pollin, 1990) make it an important area for mental health intervention. Although this volume focuses relatively little on methods specifically geared to smoking cessation, we believe that the same principles of assessment and treatment (e.g., coping with cravings and modifying beliefs) that we outline in this book are highly applicable to the patient addicted to nicotine.

Polysubstance Abuse

Individuals abusing one psychoactive substance are likely to be simultaneously abusing another substance. In fact, between 20% and 30% of alcoholics in the general public and approximately 80% in treatment programs are dependent on at least one other drug. A prevalent combination is alcohol, marijuana, and cocaine (N. S. Miller, 1991, p. 198).

N. S. Miller (1991) explains that polysubstance abuse occurs for multiple reasons. For example, some drugs enhance the effects of other drugs, while some drugs are used to avoid unwanted side effects of other drugs. Some drugs are used to treat drug withdrawal effects of other drugs and, similarly, some drugs are used as substitutes for other drugs.

The medical and psychological correlates of polysubstance abuse are numerous (N. S. Miller, 1991). They include problems associated with each individual drug (e.g., liver and heart disease associated with alcohol abuse), as well as those more commonly associated with multiple substances (e.g., interaction-induced overdose).

Dual Diagnosis: Substance Abuse and Other Psychiatric Disorders

The coexistence of substance abuse with other psychiatric disorders is also very common (e.g., Ananth et al., 1989; Brown, Ridgely, Pepper, Levine, & Ryglewicz, 1989; Bunt, Galanter, Lifshutz, & Castaneda, 1990; Davis, 1984; Hesselbrock, Meyer, & Kenner, 1985; Kranzler & Liebowitz, 1988; Nace, Saxon, & Shore, 1986; Nathan, 1988; Penick et al., 1984; Regier et al., 1990; Ross, Glaser, & Germanson, 1988; Schneier & Siris, 1987). In a survey of more than 20,000 Americans conducted by Regier et al. (1990) it was found that individuals with psychiatric disorders were 2.7 times as likely to have alcohol or other drug problems, compared to those without psychiatric disorders. In fact, 37% of individuals with substance use disorders had coexisting Axis I mental disorders.

From these data it appears that individuals with substance abuse problems should benefit most from therapeutic interventions that simultaneously address their other psychiatric disorders. Cognitive therapy is ideally suited for these individuals, since it has been developed and tested on patients with depression, anxiety, and personality disorders (see Hollon & Beck, in press, for a most recent comprehensive review). In fact, an important component of cognitive therapy involves the case conceptualization (Persons, 1989), defined as the evaluation and integration of historical information, psychiatric diagnosis, cognitive profile, and other aspects of functioning (see Chapter 5, this volume, for a detailed description of the case conceptualization). When a coexisting psychiatric syndrome is found to exist with a drug or alcohol abuse patient, for example, the therapist focuses simultaneously on substance abuse and the symptoms of the psychiatric syndrome as well as on any factors of interaction (see Chapters 14, 15, and 16, this volume, for more on the treatment of patients with dual diagnoses).

RELAPSE PREVENTION

Substance abuse and dependence are characterized both by remission and by relapse. In a classic review by Hunt, Barnett, and Branch (1971) it was found that heroin, nicotine, and alcohol were all associated with similar high rates and patterns of relapse (p. 455; see Figure 1.1). These investigators found that two-thirds of individuals treated had relapsed within 3 months. Many investigators have speculated about the meaning of these findings, most inferring

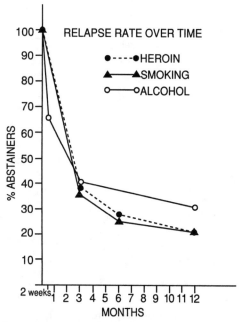

FIGURE 1.1. Relapse rate over time for heroin, smoking, and alcohol addiction. From Hunt, Barnett, and Branch (1971), p. 456. Copyright 1971 by Clinical Psychology Publishing Co., Inc. Reprinted by permission.

that they reflect common processes that underlie the addictions. In fact, since the publication of Hunt et al.'s (1971) data, addiction experts have focused on developing and testing comprehensive models of addiction that include all the psychoactive substances, as well as gambling and binge eating.

Marlatt and his colleagues (Brownell, Marlatt, Lichtenstein, & Wilson, 1986; Marlatt, 1978; Marlatt, 1982; Marlatt & Gordon, 1985) have made an important contribution to the addiction literature with their cognitive-behavioral model of relapse prevention. According to Marlatt and Gordon's (1985) model (see Figure 1.2), individuals view themselves as having a sense of perceived control or self-efficacy. When they are faced with high-risk situations, this sense is threatened. High-risk situations for the drug abuse patient might include negative or positive emotional or physical states, interpersonal conflicts, social pressure, or exposure to drug cues. Individuals faced with high-risk situations must respond with coping responses. Those who have effective coping responses develop increased self-efficacy, resulting in a decreased probability of relapse. Those who have relatively fewer coping responses or none at all may experience decreased self-

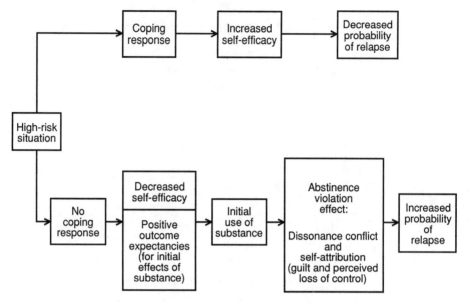

FIGURE 1.2. Model of relapse process. From Marlatt and Gordon (1985), p. 38. Copyright 1985 by The Guilford Press. Reprinted by permission.

efficacy and increased positive outcome expectancies about the effects of the drug, followed by a "lapse" or initial use of a substance. This initial use might result in what Marlatt calls an Abstinence Violation Effect (AVE; i.e., perceived loss of control) and an ultimately increased probability of relapse.

The work of Marlatt and his colleagues has had a profound effect on knowledge about addictive behaviors. In fact, most current textbooks on addictions now deal with the issue of relapse prevention in some way. Although most of the work on relapse prevention has been generated within the cognitive-behavioral model (e.g., Chiauzzi, 1991), various 12–step programs (e.g., Alcoholics Anonymous) and other advocates of the disease model have recently also increased their emphasis on relapse prevention (e.g., Gorski & Miller, 1986).

MODELS OF ADDICTION

Numerous theoretical models have been developed to explain addictive behaviors (see Baker, 1988; Blane & Leonard, 1987, for recent reviews). As previously mentioned, the dominant trend among addiction experts is toward developing comprehensive theoretical models that explain all addictions.

Cognitive Models of Addiction

A variety of related cognitive models of addiction have been developed and evaluated (e.g., Abrams & Niaura, 1987; Marlatt, 1978, 1985; McDermut, Haaga, & Shayne, 1991; Stacy, Newcomb, & Bentler, 1991; Tiffany, 1990; Wilson, 1987a, 1987b) since Bandura's (1969, 1977) classic presentations of cognitive social learning theory.

Marlatt (1985) describes four cognitive processes related to addictions that reflect the cognitive models: self-efficacy, outcome expectancies, attributions of causality, and decision-making processes. Self-efficacy refers to one's judgment about one's ability to deal competently with challenging or high-risk situations. Examples of high self-efficacy beliefs include the following: "I *can* effectively cope with temptations to use drugs" or "I *can* say 'no' to drugs." Examples of low self-efficacy beliefs might include the following: "I'm a slave to drugs," "I *can't* get through the day without drugs," or "I *can't* get what I want, so I might as well use drugs." Marlatt (1985) explains that low levels of self-efficacy are associated with relapse and high levels of self-efficacy are associated with abstinence. Marlatt (1985) also explains that self-efficacy increases as a function of success; to the extent that individuals effectively choose not to use drugs, they will experience an increased sense of self-efficacy, for example, believing that their sense of pride is greater than their need for a "high."

Outcome expectancies refer to an individual's anticipation about the *effects* of an addictive substance or activity. Positive outcome expectancies might include the following beliefs: "It will feel great to party tonight," or "I won't feel so tense if I use." To the extent that one expects a greater positive than negative outcome from using drugs, one is likely to continue using.

Attributions of causality refer to an individual's belief that drug use is attributable to internal or external factors. For example, an individual might believe the following: "Anybody who lives in my neighborhood would be a drug user" (external factor), or "I am physically addicted to alcohol and my body can't survive without it" (internal factor). Marlatt (1985) explains that such beliefs most likely would result in continued substance use, since the individual perceives his/her use to be predestined and out of control. For example, the AVE is an individual's tendency to believe that he/she is unable to control substance use after an initial lapse. That is, the AVE occurs when an individual has had a "lapse" or "slip" (i.e., has used a drug after being abstinent for some time) and attributes this lapse to a "lack of will power" (i.e., an internal causal factor). Under such circumstances, this individual is likely to *continue* using, resulting in a full-blown relapse. This is analogous to Beck's (1976) description of all-or-none thinking; for example, "I've blown it, so I might as well keep using."

Marlatt (1985) also describes substance abuse and relapse as a cognitive decision-making process. He demonstrates (with an amusing example) that substance use is a result of multiple decisions (like forks in the road) which, depending on the decisions, may or may not lead to further substance use. He further explains that some decisions initially *appear* to be irrelevant to substance use ("apparently irrelevant decisions"); however, these decisions ultimately may result in a greater likelihood of relapse because of their incremental push toward higher-risk situations. In his example, Marlatt "innocently" chooses to sit in the smoking section of an airplane after being abstinent from smoking for several months. As a result of this decision he is more vulnerable to relapse (by his exposure to other smokers, their smoke, and their offers of cigarettes to him). We see this same phenomenon in patients who claim to have had every intention of remaining abstinent from alcohol and illicit drugs, only to blithely accept an invitation to meet a friend at a local tavern, or to cavalierly choose to drive out of the way in order to go past a street corner where drugs are sold. When such patients lapse into alcohol and drug use, it is striking to see how they fail to realize the ways in which they set themselves up for a fall with their decisions that *lead up to* the actual using incident.

Unfortunately, the cognitive models of substance abuse have not been integrated adequately into many addiction treatment programs (IOM, 1990a; Miller & Hester, 1985). This volume provides a focused, step-by-step treatment based on Beck's (1976) cognitive model. It is our hope that the chapters that follow will stimulate increased application of this cognitive model to substance abuse treatment across treatment settings and modalities.

The Motivation to Change

Efforts to examine the treatment of addictions are incomplete without considering the issue of motivation. Miller and Rollnick (1991) address this issue, explaining that most addicts are genuinely *ambivalent* about changing (rather than resistant, weak-willed, or characterologically flawed). The authors view motivation as a "state of readiness or eagerness to change, which may fluctuate from one time or situation to another" (p. 14).

Prochaska, DiClemente, and Norcross (1992) provide a comprehensive model for conceptualizing patients' motivation for change. In their work, Prochaska et al. (1992) identify five stages of change: precontemplation, contemplation, preparation, action, and maintenance. In the *precontemplation* stage, individuals are least concerned with overcoming their problems and they are least motivated to change problematic behaviors. In the *contemplation* stage individuals are willing to examine the problems associated with their substance use and consider the implications of change, although they may not take any constructive action. They are also likely to respond more positively to confrontation and education, although they may still be ambivalent. In the *preparation* stage, patients wish to make actual changes and therefore desire help with their problems, although they may feel at a loss as to how to do what is necessary to become drug free. In the *action* stage individuals have made a commitment to change and they have begun to actually modify behaviors. Prochaska et al. (1992) point out that this is a particularly stressful stage, which may require considerable therapist support and encouragement. In the *maintenance* stage individuals attempt to continue the process begun in the contemplation and action stages. In recent years, with so much emphasis placed on relapse prevention, the maintenance stage has received increased attention.

Prochaska and DiClemente (1986) caution that the process of change is very complex. They explain that "most individuals do not progress linearly through the stages of change" (p. 5). Alternatively, they offer a "revolving door model" (p. 6), based on the assumption that individuals make multiple revolutions around the circle of stages prior to achieving their long-term goals. Furthermore, they observe that some individuals "get stuck" in the earlier stages of change.

In the words of Prochaska and DiClemente (1986), "Therapy with addictive behaviors can progress most smoothly if both the client and the therapist are focusing on the same stage of change" (p. 6). To use nicotine dependence as an example, a smoker in the precontemplation stage will benefit little from advice about specific strategies for quitting smoking. The same smoker, however, might respond well to general questions about health maintenance, which might lead to a discussion of the health effects of smoking, which might lead further to a discussion of the benefits of quitting, which *eventually* might lead to a discussion of specific strategies. It is clear that the field can benefit from an understanding of what makes a patient ready to seek help (Tucker & Sobell, 1992).

The Prochaska et al. (1992) stage model is a useful heuristic. However, it is important to note that patients in a precontemplative stage of change are not impossible to treat (especially if they are under court order to attend therapy). Conversely, patients in the action phase or maintenance phases are not guaranteed to succeed in treatment. The same degrees of vigilance and commitment are required of the cognitive therapist regardless of the substance abuse patient's stage of change.

Treatment Outcome Goals

Some models of addiction (e.g., Alcoholics Anonymous and other disease-model programs) view total abstinence as the only acceptable goal of treatment. Proponents of these models view addiction as an all-or-nothing phenomenon, with any use seen as pathological and abstinence considered a state of "recovering" (rather than "recovered"). Alternatively, proponents of cognitive-behavioral models are more likely to view light or moderate use (i.e., "controlled drinking") as an acceptable goal of treatment in some cases.

At one time controlled drinking was extremely controversial (Marlatt, 1983). Presently, however, it is generally accepted that the goals of treatment should vary according to the patient's needs, problems, and previous response to treatment. Sobell, Sobell, Bogardis, Leo, and Skinner (1992), for example, surveyed problem drinkers to determine their preference for self-selected versus therapist-selected treatment goals (e.g., abstinence vs. controlled drinking). They found that most respondents preferred setting their own goals and believed that they would be more likely to achieve them; respondents with more serious drinking problems were even more likely to favor self-set goals. In general, we favor a collaborative approach in setting goals with patients. Therefore, to the extent that allowing severely addicted patients to set the modest goal of substance use *reduction* succeeds in getting otherwise resistant patients engaged in a more complete course of therapy, we are in favor of a controlled substance use approach. In the long run, however, we *strongly* advocate assisting patients in becoming drug- and alcohol-free.

THE TREATMENT OF SUBSTANCE ABUSE AND DEPENDENCE

In reality, most substance abuse treatment programs are eclectic in theory and practice, and they include varying degrees of inpatient and outpatient services, 12-step program attendance, education, psychotherapy, family therapy, support groups, pharmacotherapy, and so forth. In our view, cognitive therapy can be compatible with any of these approaches. In fact, many of our drug and alcohol abuse patients attend support groups, have had inpatient detoxification, and take medication. The special strengths that cognitive therapy *adds* to this battery of approaches are its emphasis on (1) the identification and modification of *beliefs* that exacerbate cravings, (2) the amelioration of negative affective states (e.g., anger, anxiety, and hopelessness) that often trigger drug use, (3) teaching patients to apply a battery of cognitive and behavioral skills and techniques, and not just willpower, to become and remain drug-free, and (4) helping patients to go beyond abstinence to make fundamental positive changes in the ways they view themselves, their life, and their future, thus leading to new *lifestyles*.

In the following section we present a brief overview of more traditional treatments of substance abuse and dependence.

Alcoholism Treatment

Miller and Hester (1980, 1986) have conducted exhaustive reviews of the alcoholism treatment literature. These authors have examined nine major classes of interventions. The four most common were pharmacotherapy, psychotherapy or counseling, Alcoholics Anonymous, and alcoholism education. The five less commonly employed approaches included family therapy, aversion therapies, operant methods, controlled drinking, and broad spectrum treatment.

Miller and Hester (1986) conclude from their reviews that alcoholism treatment is best approached as a two-stage process, requiring different interventions at each stage. The first set of interventions should be focused on changing drinking behaviors to abstinence or moderation (e.g., behavioral self-control training). The second set of interventions should be focused on maintenance of sobriety (e.g., social skills training in order to increase confidence in relating to drug-free people).

Miller and Hester (1986) also draw some disturbing conclusions, however, about the poor relationship between empirical research and traditional inpatient treatment approaches. Treatment methods that are supported by controlled research include aversion therapies, behavioral self-control training, community reinforcement, marital and family therapy, social skills training, and stress management, whereas approaches actually currently employed as standard practice in alcoholism programs include Alcoholics Anonymous, alcoholism education, confrontation, disulfiram, group therapy, and individual counseling. They point out that there is little apparent overlap between these lists: Alcoholism treatment programs in the United States do *not* tend to use treatment methods that have been validated by controlled outcome studies. Furthermore, Miller and Hester (1986) point out that traditional inpatient treatment programs are very expensive, "despite clear evidence that they offer no advantage in overall effectiveness" (p. 163). Concurring in this, McLellan et al. (1992) note that standard detoxification and "28–day programs" (in spite of their high costs) are insufficient to deal with long-term issues. Clearly, to help drug and alcohol patients deal with more enduring issues, these treatments need to be supplemented with ongoing outpatient treatment that focuses on attitude change and skills acquisition.

The Institute of Medicine recently commissioned a National Academy of Sciences committee to make an exhaustive critical review of the research literature on treatment for alcohol problems (1990b). The committee discovered that interventions included "a broad range of activities that vary in content, duration, intensity, goals, setting, provider, and target population" (p. 86). The committee's assessment was that "no single treatment approach or modality has been demonstrated to be superior to all others" (p. 86). Its conclusions, published in *Broadening the Base of Treatment for Alcohol Problems* (1990a), included the following:

1. There is no single treatment approach that is effective for all persons with alcohol problems.
2. The provision of appropriate, specific treatment modalities can substantially improve outcome.
3. Brief interventions can be quite effective compared with no treatment, and they can be quite cost-effective compared with more intensive treatment.
4. Treatment of other life problems related to drinking can improve outcome in persons with alcohol problems.
5. Therapist characteristics are partial determinants of outcome.
6. Outcomes are determined in part by treatment process factors, posttreatment adjustment factors, the characteristics of individuals seeking treatment, the characteristics of their problems, and the interactions among these factors.
7. People who are treated for alcohol problems achieve a continuum of outcomes with respect to drinking behavior and alcohol problems and follow different courses of outcome.
8. Those who significantly reduce their level of alcohol consumption or who become totally abstinent usually enjoy improvement in other life areas, particularly as the period of reduced consumption becomes more extended (pp. 147–148).

The findings of the Institute of Medicine (1990a) coupled with those of Miller and Hester (1986) make it apparent that there is still a profound need for effective alcoholism treatment interventions. It is hoped that the principles introduced in this text will be integrated into, and evaluated in, traditional treatment programs in order to move toward more effective and appropriate alcoholism treatment programs.

Illicit Drug Treatment

In addition to its report on alcohol treatment programs, the Institute of Medicine appointed a separate committee (1990a) to review the treatment of drug problems in the United States. Specifically, the committee divided treatments into four classifications: methadone maintenance, therapeutic communities, outpatient non-methadone programs, and chemical dependency programs.

These findings (1990a) were similar to those of Miller and Hester (1986). The most empirically validated programs have been methadone maintenance clinics for opioid dependency. Some evidence also supported the efficacy of therapeutic communities and outpatient nonmethadone treatment. Nonetheless, "Chemical dependency is the treatment with the highest revenues, probably the second largest number of clients, and the smallest scientific basis for assessing its effectiveness" (IOM, 1990a, p. 18). The Institute of Medicine acknowledges that most of the studies on methadone maintenance were conducted in the 1970s and early 1980s, however. As a result, research has insufficiently addressed the growing cocaine problems in this country. By contrast, this volume *will* focus heavily on the cognitive therapy of cocaine and crack cocaine addiction.

Smoking Cessation Interventions

In a report published by the National Cancer Institute, Schwartz (1987) critically reviewed the literature on smoking cessation interventions. He divided the various methods into 10 categories: (1) self-care, (2) educational approaches/groups, (3) medication, (4) nicotine chewing gum, (5) hypnosis, (6) acupuncture, (7) physician counseling, (8) risk factor preventive trials, (9) mass media and community programs, and (10) behavioral methods. Schwartz (1987) found considerable variability in cessation rates among these methods.

Approximately 1 million Americans per year quit smoking, and most do so on their own through "self-care." In fact, three-fifths of all smokers would *prefer* to quit on their own, rather than seek group quit-smoking programs (Schwartz, 1987). There are many self-help aids for those wishing to quit smoking, including books, pamphlets, audio cassettes, drug store preparations, correspondence courses, and so forth. Almost all self-care efforts and aids involve some cognitive techniques. In fact, those who successfully quit on their own have higher levels of success expectancy and self-efficacy (areas strongly affected by cognitive interventions) than those who are unsuccessful. Approximately 16%–20% of smokers who quit on their own are abstinent at 1 year (Schwartz, 1987).

For those who wish to receive assistance with smoking cessation, there are nonprofit and commercial clinics and groups available. Most of these utilize cognitive methods, including education, self-monitoring, and modifying attitudes about smoking. In a review of 46 group smoking cessation programs, Schwartz (1987) found median cessation rates ranging from 21% to 36%, depending on the length of follow-up and the time the study was conducted.

A number of medications have also been tried as aids to smoking cessation over the years. These have included lobeline, meprobamate, amphetamines, anticholinergics, sedatives, tranquilizers, sympathomimetics, anticonvulsants, buspirone, propranolol, clonidine, nicotine polacrilex, and most recently transdermal nicotine. Of these, the most promising medications have been those that replace the nicotine from cigarettes with prescription nicotine (i.e., nicotine gum and transdermal nicotine). In fact, the median cessation rates for nicotine gum at 6-month and 1-year follow-ups were 23% and 11%. These rates were substantially higher when the gum was used in conjunction with cognitive-behavioral smoking cessation programs: 35% and 29% (Schwartz, 1987). At the time this book was being written, transdermal nicotine delivery systems had just been approved by the Food and Drug Administration. Hence, substantial field trials of these "patches" have not been conducted.

Both hypnosis and acupuncture have been of interest to the general public as smoking cessation techniques. However, empirical validation of these methods has been weak and further controlled studies are necessary prior to assuming their efficacy (Schwartz, 1987).

SUMMARY

Huge numbers of people in the United States are affected by substance abuse. Thousands of books and articles have been written and millions of dollars have been spent on research on the addictions. Nonetheless, there is a noticeable paucity of reliably effective substance abuse treatment strategies. For years, however, it has been noted that there are underlying cognitive processes common to the addictions. (Even Alcoholics Anonymous warns alcoholics about "stinkin' thinkin.'") We believe strongly that understanding and working with these cognitive aspects more explicitly will help to resolve some of the uncertainty plaguing the field of substance use treatment.

In the chapters that follow we strive for a high degree of specificity in describing the procedures that comprise this approach. A preliminary version of this book currently serves as a therapist manual in an ongoing National Institute on Drug Abuse pilot study comparing cognitive therapy, supportive-expressive therapy, and general drug counseling treatment outcomes for cocaine abusers. Our hope is that *Cognitive Therapy of Substance Abuse* will continue to serve as a training guide for further clinical and empirical tests.

CHAPTER **2**

Cognitive Model
of Addiction

WHY DO PEOPLE USE DRUGS (AND/OR ALCOHOL)?

Some individuals are "generalists" and may use a wide variety of addictive substances almost randomly or depending on their availability. Others are "specialists" and their drug of choice may depend on its specific pharmacological properties as well as its social meanings (e.g., alcohol is often viewed as manly and associated with sports, whereas cocaine is associated with group acceptance and sexual activity). Cocaine may be used because of its stimulant properties—producing a rapid "high," for example. Similarly, amphetamines may be chosen as psychic energizers. In contrast, barbiturates, benzodiazepines, and alcohol may be preferred because of their relaxing effect and, perhaps, their presumed relief of inhibitions. Hallucinogens are attractive to some to relieve boredom and "expand consciousness." Most people addicted to cocaine have also abused other drugs and/or alcohol (N. S. Miller, 1991; Regier et al., 1990; Stimmel, 1991).

There are numerous explanations for why people use—and become addicted to—psychotropic substances. In general, the process of addiction can be understood in terms of a few simple, perhaps obvious, formulas. A basic reason for starting on drugs or alcohol is to get pleasure, to experience the exhilaration of being high, and to share the excitement with one's companions who are also using (Stimmel, 1991). Further, there is the expectation that the drug cocaine, for example, will increase efficiency, improve fluency, and enhance creativity.

How do people progress from recreational or casual use to regular use? In time, additional factors may contribute to becoming dependent on the drug. Some people find that drug taking—for example, heroin, benzodiazepines (such as Valium), or barbiturates—provides temporary relief from anxiety, tension, sadness, or boredom. These individuals soon develop the belief that they can weather the frustrations and stresses of life better if they can turn to drugs and/or alcohol for a period of escape or oblivion. People with adverse life circumstances are more likely to become addicted than are those with more sources of satisfaction (Peele, 1985). For a while, real-life problems fade into insignificance and life itself seems more attractive. As one patient put it, "If I take coke, my bad thoughts go away." Further, people whose self-confidence is low may find that the drug or alcohol boosts their morale—in the short run. Finally, many individuals discover that using drugs provides new social groups in which the only requirement for admission and acceptance is that they are users.

If drug using has so many advantages, why should we be concerned with getting people off the "drug habit"? The profound implications of breaking the law by using illegal drugs (and selling them in order to support their habit) are so obvious that they do not need further elaboration. Regardless of whether the drugs are legal, such as alcohol, or illegal, substance abuse creates serious personal, social, and medical problems (Frances & Miller, 1991; Kosten & Kleber, 1992).

A major problem is that the drug seems to take control of addicted individuals. Their goals, values, and attachments become subordinate to the drug using. They cannot manage their lives effectively. They become subject to a vicious cycle of craving, precipitous drops in mood, and greater distress that can be relieved immediately only by using drugs again.

The web of external and internal problems leading to and, later, maintaining compulsive drug use is a defining characteristic of addiction. Far from soothing life's pains, the drugs create a new set of problems—enormous financial outlays (for illegal drugs), threat of or actual loss of employment, and difficulties in important personal relationships, such as marriage. The individual also becomes stigmatized by society—as a "lush" or a "junkie." Finally, of course, chronic use may cause serious medical problems and even death.

As pointed out by Peele (1989), the compulsive use of psychotropic agents depends on a wide variety of personal and social factors. If the environment is malevolent and there is group support for drug use—as in the case of U.S. soldiers in Vietnam—widespread drug use is more likely. When the environment is comparatively less stressful (as when veterans return to civilian life), individuals do not continue excessive use—except for those who had been heavy users prior to military service (Robins, Davis, & Goodwin, 1974).

A number of characteristics distinguish addicted individuals from casual users. A major difference, as pointed out by Peele (1985), is that while addicted individuals subordinate important values to drug using, casual users prize other values more highly: family, friends, occupation, recreation, and economic security, to name a few. In addition, drug users may have certain characteristics, such as low frustration tolerance, nonassertiveness, or poor impulse control, that make them more susceptible. Thus, psychological and social factors may be the determinative factors—rather than the pharmacological properties per se—in converting a drug user into a drug abuser. Supporting this hypothesis is the commonly encountered phenomenon in hospital settings where "patients who take opioids for acute pain or cancer pain rarely experience euphoria and even more rarely develop psychic dependence or addiction to the mood-altering effects of narcotics" (*Medical Letter on Drugs and Therapeutics*, 1993, p. 5). If drug addiction were merely a biological process, we would not expect this to be the case.

The sequence of using or drinking is illustrated in Figure 2.1. An addicted individual who is feeling anxious or low decides to have a smoke or a snort. The short-term relief is followed by delayed, longer-term negative consequences: problems about breaking the law, serious financial problems, family difficulties, and possibly medical problems. These problems lead to realistic fears of being apprehended, becoming bankrupt, losing a job, disrupting close relationships, and becoming ill. These fears generate more anxiety and lead to craving and further using or drinking to neutralize the anxiety. Thus, a vicious cycle is established.

Many other kinds of vicious cycles, which are described in Chapter 3 (this volume), may be created. These involve a number of psychological factors such as low self-esteem, emotional distress, and hopelessness.

WHY NOT STOP IF DRUGS
OR ALCOHOL CREATE PROBLEMS?

By definition, addicts are people who have difficulty in stopping permanently. They may have started to use voluntarily, but they either do not believe that they can stop or they do not choose to stop voluntarily. At the first sign of medical, financial, or interpersonal problems, many users ignore, minimize, or deny the problems

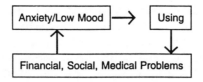

FIGURE 2.1. Simple model of vicious cycle.

or attribute them to something other than drugs (e.g., they may blame their spouse for domestic problems). Others may be aware of the problems, but they evaluate the advantages of using as greater than the disadvantages. Much of this evaluation is based on avoiding a true assessment of the disadvantages (Gawin & Ellinwood, 1988; Gawin & Kleber, 1988). As the problems increase, many users become more ambivalent and begin to vacillate in their decision to use.

One factor in maintaining drug use is the common belief that withdrawing from the drug will produce intolerable side effects (Horvath, 1988, in press). However, these effects vary enormously from person to person—and from substance to substance—and the impact is greatly enhanced by the psychological meaning attached to the withdrawal symptoms. These meanings are often more salient than the actual adverse physiological sensations in determining the intensity of withdrawal symptoms. Most cocaine abusers participating in detoxification programs, for example, feel better in the early stages after they stop using (Ziedonis, 1992).

A major obstacle to eliminating using or drinking is the network of *dysfunctional beliefs* that center around the drugs or alcohol. Examples of these beliefs are: "I can't be happy unless I can use," and "I am more in control when I've had a few drinks." An individual who is contemplating eliminating the use of drugs or alcohol may feel sad or anxious. Termination of reliance on drugs or alcohol is seen as a deprivation of satisfaction and solace or a threat to well-being and functioning (Jennings, 1991). Stopping may mean, for some, removing the "security blanket" used to cushion dysphoria.

Addicted individuals often try on their own to stop using or drinking. However, when they experience the craving (often stimulated by low mood or exposure to the drugs or related stimuli), they feel disappointed if they restrain themselves from using or drinking. They perceive their feelings of disappointment and distress as intolerable; the thought, "I can't stand this feeling," upsets them even more. Hence, they feel driven to yield to the craving in order to dispel the sense of loss and relieve their distress. Patients often have a cluster of beliefs that seem to become stronger when they decide to stop using. These center around the anticipated deprivation: "If I can't use, I won't be able to bear the pain (or boredom)," "There is nothing left in life for me," "I will be unhappy", or "I will lose my friends." These beliefs are elaborated more in the section on low frustration tolerance (Chapter 15, this volume).

Another set of beliefs centers around the addicted individual's sense of helplessness in controlling the craving: "The craving is too strong," "I don't have the power to stop," or "Even if I do stop—I will only start up again." These beliefs become self-fulfilling prophecies. Since the patients believe they are incapable of controlling their urges, they are less likely to *try* to control them and, thus, confirm their belief in their helplessness in overcoming their addiction.

WHY DO PEOPLE WANT HELP?

There are roughly five stages people go through in seeking help (Prochaska et al., 1992). In the *precontemplative* stage, they do not even acknowledge to themselves that they have a problem (or else they consider using more important than the problems it causes). In the *contemplative* stage, they are willing to consider their problems, but are still unlikely to stop using on their own. Individuals in the *preparation* stage *intend* to take action to cease their drug and alcohol use, but are uncertain about being able to follow through. In the *action* stage, patients behaviorally *demonstrate* a decrease in their drug-taking behaviors and a therapeutic modification in their drug-taking beliefs. Those who are successful enough to reach the *maintenance* stage have already taken great strides toward a drug-free and alcohol-free life, and are actively working to maintain consistency in this endeavor over a period of months and years.

People come to therapy for a variety of reasons. Some users have been arrested for "dealing" or possession and are referred by the courts. Others see their lives deteriorating as a result of the financial, psychological, and interpersonal consequences of using or drinking. Still others are pressured by friends or family. By the time these patients are labeled drug abusers, addicts, or alcoholics, they have often hit a low point in terms of any combination of the following: health, social adjustment, employment and economic status, and psychological well-being.

Many people with drug and alcohol problems have tried repeatedly to "break the habit," only to relapse eventually. Others suffer from a personality disorder (e.g., Mirin & Weiss, 1991; Nace, Davis, & Gaspari, 1991; Regier et al., 1990) and/or a psychiatric syndrome such as chronic anxiety (e.g., Kranzler & Liebowitz, 1988; LaBounty, Hatsukami, Morgan, & Nelson, 1992; Walfish, Massey, & Krone, 1990) or depression (e.g., Hatsukami & Pickens, 1982; Rounsaville & Kleber, 1986). For some, drug use is simply a manifestation of their manifold difficulties. For others, drugs represent a form of self-medication (Castaneda, Galanter, & Franco, 1989; Khantzian, 1985) to relieve their feelings of distress, sadness, or anxiety.

Given the consequences of sustained drug use, it is important to consider the problem in terms of its sociological, interpersonal, and psychological dimensions, in addition to the strictly pharmacological properties of drugs. In fact, substance abuse or addiction could be defined as compulsive use leading to a web of entanglement involving social, economic, and legal problems over which the patient no longer has control. Given their acknowledgment that they are addicted, many of these individuals come to the conclusion that the only way they can manage or even salvage their lives is to receive assistance, professional or otherwise.

HOW CAN COGNITIVE THERAPY HELP?

Cognitive therapy is a system of psychotherapy that attempts to reduce excessive emotional reactions and self-defeating behavior by modifying the faulty or erroneous thinking and maladaptive beliefs that underlie these reactions (Beck, 1976; Beck, Rush, Shaw, & Emery, 1979).

The approach to a particular patient is derived from a thorough conceptualization of the particular case. The specific case formulation, in turn, is based on the cognitive model of that disorder. The thorough case conceptualization, including the relationship of early life patterns to current problems, at the beginning stages of treatment differentiates cognitive therapy from some of the other forms of therapy. The approach is (1) collaborative (builds trust), (2) active, (3) based on open-ended questioning to a large degree, and (4) highly structured and focused.

As applied to substance abuse, the cognitive approach helps individuals to come to grips with the problems leading to emotional distress and to gain a broader perspective on their reliance on drugs for pleasure and/or relief from discomfort. In addition, specific cognitive strategies help to reduce their urges and, at the same time, establish a stronger system of internal controls. Moreover, cognitive therapy can help patients to combat their depression, anxiety, or anger, which frequently fuels addictive behaviors.

A major thrust of cognitive therapy of substance abuse is to help the patient in two ways: (1) to reduce the intensity and frequency of the urges by undermining the underlying beliefs, and (2) to teach the patient specific techniques for controlling or managing their urges. In a nutshell, the aim is to reduce the pressure and increase control. When the patient's addiction is related to a coexisting psychiatric disorder, that condition also needs to be addressed by the cognitive therapist.

Cognitive therapy is carried out in several ways. The therapist helps the patient to examine the sequence of events leading to drug use and then to explore the patient's basic beliefs about the value of drugs, alcohol, and nicotine. At the same time, the therapist trains the patient to evaluate and consider the ways in which faulty thinking produces stress and distress. Therapists help patients to modify their thinking so that they can gain a better grasp of their realistic problems and can disregard pseudo-problems derived from their faulty thinking. In addition, through rehearsal and practice, patients are trained to build up a system of controls to apply when confronted with strong urges.

The techniques the therapist uses include a painstaking evaluation of the short-term and long-term benefits and disadvantages of using: the cost–benefits analysis (also called the advantages–disadvantages analysis; see Chapters 9 and 10, this volume). The therapist also helps the patient to find more satisfactory ways of coping with realistic problems and unpleasant feelings without turning to drugs or alcohol for relief. They also work together to structure the patient's life so that other sources of pleasure are made available (cf. Havassy, Hall, & Wasserman, 1991). Since many patients have a low frustration tolerance (Ellis, McInerney, DiGiuseppe, & Yeager, 1988), they are shown how their self-defeating attitudes about themselves and their capabilities lead to overreacting when they encounter obstacles, delays, or thwarting (Chapter 15, this volume). The therapist also demonstrates how patients can approach these obstacles as problems to be solved rather than as barriers to their goals.

Many patients who suffer from difficulties in asserting themselves in an appropriate way are likely to be dominated and even exploited by other people, and thus are prone to experience frequent impatience, anger, and disappointment. By learning new interpersonal skills, the patients are able to assert their rights more effectively. The same type of assertion can help them to refuse when others coax them to start using. Refusal can take on a new meaning for them—standing up for themselves, putting long-term interests before short-term gains, and becoming desensitized to derogatory or profane epithets.

One of the main features of cognitive therapy is the use of "Socratic questioning." By skillfully asking questions, the therapist leads the patient to examine areas that the patient has closed off from scrutiny, for example, the true frequency and quantity of drug use, the actual losses from the addiction, and the quality and effects on interpersonal relations. Also, questioning leads patients to generate options and solutions that they have not considered. Finally, this approach puts patients in the "questioning mode" (as opposed to the "automatic impulse" mode) so that they will start to evaluate more objectively their various attitudes and beliefs.

In a sense, stopping drug use or drinking is a technical problem. The patients coming for help would like to stop using but they do not know how. Many of them have tried to stop many times but have been unsuccessful. Cognitive therapy provides them with tools that will enable them to stop and maintain the abstinence from drugs or to moderate their drinking and smoking. Moreover, they can apply these same useful techniques to their daily problems and thus have a more enjoyable, more fulfilling life.

DO SUBSTANCE ABUSERS HAVE ADDITIONAL PSYCHIATRIC PROBLEMS?

Many of the patients seeking—or referred for—treatment of addictions have a "dual diagnosis" (Mirin & Weiss, 1991; Regier et al., 1990). By this we mean that in addition to their diagnosis of addiction, they also have a syndromal diagnosis (Axis I), such as depression, or a diagnosis of personality disorder (Axis II), or a combination of both. A good conceptualization takes into account the various ways in which the patients' psychological problems play themselves out. For example, a patient with a dependent personality disorder centered around a poor self-concept may become depressed following a rejection and seek to counteract the depressed feelings through using and/or drinking. Linking these behaviors may be a common thread, such as "I am too weak or fragile to make it on my own." This belief may lead to clinical depression when interpersonal supports are removed. The same belief promotes using or drinking when the patient is confronted with a difficult problem or a stressful situation: "I can't handle this without a drink (or drug)."

WHY DO PEOPLE RELAPSE AFTER NOT
USING FOR A SUBSTANTIAL PERIOD?

Many individuals handle the withdrawal symptoms, if present, and go for significant periods without using but then relapse—sometimes, for no apparently compelling reason (Carroll, Rounsaville, & Keller, 1991; Tiffany, 1990). The problem seems to lie in the fact that these individuals have not become "inoculated" to the external or internal conditions that can trigger the craving and undermine the control. These circumstances fall into the category of "people, places, and things," which is described in 12-step programs. This category includes situations such as associating with companions or sex partners who urge one to have a "hit" or drink, visiting a place where one has previously used or drunk, seeing drug paraphernalia, or receiving one's paycheck. These individuals also may experience a craving for the substance if they are feeling sad, bored, or anxious. Some individuals have a lapse when an unusual stressful situation occurs: death of a friend or relative, serious argument with a spouse, or loss of a job.

One of the underlying reasons why recovering addicts are still prone to react with powerful urges to various stimulus (high-risk) situations is that their basic beliefs regarding the relative advantages and disadvantages of drug taking have not changed substantially. They may have acquired a number of strategies for controlling their drug-taking behavior, but *they have not significantly modified the attitudes that help to fuel the craving.* Consequently, when their controls are weakened, perhaps as a result of stress, and their urges are stimulated, for example by exposure to a high-risk situation (a situation that activates their drug-using beliefs), they are vulnerable to lapse by using or drinking a minimum or moderate amount. This lapse is accentuated by a sense of helplessness or hopelessness: "It proves I can't control my urges"; "I will never be able to beat this problem."

As they are swept back into the drug-using cycle, the lapse becomes a relapse. Sometimes, patients may lapse for no discernible reason—that is, they have not been exposed to a high-risk situation (Tiffany, 1990). The probability of such a lapse is increased any time the ratio of the perception of control to the intensity of craving is decreased; that is, when control is weakened by fatigue and a gradual slippage of the constructive beliefs (anti-indulgence beliefs) and/or an increase in the desire to use or drink, based, for example, on transient unpleasant feelings. The degree of commitment to abstinence may simply decrease with the passage of time—perhaps because of fading of memories of the bad effects of using or drinking (Gawin &

Ellinwood, 1988; Velten, 1986). At this time, a "normal" degree of craving may lead to a lapse. If the patient's reaction is, "My control must be pretty poor if I give in to such mild craving," he/she may progress into a relapse.

The basic beliefs that have been dormant but become stimulated by exposure to the stimulus (high-risk) situations include notions such as "If I use, I can handle my problems better," "Having a smoke or hit will make life more enjoyable," or "I need a drink to overcome my anxiety." As soon as these beliefs are activated, the individual experiences an exacerbation of craving. The patient's attempts at self-control are undermined by permission-related thoughts (stemming from the beliefs) such as "I can do it this once and stop," or "There's no reason why I should continue to deprive myself." There is, thus, a continuing conflict between the attitudes concerned with controlling the urge and those attitudes favoring yielding to the temptation (or, more strictly, initiating the behavior that would satisfy the urge).

PHENOMENA OF ADDICTION

Cravings and Urges

In helping patients deal with their substance use problems, it is crucial to have a full understanding of the phenomena associated with drug use. *Craving* refers to a desire for the drug, whereas the term *urge* is applied to the internal pressure or mobilization to act on the craving (Marlatt, 1985, and Horvath, 1988, use the terms in a similar way). In short, a craving is associated with *wanting* and an urge with *doing*. The two terms are often used interchangeably, but it is useful to separate them.

Cravings represent a strong desire for a particular type of experience, for example, the pleasure from eating, relaxation from smoking, or the gratification from sex. The fulfillment of the wish may be labeled the consummation and the means, the consummatory act. When one form of consummation is not available, an individual may turn to another form. For example, if there is no satisfaction in sight for yearning for affection, an individual may reach for a sweet or a beer instead.

An urge is the instrumental sequel to a craving. A person desires to experience a "high" or relief from discomfort and feels a pressure to act to obtain this experience. Marlatt and Gordon (1985) define an urge as a behavioral intention to engage in a specific consummatory behavior. Urges may be regarded as compulsions when the individual feels incapable of resisting them. Thus, an urge may be instigated by an unpleasant feeling state (such as anger or anxiety) or the anticipation of an unpleasant stressful event. The ultimate goal of consummating the urge is a reduction of the instigating state, whether it be a craving for excitement or a desire to relax.

The delay between the experience of craving and implementation of the urge does provide an interval for a therapeutic intervention—for the technical application of control or what is called, in common parlance, "will power," which we define as an active process of applying self-help techniques, not simply a passive enduring of discomfort. Additionally, fostering a delay between the craving and the use of drugs allows for the natural diminishing of the acute craving episode (Horvath, 1988), thus lowering the chances that the patient will act on the craving (Carroll, Rounsaville, & Keller, 1991).

Urges are governed by the anticipated consequences, for example, reward for doing something or pain for not doing it. The urge may be accompanied by a positive feeling when it is driven by a positive expectation or a negative feeling when it is driven by expectation of unpleasantness unless the urge is consummated. Some people confuse urge with "need." They will say "I *need* a smoke" or "I *need* a drink" as though they cannot survive, or at least function, without it. Such a belief is, of course, spurious and becomes a focus for therapeutic interventions.

Cravings and urges tend to be automatic and may become "autonomous"; that is, they can continue even though the individual tries to suppress or abolish them. They may become imperative and are not easily dissipated even if blocked from being carried out. At this point, the word "compulsion" seems most appropriate to describe cravings and urges. We see compulsions most clearly in obsessive–compulsive disorder, in which the individual experiences strong pressure to engage in a repetitive act in order to ward off some feared event. Addictive behaviors incorporate some of the same characteristics.

The Role of Beliefs

Dysfunctional beliefs play a role in the generation of urges. The beliefs help to form the expectation, which then molds the urge. For example, a patient with a serious drinking problem had the following beliefs: "If I am 'amusing and friendly' I will receive lots of praise" and "If I have a drink I will be more entertaining." He translated these beliefs into a specific expectation for receiving praise when an opportunity arose for entertaining people. The expectation, then, led to the urge to "show off." However, he was uncertain of his success unless he had crack cocaine first. His expectation of success was enhanced by his belief in the stimulating or disinhibiting effect of cocaine. As it happened, he would usually "overshoot the mark" and become so excited that people considered him "pathetic."

Following Bandura (1982), Marlatt and Gordon (1985) have refined the concept "beliefs about the positive effect of using" into "positive outcome expectancies." Research by Brown, Goldman, Inn, and Anderson (1980) has shown that the expectancies of alcoholics fall into six factors: that drinking will (1) transform experiences in a positive way, (2) enhance social and physical pleasure, (3) increase sexual performance and satisfaction, (4) increase power and aggression, (5) increase social assertiveness, and (6) decrease tension. A similar set of expectations is associated with drug use (see Drug Belief Questionnaire in Appendix, this volume).

The "Drug Habit"

The habit of taking substances for relief or pleasure differs from the way the term "a bad habit" is generally understood. A particular "habit," such as grimacing when frustrated or leaving clothes on the floor, is a repetitive pattern—but it is not experienced as a craving or a need. For the drug abuser the immediate response to a relevant situation is subjective, namely, a craving or an urge. There is a delay between the stimulus and the consummatory act, such as preparing the syringe or the powder. What are chained to the stimulus, thus, are the cravings and urges. Through continual repetition, the chain becomes stronger. In contrast to the habits involved in skilled acts such as driving, the pattern of drug taking is compulsive and dysfunctional. In addition, the skilled acts are based on voluntary decisions, whereas drug-taking cravings are involuntary (even though the *control* of the urges is voluntary). Because of the difference between using and the habits of everyday life, the term "drug habit" is probably a misnomer.

Through a process of "stimulus generalization," the addicted individual is likely to respond with craving to an increasingly broader range of stimulus situations. Whereas originally the individual might have felt the craving for a drink or smoke only in a group, he or she now may experience it when upset, bored, or lonely. With the binding of the craving to more and more stimuli, there is a concomitant expansion of the dysfunctional beliefs about drug use. Whereas initially the belief might be "I should take a smoke to be part of the group," the beliefs may build up to "I need a smoke to be accepted" and later to "I have to take a snort to relieve my loneliness and dis-

tress." The urges, thus, become more generalized and more imperative in keeping with the broadening content of the beliefs.

Furthermore, the rebound dysphoria experienced particularly after
a "cocaine crash" (Karan et al., 1991; Ziedonis, 1992), for example,
leads to a renewal of the craving in order to counteract this low feeling. The consequence of the repetition of *emotional distress* leading
to *craving* to *indulgence* to *temporary relief of dysphoria* is the development of beliefs such as "I need a hit in order to feel better." When a
drug or alcohol is taken to relieve stress-related or naturally occurring tension, anxiety, or sadness, it tends to reinforce the belief "I
need the drug," as well as "I can't tolerate unpleasant feelings."

The Control/Urge Equation

There is a common belief that addicted individuals
have little or no control over their urges and behavior or that the
craving is irresistible. On the surface, this seems to be true because
these people seem to be driven by such a powerful force that they
engage in addictive behavior even though they recognize its destruc-
tiveness; many make repetitive abortive attempts to control their
behavior and will say that they know they want to control their behavior but simply cannot. This common observation of their cravings and
urges overwhelming any resistance has led to the principle expressed
by Alcoholics Anonymous: "I recognize that I am powerless."

Their perception of "being out of control" has the positive benefit of inducing addicted people to seek professional help rather than
continuing to waste energy in futile attempts to exercise control—often
followed by self-castigation for not successfully counteracting the urge.
Developing control is a technical problem to a large extent. Learning
specialized techniques for reducing craving and establishing some
measure of control is generally necessary for those who are truly
addicted. On the one hand, the sources of craving need to be explored.
On the other hand, the notion of total loss of control is simplistic
and does an injustice to the potential internal resources available to
the individual. In actuality, most people who abuse drugs do exercise control most of the time. When the urge is not strong or the
substance is not currently available, they are able to abstain. They do
not necessarily go off in wild pursuit of the drug at the first sensation of craving. There is a qualitative difference between the wish to
use (to experience "benefits" of the drug) and the wish to control the
urge.

The craving activates a drug-taking routine: The individuals'
sources for consummating the urge are scanned, a plan emerges, the
body becomes mobilized to act, and the physiology shifts to a recep-

tive state (e.g., the parasympathetic nervous system goes into an activated state). Since craving is an "appetitive state," it is accompanied by a variety of bodily sensations somewhat akin to hunger or an unpleasant yearning for someone or something. This kind of appetite operates according to the *pleasure principle*, in contrast to the wish to control the urge, which operates according to the *reality principle*.

The wish *not* to use, thus, to control, is not expressed in visceral terms (as is craving) but is experienced as a sort of mental state. It has a strong cognitive component, specifically, decision-making. What powers the decision-making is a sense of resolution or commitment that is felt in the musculature (in contrast to craving, which is more visceral). Thus, the two opposing motivations—craving and self-control (or will power)—are qualitatively different.

Parallel to the decision not to use (refusal state) is the decision to indulge (permission giving). Permission giving and permission refusal are akin to gatekeepers. Their relative 'strength determines whether the gates will open or close. There is more conscious (voluntary) participation in the gatekeeping than in the craving; therefore, the individual can reflect and decide whether or not to indulge. If the craving is strong, the decision to refuse/abstain may be too weak to control it. If the balance favors refusal, the using does not occur.

Even when the urge is strong, addicted individuals can abstain at times, particularly if the drug is not immediately available. It is important to recognize that addictive behavior is related to the *balance* of control versus urge. Put in more abstract terms, the ratio of the strength of the control to the strength of the urge influences whether the individual will abstain or use. The formula or ratio *power of control/power of urge* may be used as a guide for intervention. Treatment is focused on increasing this ratio. It does not require a superhuman effort to change the relative strengths. It may simply involve reducing the denominator (urge) or increasing the numerator (control) or, preferably, doing both.

Beck et al. (1979) have used the analogy of the votes in Congress for a declaration of war to illustrate how suicidal behavior may be modified. A somewhat similar analogy may be applied to a decision to use. To declare war requires a simple plurality, a margin of one vote of the yeas over the nays. However, just as in the case of suicide, if the decision is postponed or the relationship of yea to nay votes is changed in favor of the nays, the progression to action is arrested. In the case of declaration of war, lobbying for a few votes for peace may forestall the fateful action; in the case of addiction, strengthening the votes for abstinence can reverse the tendency to use. In the long run, however, it is necessary to build a solid "majority" to forestall relapse.

The point to this analogy is that it is not necessary to eliminate cravings totally or to institute absolute control. It is sufficient to change the relative strengths of the two parts of the equation. A change involving reduction of craving or increase in control may interrupt the drug-using progression in the short run. Since the goal is usually permanent abstinence, a durable improvement requires enough lasting change in the ratio to provide a sufficient margin of safety. Treatment, thus, is directed toward both halves of the equation: increasing control and reducing craving.

Increasing Control

Many addicted individuals simply have not developed the skills to control temptation. If such a skill deficit exists, one part of the therapy is directed toward increasing self-control skills. A variety of methods can be used to increase control. These techniques can be practiced in the therapist's office. The basic procedure is to reproduce stimulus conditions that will elicit craving and then to rehearse control behaviors as the craving is stimulated. For example, the individual is asked to imagine a situation in which she is offered crack cocaine. She then imagines ways in which to refuse the offer. Or she might imagine feeling blue or anxious and then desiring relief from the discomfort. She then pictures what she will do when craving occurs: divert herself by calling a friend, become engaged in some pleasant activity, or read a flashcard detailing rational responses to cognitions related to craving.

Another approach involves dealing directly with permission-giving thoughts. This exercise is carried out in the form of a debate. The patient mentally verbalizes or rehearses reasons for giving permission to indulge and, at the same time, presents a rebuttal to this argument. At some point, however, it is necessary to identify and evaluate the underlying beliefs regarding permission giving and permission refusing. Ultimately, of course, the therapist needs to help the patient reduce the craving by dealing with its various psychological and social sources. These sources may cover very broad domains of the patient's life ranging from low frustration tolerance to marital problems.

"Will Power"

In the context of drug using, "will power" refers to a deliberate conscious decision (plus sufficient drive and technical self-help know-how to enforce it) to halt or delay the implementation of an urge. When the urge to use is low or absent, the individual's drive to abstain from further use may appear to be quite strong. However, when the temptation is strong, the will power may become attenuated. Marlatt and Gordon (1985) consider will power in terms of the strength of the *commitment* not to use or drink. Commitment means attaching a value to a particular goal so that it supersedes other contradictory goals. Thus, the allocation of importance to abstinence can power the resolve to resist cravings.

The successful application of will power when cravings and urges are aroused depends on a number of factors. An individual may make a serious commitment to stop smoking, drinking, or using but may not have the technical skills to fulfill the commitment. The application of this technical knowledge can greatly increase the amount of leverage when the resolve to abstain is opposed to cravings and urges. Further, core beliefs about oneself (e.g., whether one is effective or helpless) may affect one's capacity to apply will power to controlling urges. We must caution that patients tend to misconstrue the meaning of will power, seeing it as an almost masochistic battle to maintain an unceasing state of discomfort in the face of drug urges (Tiffany, 1990). Clinicians must emphasize to patients that they will be taught to modify their beliefs and behaviors (cf. Washton, 1988) so that positive self-image and lifestyle changes will take place. This, along with the natural dissipation of cravings over time (Horvath, 1988), will help patients to feel good about resisting drug use in the long run, as opposed to feeling deprived and in pain.

According to the myth of the "rational man" (e.g., in jurisprudence or economics), an individual weighs the risks and benefits of a given action and makes a rational decision. In the case of the addicted individual, however, the objective cost–benefit analyses, or advantages–disadvantages calculations, are thrown off by the momentary appeal of using, drinking, or smoking. The immediacy and reliability of the effect of the drug and the subjective certainty that some desired effect will be achieved right away contrasts with an uncertain, possibly undesirable consequence in the future. Some individuals become oblivious to the negative consequences when they experience the craving (Gawin & Ellinwood, 1988). Others simply shrug off the long-range effects with the attitude "I'll take my chances," or rationalize, "It won't hurt if I give in this one time."

On the other hand, a number of individuals are able to summon up, on their own, arguments and unpleasant memories that deter them from yielding to the temptation. In any event, there is always a conflict when individuals try to utilize will power to forestall yielding to their urges. On the one hand, for example, an individual experiences the craving (and the anticipated relief or pleasure) and, on the other, the voice of reason and restraint (and the anticipated deprivation and distress). After many unpleasant experiences, one may be able to issue oneself warnings of the dangers of indulgence when exposed to a high-risk situation or when aware of the lowering of one's resistance. Whether one will be able to heed these warnings to oneself depends to a large extent on one's access to techniques to implement them.

Addictive Beliefs

In our work, we have been impressed by the commonality of certain beliefs across various types of addictions (cocaine, opiates, alcohol, nicotine, and prescription drugs) and various addicted individuals. Even individuals susceptible to binge eating or generalized overeating show these types of dysfunctional beliefs (Heatherton & Baumeister, 1991; Lingswiler, Crowther, & Stephens, 1989; Zotter & Crowther, 1991). The addictive beliefs characterize those individuals after they have become addicted (i.e., they are characteristic of the disorder), however, and cannot in themselves be considered predispositional to addiction. Nonetheless, the addictive beliefs do contribute to maintaining the addiction and provide the groundwork for relapse.

Addictive beliefs may be considered in terms of a cluster of ideas centering around pleasure seeking, problem solving, relief, and escape. The specific items will vary depending on the type of preferred substance. Among the dysfunctional ideas are (1) the belief that one *needs* the substance if one is to maintain psychological and emotional balance; (2) the expectation that the substance will improve social and intellectual functioning; (3) the expectation that one will find pleasure and excitement from using; (4) the belief that the drug will energize the individual and provide increased power; (5) the expectation that the drug will have a soothing effect; (6) the assumption that the drug will relieve boredom, anxiety, tension, and depression; and (7) the conviction that unless something is done to satisfy the craving or to neutralize the distress, it will continue indefinitely and, possibly, get worse.

In addition to these expectations/beliefs, the patients have a variety of beliefs relevant to justification, risk taking, and entitlement. These attitudes fall into one category of *"permission-giving beliefs,"* such as "Since I'm feeling bad, it's OK to use," "I've been having a hard time; therefore, I'm entitled to relief," "If I take a hit, I can get away with it," "The satisfaction I get is worth the risk of relapsing," or "If I give in this time, I will resolve to resist the temptation next time."

Predispositional Characteristics

A number of characteristics of the drug abuser, however, may have existed prior to drug use and thus may be considered predispositional. These characteristics center around (1) general sensitivity to their unpleasant feelings or emotions—for example, they have a low tolerance for the normal cyclical changes in mood; (2) deficient motivation to control behavior—thus, instant satisfaction is more highly valued than control; (3) inadequate techniques for controlling behavior and coping with problems—therefore, even when motivated to exert restraint, they do not have the technical knowledge to follow through with it; (4) a pattern of *automatic*, nonreflective yielding to impulses; (5) excitement seeking and low tolerance for boredom; (6) low tolerance for frustration (low frustration tolerance in itself rests on a complex set of beliefs and cognitive distortions); and (7) relatively diminished future time perspectives, such that the individual's attention is focused on here-and-now emotional states, cravings, and urges and on the actions for relieving or satisfying them. None of the attentional resources are devoted to the *consequences* of these actions.

Low frustration tolerance (LFT) seems to be an important precursor to drug using (Chapter 15, this volume). Specifically, a number of dysfunctional attitudes magnifying the usual everyday sources of frustration lead to excessive disappointment and anger. Among the components of this belief complex are attitudes such as (1) things should always go smoothly for me *or* things should not go wrong; (2) when I am blocked in what I am doing, it is awful; (3) I cannot stand being frustrated; (4) other people are to blame for my being thwarted, and they should be punished; and (5) people deliberately give me a hard time.

When individuals with LFT find that their activity is blocked or their expectations are thwarted, they are likely to (1) greatly exaggerate the degree of loss resulting from thwarting, (2) exaggerate the long-range consequences of this loss, (3) blame whomever they think might be responsible for thwarting, (4) experience excessive anger, (5) have a strong desire to punish the offender, and (6) importantly, overlook other ways of achieving their goal, such as problem solving.

The result of this sequence of events is that an individual becomes overmobilized to attack the offender. Since there is rarely a legitimate avenue for expressing the hostile impulses, the individual is left in a highly energized state, full of tension and anger. At some point, such individuals find that drug taking may reduce the highly volatile state and relieve the pent-up tension. Of course, the use of drugs for this purpose is at best only a temporary remedy and in the long run is self-defeating because the individual never learns ways of coping directly with frustration and solving the contributing problems. Consequently, LFT is perpetuated, as are the beliefs regarding helplessness.

SUMMARY

Many addicted individuals have characteristics that predispose them to drug abuse. These predispositional factors include (1) general exaggerated sensitivity to unpleasant feelings, (2) deficient motivation to control behavior, (3) impulsivity, (4) excitement seeking and low tolerance for boredom, (5) low tolerance for frustration, and (6) in many cases, insufficient prosocial alternatives for gaining pleasurable feelings, and a sense of hopelessness in ever achieving this goal. LFT is characterized by exaggeration of the degree of loss resulting from thwarting, blaming other people for any frustration, a strong desire to punish the offender, and overlooking other ways of problem solving. Each of these predispositional factors is addressed in the course of cognitive therapy.

The sequence of addiction often follows a vicious cycle proceeding from anxiety or low mood to self-medication by using or drinking. This behavior, in turn, produces and/or exacerbates financial, social, and/or medical problems, which lead to further anxiety and low mood. Patients often ascribe their drug and alcohol use to "uncontrollable cravings and urges." However, certain dysfunctional beliefs tend to fuel these cravings. Abusers tend to ignore, minimize, or deny the problems resulting from their drug use or attribute these problems to something other than the drugs or alcohol. An important factor in maintaining psychological dependency is the belief that withdrawal from the drug will produce intolerable side effects. In actuality, through careful clinical management these side effects generally turn out to be tolerable. Another important set of core beliefs centers around the addicted individual's sense of helplessness in controlling the craving.

Cravings are associated with wanting gratification or relief, whereas urges are concerned with doing something to provide a gratification or relief. The delay between the experience of craving and the implementation of the urge provides an interval for therapeutic intervention. Cravings and urges tend to be automatic and may become autonomous; the thrust of therapy is to provide voluntary methods for managing them. Patients tend to equate the strong craving with an imperative "need" and an uncontrollable urge. Although the craving leading to drinking and using is involuntary, controlling the urge is voluntary and can be adopted even though the patient may feel helpless. Increasing the ratio of the subjective power of control to the subjective power of the urge may be used as a guide for intervention.

Cognitive therapy is a system of psychotherapy that attempts to reduce self-defeating behavior by modifying erroneous thinking and maladaptive beliefs and teaching techniques of control. In the cognitive therapy of drug abuse, the specific case formulation forms the basis for the therapeutic regimen. This formulation, in turn, is based on the cognitive model of addictions.

The therapeutic approach consists of undermining the urge by weakening the beliefs that feed into the urge and, at the same time, demonstrating to the patient various ways of controlling and modifying their behavior. Cognitive therapy of substance abuse is characterized by the following: (1) It is collaborative (builds trust), (2) it is active, (3) it is based, to a large degree on guided discovery and empirical testing of beliefs, (4) it is highly structured and focused, and (5) it attempts to view the drug or drinking problem as a technical problem for which there is a technical solution.

CHAPTER 3

Theory and Therapy of Addiction

According to the cognitive perspective, the way people interpret specific situations influences their feelings, motivations, and actions. Their interpretations, in turn, are shaped in many instances by the relevant beliefs that become activated in these situations. A social situation, for example, may activate an idiosyncratic belief such as "Cocaine makes me more sociable" or "I can be more relaxed if I have a beer (or a cigarette)," and lead to a desire to use, drink, or smoke. Specific beliefs such as these constitute a vulnerability to substance abuse. Activated under particular predictable circumstances, the beliefs increase the likelihood of continued drug or alcohol use (i.e., they stimulate craving).

Beliefs also shape the individual's reactions to the physiological sensations associated with anxiety and craving (Beck, Emery, with Greenberg, 1985). Beliefs such as "I cannot tolerate anxiety" or "I must give in to this hunger" will influence the person's reactions to these sensations. Individuals with such beliefs are likely to be hyperattentive to these sensations. Even a low-level degree of anxiety or craving can elicit a substance-using belief such as "I must take a hit (or drink) to relieve my anxiety (or satisfy my craving)."

The activation of substance-using beliefs is illustrated in the experience of Les, a chronic cocaine user, who experienced a sudden craving for cocaine while attending a party. In this scenario, his acute urge to use was related to his sense of social isolation within a group. His underlying belief, "I can't stand it without cocaine," was activated by his sad feelings at seeing other people having a good time using drugs. Les lived in a rundown neighborhood in which there was a great deal of drug traffic. He had a longstanding belief, "I'll never get out of this awful environment." This belief (not the environment per se) led to chronic feelings of sadness and hopelessness. The belief underlying his chronic urge to use cocaine was "I need some coke to get through the day." This case illustrates the coexistence of *acute* cravings and urges related to a specific situation with more *chronic* urges related to the patient's general life situation. The combination of these beliefs made Les prone to addiction.

LAYERS OF BELIEFS

There were several levels of beliefs underlying Les's addictive behavior: (1) his more general basic belief that he was "trapped" in a noxious environment; (2) his belief that the only way he could escape from his environment and his unpleasant feelings was to take drugs; and (3) the belief that he "needed" drugs to relieve any unpleasant feelings. Added to these drug-related beliefs was a basic belief that he did not belong and was not accepted as a member of his peer group. This cluster of beliefs made Les vulnerable to addictive behavior; that is, they fed into a compulsive urge to relieve his distress through drug taking.

The essence of a large proportion of addictive behaviors, consisting of the types of general and specific beliefs held by this patient, are illustrated in Figure 3.1.

The addictive beliefs (Chapter 2, this volume) seem to derive from either one or a combination of *core beliefs* (sometimes referred to as "core schemas"). The first set of dysfunctional core beliefs has to do with personal survival, achievement, freedom, and autonomy. Depending on the precise nature of the patient's vulnerability, the core belief that is expressed may have a content such as any of the following: "I am helpless, trapped, defeated, inferior, weak, inept, useless, or a failure." The second set of dysfunctional core beliefs is concerned with

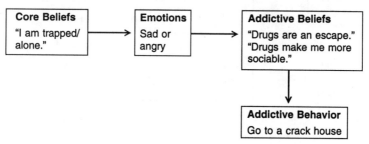

FIGURE 3.1. Sequence of core beliefs and addictive beliefs.

bonding with other individuals or to a group. This set of beliefs is concerned with lovability or acceptability. The various permutations of the core belief may take the following form: "I am unloved, undesirable, unwanted, repulsive, rejected, different, socially defective." Such core beliefs constitute a specific sensitivity or vulnerability: When circumstances (e.g., social rejection) that are relevant to the core belief arise, they trigger the belief (e.g., "I am defective") and lead to distress.

Les had a double set of core beliefs revolving around the notions "I am helpless" and "I am undesirable." When he noted the difficult conditions in his neighborhood, the first belief was triggered and took the form "I am trapped." Once this notion took hold, he believed himself incapable of improving his lot, saw the future as hopeless, and felt frustrated and sad. The specific *addictive belief* was then triggered: "The only way to get relief is to take a hit."

In a group situation his automatic thought was "I don't belong." This thought stemmed from his other core belief, "I am unacceptable." These beliefs converged on the addictive belief: "The only way to get accepted is to use coke." The relation between his two core beliefs, his automatic thought, his addictive belief, and his craving is illustrated in Figure 3.2.

The same sort of constellation of core belief, addictive belief, and craving may apply whatever the instigating factor and whether the form of relief is alcohol, illegal drugs, legal drugs, or tobacco. The sequence generally proceeds from (1) a core belief, such as a negative view of the self (helpless, undesirable) and/or a negative view of the environment (noxious, oppressive), and/or a negative view of the future (hopeless), to (2) unpleasant feelings, such as dysphoria or anxiety. From there, the addiction-prone individual experiences (3) craving and psychological dependency on drugs (e.g., "I *need* cocaine to make me feel better).

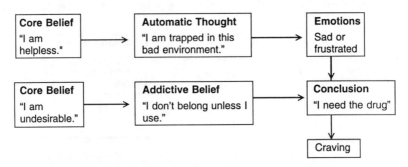

FIGURE 3.2. Interaction of multiple beliefs.

It is important to note that the perception of a noxious environment is not limited to inner-city individuals. Privileged individuals who perceive their job, family, or marital situation as inimical, who experience the same sequence of discouragement over life circumstances and have negative views of themselves and their future, may turn to drugs as a form of escape. In depression (Chapter 14, this volume), the negative view of the self, the current circumstances, and the future often is exaggerated. After patients modify their depressive thinking, the therapist often finds that compulsive drug use is diminished (Woody et al., 1983).

Individuals like Les become habitual users because they regard using as a way of gaining or maintaining social acceptance. They have addictive beliefs such as "I can't let my friends down . . . they will reject me if I don't use." (This fear, of course, may be realistic and one of the goals of therapy may be to help the patient to develop friendships with nonusers.) One patient greatly admired his cousin who was addicted to cocaine. The patient constantly used crack when he was with his cousin. The instigating factor each time was a desire to please his cousin. Eventually, using became embedded in his system of coping with his fear of becoming socially ostracized.

SEQUENCE OF BELIEFS

Although the core beliefs represent the background of the addictive beliefs, they are not immediately apparent unless the patient is depressed (Chapter 14, this volume). The addictive beliefs may be more accessible. These addictive beliefs are activated in a specific sequence. First in the sequence are *anticipatory beliefs*. Initially these take a form such as "It will be *fun* to do this . . . It's okay to try it occasionally." As the patient gains satisfaction from using, he/she often develops romanticized beliefs predictive of gratification or escape: "I will have an hour or so of sheer pleasure . . . I will feel less sad/anxious . . . It will be a sweet oblivion." Some beliefs are predictive of increased efficacy or socialization: "I will perform better . . . I will be more entertaining and will be accepted into the group."

As the individuals start to rely on the drug to counteract feelings of distress, they develop relief-oriented beliefs, such as "I need cocaine in order to function . . . I can't continue without it . . . I will feel well again if I use . . . I *need* the drug . . . I can't control the craving . . . I must have it or I'll fall apart." Note the imperative quality of these beliefs: "I must have a smoke to make it through the day." The activation of these beliefs then leads to cravings.

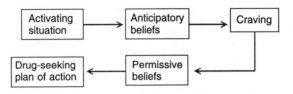

FIGURE 3.3. Sequence of anticipatory and permissive beliefs.

Since addiction-prone individuals may have some conflict about using (e.g., medical, financial, social, or legal consequences of using), they generally develop a *facilitating* or *permissive belief*, such as "I deserve it" or "It's all right, I can handle it . . . Since I'm feeling bad, it's all right to use . . . Nothing else is going right; this is the only right thing in my life." The relation of these beliefs is illustrated in Figure 3.3.

The sequence of these beliefs formed by Les is illustrated in Figure 3.4. His uneasiness in a social situation triggers the anticipatory belief "I will feel better if I use," which is immediately followed by a craving and then the plan of action to call his cousin for a "hit."

CONFLICTING BELIEFS

In the various stages of cocaine use the patient can have conflicting sets of beliefs, such as "I should not use cocaine" versus "It's OK to use this one time." Each belief can be activated under different circumstances or even at the same time. *The balance between the relative strength of each belief at a given time will influence whether the patient uses or abstains.* (Of course, the availability of the drug will also be a determining factor.)

Sometimes the individual experiences a conflict between the desire to use and the desire to be free of drugs. This ambivalence may be formulated as a conflict between two beliefs: "It's OK" (permissive) versus "It's not OK" (abstinent). The conflict between these beliefs results in discomfort or may increase the individual's current discomfort. Paradoxically, the individual may experience an even greater pull toward using in order to relieve the uneasiness produced by the conflict. The belief "I need relief from this feeling" becomes more potent and may tip the scales in favor of using.

In therapy, patients learn skills to cope with the discomfort and to test out and restructure their belief that using or drinking is the most useful way of dealing with discomfort.

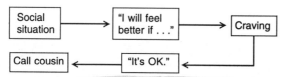

FIGURE 3.4. Simple model of Les's substance use (maps onto Figure 3.3).

ACTIVATION OF BELIEFS
IN STIMULUS SITUATIONS

Drug-using beliefs and desires typically are activated in specific, often predictable, circumstances, which we term "stimulus situations." These are also labeled "cues" (Moorey, 1989). However, depending on the patient's current mood and self-control, the degree of riskiness of a situation may vary considerably from time to time. That is, a situation that is manageable at one time may be stimulating enough to promote drug use at another time. These circumstances, which can be external or internal, correspond to what Marlatt and Gordon (1985) term "high-risk situations." These situations stimulate the craving to "smoke, shoot, snort, or swallow drugs."

Examples of *external* stimulus situations are a gathering of friends using cocaine, contact with a drug dealer, or receiving a weekly paycheck. *Internal* circumstances (or cues) include various emotional states such as depression, anxiety, or boredom, which can trigger drug-using beliefs and, consequently, craving for the drug.

As shown in Figure 3.5, drug use may be regarded as representing the final common pathway of the activation of the cluster of the aforementioned beliefs. Cognitive therapy is aimed at modifying each of the categories of beliefs: anticipatory and permissive, as well as the underlying core beliefs (e.g., "I am trapped") that potentiate these drug-

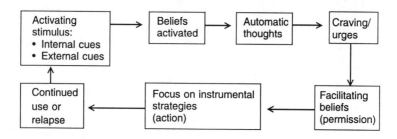

FIGURE 3.5. Complete model of substance use.

related beliefs. The therapist attempts to introduce or reinforce more adaptive beliefs relevant to each of the classes of beliefs. Other techniques are concerned with dealing with major life problems (see Chapters 12 and 13, this volume) or personality difficulties or disorders (see Chapters 14, 15, and 16, this volume) leading to drug use.

As shown earlier, craving is aroused in a specific situation and seems to arise as a reflex reaction to the stimulus. However, the situation does not directly "cause" the craving: Interposed between the stimulus and the craving is a drug-related belief that is activated by the situation and an automatic thought derived from this belief. For example, when he was feeling sad, Les would get the thought "If I take a hit now, I will feel better." His underlying belief was: "I can't stand discomfort . . . I need a fix to make the discomfort go away." The sequence then proceeded to craving, to facilitating beliefs ("It's OK this time"), to an actual plan for obtaining the drug, and finally to using. These beliefs can be ascertained by direct questioning and the use of inventories (see Appendix, this volume).

The sequence proceeds so rapidly that it is often viewed as a "conditioned reflex" (O'Brien, 1992). The automatic thought, in particular, seems to be almost instantaneous and can be captured only if the patient learns to focus on the chain of events.

Figure 3.6 illustrates the sequence from the activating stimulus to the implementation of the plan to get the drug. It should be noted that each step offers an opportunity for a cognitive intervention. Using the method of guided discovery (Beck et al., 1979), for example, the cognitive therapist questions the *meaning* attached to the activating stimulus, the relief-oriented belief that taking a fix is the most desirable solution, the permission-giving belief ("I can do it without harm"), and the implementation plan (the decision to look around for money).

Les had a very low tolerance for unpleasant feelings, whether sadness, anxiety, or sheer boredom. His belief regarding the necessity for alleviating feelings of distress was activated when he attended a party. His drug-taking beliefs centered on the anticipation of relief

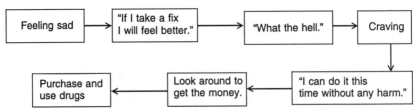

FIGURE 3.6. Example of Les's drug-using sequence (maps onto Figure 3.5).

from any negative feelings. Other examples of his anticipatory relief-oriented beliefs were: "There is only *one way* for me to have fun," "I can't stand the withdrawal symptoms," "I feel better knowing it's there," and "If I don't take a hit regularly, I will feel much worse."

It should be noted that the patient's permissive thoughts about the harmlessness of drug taking stemmed from a simplistic (and deceptive) set of beliefs. He believed that since he only *snorted* cocaine, he could not be addicted: He saw himself as being safe from addiction provided he did not *smoke crack*. In fact, one of his typical permissive thoughts was, "I'm OK since I don't smoke crack."

"Spontaneous craving" (i.e., craving in the absence of an obvious external stimulus) is also often observed. For example, a patient with a 5-year history of cocaine use reported having a dream about using cocaine. Upon awakening, he "felt high." Next, he started daydreaming about the last time he had used cocaine. This imagined scenario in turn activated the belief, "Life is more fun when I use," and was followed by the automatic thought, "I love this stuff." A permission-giving belief was also activated, "There is no harm in this." His attention then focused on checking to see whether he had enough money to buy cocaine. Although the craving appeared to be spontaneous in this case, the patient's mental state during the dream and upon awakening set the stage for daydreaming about using. This imagery served as a catalyst for the permission-giving thoughts. His attention then focused on implementing his craving and shut out any consideration of the ill effects of using.

INFORMATION PROCESSING: MEANING, SYMBOLISM, AND RULES

In referring to the kinds of circumstances (external or internal) that excite the craving–using cycle, we generally use the term "stimulus situations" or "triggers" rather than "high-risk situations" introduced by Marlatt and Gordon (1985). Although many situations have a high probability of setting the craving–using pattern into motion, their effect varies from person to person and even for the same person over time. By conceptualizing these situations in terms of their stimulus properties and meanings, we can align our concept of drug use and abuse with concepts regarding stress (Beck, 1993), syndromal disorders (e.g., depression; Beck et al., 1979), and personality disorders (Beck, Freeman, & Associates, 1990).

While the term "high-risk situation" fits nicely into a descriptive model, the formulation in more cognitive terms can fit our observation into an explanatory model. This model, encompassing concepts of the activation of beliefs, symbols, information processing, and motivation, provides a broader framework for understanding and psychological intervention.

Although we use the terms "stimulus situations" and "stimulus properties," it should be noted that the actual situation is neutral. It becomes a stimulus if a person attaches a special meaning to it. For example, an addicted individual looks at a cocaine pipe and other paraphernalia and becomes excited and experiences craving. Another person, indifferent to drugs or not knowledgeable about the paraphernalia, simply sees a pipe. For the first person, the pipe is a symbol, a coded message, packed with meaning. The meaning is not inherent in the pipe but in the individual's personal symbolic code (embedded in his or her information or cognitive processing system). The individual automatically applies this code when he/she perceives the paraphernalia, for example, and consequently experiences pleasure and craving.

The therapist's task is to help the patient to decode the symbol. If one "unpacks" its meaning, it would read something like this: "The pipe means taking a hit, which will give me pleasure." The pipe and the concept of pleasure have become fused so that the expectation of pleasure in the future gives pleasure now and leads to craving.

The drug abuser may seem to be stimulus bound. Any depiction of or reference to drugs on television, radio, or magazines, for example, may be sufficient to excite the individual. The addicted person is actually "schema driven"; that is, Les's reactions are produced by internal cognitive structures, labeled schemas, that contain the code, formulas, or beliefs that attach meaning to the situation (see Beck, 1967, for a complete description of schemas). Thus, a schema containing the belief "Using is necessary for my happiness" will be primed when the person is exposed to a relevant situation.

Similarly, a schema containing the belief "I cannot be happy unless I am loved" will be activated if the person perceives that he or she has been rejected by a lover and, thus, will feel sad. The experience of the sad affect will, in turn, be processed cognitively by beliefs such as "I can't stand sadness," "I need relief by using." The individual then experiences craving.

The therapeutic application of this explanatory model involves attaching more importance to modifying the individual's belief system than to simply getting him to avoid or cope with high-risk situations. Since some "situations" (such as internal states) are unavoidable and other situations (e.g., exposure to drug-related situations) may be inevitable (Childress, Hole, & DePhilippis, 1990; Moorey, 1989;

O'Brien, McLellan, Alterman, & Childress, 1992; Shulman, 1989), the best outcome can be derived from changing the beliefs that make these situations risky.

Les, for example, often compared himself with other people more successful than he. When he saw such a person, his negative beliefs ("I'm inferior" and "I'm no good") were activated. Thus, the meaning attached to the perception of the other person was a self-devaluation, leading to sadness. He also attached a meaning to sadness: "My life is intolerable . . . I can't stand the pain." Following the activation of the belief "I need dope to ease the pain," Les experienced craving. In therapy, each of these beliefs was explored.

The proposed mechanism for therapeutic change consists of aligning the belief system more closely with reality. Since the beliefs are maladaptive (e.g., "I need the drug [or alcohol] in order to function"), it is necessary either to modify these beliefs or to substitute more functional beliefs (or both).

The process of change, however, involves more than simple modification of the beliefs. The therapist and patient need to work together to improve the patient's system of controls (e.g., by practicing delay of gratification) and to learn coping techniques such as anticipating and solving problems.

Thus, the therapeutic goals are (1) conceptual change and (2) technical development of proficiency in coping.

Cognitive Blockade

When they are not experiencing craving, patients are generally able to recognize the disruptive effects of the drug on their lives. However, once the drug-taking beliefs are activated, a "cognitive blockade" inhibits awareness of or attention to the delayed long-term consequences of drug use (Gawin & Ellinwood, 1988; Velten, 1986) and increases the focus on immediate instrumental strategies, such as searching for money to buy drugs. As these beliefs become hyperactive, recognition of the drawbacks of drug use become attenuated. When Les was not feeling sad, he was convinced that using cocaine was bad for him, but once his craving was stimulated, he had difficulty in remembering his reasons for not using. His attentional processes were predominantly allocated to using. The immediacy of the stimulus and the activated meanings shut out serious consideration of long-range consequences.

This kind of "tunnel vision," in which the individual's attentional resources are devoted almost totally to the immediate situation, has been demonstrated in cognitive psychology experiments (Beck, 1991).

For example, very hungry individuals will be hypersensitive to stimuli relevant to food or eating and will be relatively insensitive to other signals. The introduction of danger stimuli, however, will shift the attention to the danger stimuli and away from food stimuli. Clinical states show the same type of phenomenon. Information that is congruent with the clinical condition will be processed very rapidly and memories congruent with the state can be rapidly recalled, but the patient has trouble gaining access to stored information that is not congruent with the clinical condition. Depressed patients, for example, quickly assimilate negative information about themselves but block out positive information. Also, they recall negative information much better than positive information (Beck, 1991). Similarly, patients having a panic attack readily respond to suggestions that they are experiencing a serious condition but have problems in recalling benign explanations for their attacks or even in applying reason to counteract the catastrophic interpretations they are making (Beck, 1986).

A somewhat similar phenomenon may be observed among many individuals addicted to drugs, alcohol, or nicotine. Although when sober they may be quite adept at reeling off (with sincerity and conviction) the reasons for not using, drug users have difficulty in recalling or attaching the same significance to these reasons once they are in the throes of a specific drug-using episode. Since all their attention is focused on the mechanics of obtaining the drug, the reasons for using at that time become very salient and the contradictory reasons become inaccessible or insignificant.

This phenomenon is termed the "cognitive blockade" because of blocking out the incongruent (i.e., the corrective, realistic) information. The therapeutic task is to lift the blockade, as it were, through a variety of tasks. One approach is to deliberately activate the craving cycle in the office (e.g., through imagery) and, while the craving is strong, review the reasons for not using. Of course, sufficient time must be allotted for this maneuver to preclude the craving's being maintained following the session (Childress et al., 1990). A similar strategy involves the preparation of flashcards (listing reasons for not using) which patients will read when they experience craving in the natural environment.

SUMMARY

At the core of the problem of the addicted individual is a set of addictive beliefs which appear to be derived from core beliefs such as "I am helpless," "I am unlovable," or "I am vulnerable." These core beliefs interact with life stressors to produce excessive anxiety, dysphoria, or anger. These stressful or stimulus situations do not directly "cause" craving, but they activate the drug-related beliefs that lead to the craving. Although we use the term "stimulus situation," it should be noted that the situation itself is neutral. The *meanings*, derived from the beliefs, that are attached to a situation are what cause the individual's craving. Individuals with beliefs that they cannot tolerate anxiety, dysphoria, or frustration, for example, will tend to be hyperattentive to these sensations and may build up expectations that they can relieve the sensations only through using or drinking. Thus, when an unpleasant affect arises, the individual attempts to neutralize it by using or drinking.

A specific sequence of drug-related beliefs leading to drinking or using may be delineated. First is the activation of *anticipatory beliefs* relevant to obtaining pleasure from using or drinking. These antici- patory beliefs usually progress to relief-oriented imperative beliefs, which define using or drinking as a dire necessity and stipulate that the craving is uncontrollable and must be satisfied. The anticipation of pleasure or relief leads to the activation of craving and *facilitating* or *permissive beliefs*, such as "I deserve it" or "It's OK this time," which legitimize using or drinking. Finally, the instrumental plans, which have to do with plans or strategies for obtaining drugs or alcohol, are propelled by the imperative craving.

Many individuals have conflicting beliefs regarding the pros and cons of using. At times they are locked in such an unpleasant struggle between these opposing beliefs that, paradoxically, they may seek drugs simply to relieve the tension generated by the conflict.

The therapeutic application of this model, consisting of modify- ing the individual's belief system, goes beyond teaching the individual to avoid or cope with "high-risk situations."

CHAPTER 4

The Therapeutic Relationship and Its Problems

A collaborative relationship between the therapist and the patient is a vital component of any successful therapy. The most brilliantly conceived interventions will be reduced in effectiveness if the patient is not engaged in the process of treatment. All the support and effort that the therapist may put forth in an effort to help the patient will make little impact if the therapist has not gained some measure of the patient's trust.

While this seems to be relevant to almost every type of patient, it is most especially true of the substance-abusing population. Numerous potential factors interact to create an almost adversarial relationship between the therapist and the drug-abusing patient at the beginning of therapy and during the course of treatment. These factors include:

1. Drug-abusing patients often do not enter treatment on a voluntary basis.
2. Patients often maintain highly dysfunctional presuppositions about therapy.
3. Patients often are not very open and honest, at least at the start of therapy.
4. Patients may be currently involved in felonious activities, thus presenting confidentiality dilemmas.
5. Patients view their therapist as part of the "system," and not as an ally.

6. Patients have a difficult time believing that their therapist really cares about their problems.
7. Patients look askance at therapists whom they perceive to differ from them markedly in terms of demographics and attitudes.
8. Therapists may maintain negative presuppositions about drug-abusing patients.

Many of these patients do not come into therapy of their own volition. Some are given an ultimatum by their significant others (e.g., spouse, children, or parents) or employers, while others are remanded by the courts following criminal legal proceedings (Frances & Miller, 1991). Consequently, the drug-abusing patient may enter the therapist's office with any number of counterproductive automatic thoughts, such as "I don't want to be here; I'm only here so my wife will get off my back," "I'll just tell this doctor what he wants to hear, and then I'll blow out of here," "This whole therapy thing is like doing real easy time compared to prison; I'll just go along with this and do what I want to do anyway," "I don't really have a problem; maybe I'll show up for therapy, and maybe I won't," and "I'm not going to tell this shrink anything that can be used against me; my life is nobody's business but my own." The list could go on and on.

To complicate matters further, drug-abusing patients typically enter therapy playing their cards close to their vests, and therefore conceal the kinds of automatic thoughts listed above. The therapist must actively probe for them, as the patients often will not divulge them in an unsolicited fashion (Covi et al., 1990).

Another factor that militates against the ready formation of a positive therapeutic relationship is that substance abuse often represents felonious behavior. As such, patients are highly motivated to be dishonest in self-reporting their substance abuse activities. Although the vast majority of therapeutic interactions represent privileged communications between therapist and patient, drug-abusing patients are typically well schooled in covering their tracks. As the stakes are high, such patients may simply decide it is best to take no chances, and therefore will not readily admit to drug-abuse-related behaviors. Furthermore, some actions of the patients may be serious enough threats to themselves or to the general public that the therapist may legally and ethically be required to contact the authorities (e.g., when the patient admits that a drug-related murder has been arranged, or when the patient calls the therapist and claims to have taken a drug overdose in order to attempt suicide).

Since therapists should inform their patients about the limits of confidentiality at the outset, drug-abusing patients will come to know what information they cannot safely reveal. If they do come forth with such sensitive material, the therapist is placed in the uncomfortable position of having to serve as society's watchdog, and may in the process completely discourage the patient from continuing with much needed treatment.

This point highlights another more general factor that adds to the difficulty in forming a working alliance with drug-abusing patients—namely, that such patients often view the therapist as an agent of the police, the courts, "the system," or a more privileged socioeconomic class. Such patients find it hard to believe that their therapists will sincerely try to help them with their problems, or will treat them with honesty, respect, and positive regard. As a result, the patients tend to dread and avoid therapy sessions. They may take confrontational statements from the therapist as confirmation that the therapist is working against them, while positive statements from the therapist may be seen as naive, manipulative, insincere, or patronizing. This places the therapist in a "damned if I don't, damned if I do" position, which, left unaddressed, may sabotage therapy before it gets started.

Yet another stumbling block to the formation of a healthy therapeutic relationship is the perceived demographic and/or attitudinal differences between therapist and patient. For instance, the patient might think, "This doctor is probably rich and has everything she wants in life. There's no way that she could possibly understand what it's like to struggle every day of your life like I do. How in the world can she help me? The rules of her world just don't apply to mine. Whatever she says is just bullshit." Another thought might be, "I wonder if this therapist ever used drugs. If he did, then he's no better than me, so why should I listen to him? If he didn't, then how can he know what it's like to be hooked? Only someone who's been there could know what he's talking about."

Similarly, the therapist may have maladaptive beliefs about the patient, such as "This guy is a low-life. At best he's going to waste my valuable time, and at worst he's going to be a liability or a threat to my personal safety," or "These types of patients are beyond help. They have a chronic disease for which there is little hope for cure or rehabilitation. Therefore, there's not much point in investing too much of my time or energy," or "I can't relate to this patient at all. I wouldn't associate with him (or her) in 'real life' so I don't think I'll be able to form a working bond with this patient here in the office either."

Admittedly, working with drug-using patients can be highly stressful; therefore we strongly encourage therapists to engage in regular peer supervision with colleagues in order to receive professional support and objective advice. Such consultations can help therapists to avert burnout, and to combat their own dysfunctional beliefs pertinent to working with the drug-abusing populations (cf. Weiner & Fox, 1982).

We acknowledge that the obstacles are formidable. However, based on extensive clinical experience, we believe it is possible to establish a positive, collaborative therapeutic relationship with the substance abuser. We consider this to be the case even when such patients exhibit severe concomitant Axis II disorders, such as paranoid, narcissistic, and/or antisocial personalities (see Chapter 16, this volume). To be sure, the task is difficult, and frequently trying. At the same time, treating the substance-abusing patient can be reframed as representing a growth-enhancing challenge for the therapist. The skills of developing therapeutic alliances with difficult populations (e.g., substance abusers and borderline patients), comprise the "art" of therapy, and as such are very much a measure of the competency of the mental health professional.

This chapter presents guidelines for facilitating the formation and maintenance of an adaptive and functional therapeutic relationship with the drug-abusing patient. Case illustrations are provided in order to highlight various techniques and strategies, as well as to demonstrate how things can go awry. The central messages of this chapter are that (1) a positive therapeutic relationship does not occur by chance—it can be actively constructed, (2) treating the drug-abusing patient requires careful and vigilant attention to the vicissitudes of the interactions between the therapist and the patient, and (3) the management of the therapeutic relationship with the drug-abusing patient is neither a straightforward nor an overwhelming task.

ESTABLISHING RAPPORT

The initial interactions between the patient who is just entering therapy and the therapist are extremely important. Even when drug-abusing patients are self-referred, they often have a great deal of ambivalence about seeking ongoing contact with a therapist (Carroll, Rounsaville, & Gawin, 1991; Carroll, Rounsaville, & Keller, 1991; Havassy et al., 1991; Institute of Medicine, 1990b). From the very start, such patients will be sizing up their therapists to determine if they can be trusted and if they know what they are doing (Perez, 1992). A perceived negative experience with the therapist can lead such patients to choose never to return for further sessions. For those patients who are constrained to continue with therapy as per the terms of their parole or probation, the lack of a positive start to treatment may lead to the kinds of negative expectations that foster passive resistance or contentious behavior in session.

The introductory session in cognitive therapy typically involves the dual aims of establishing rapport with the patient, and socializing the patient into the cognitive model. We suggest that the therapist adhere to both these aims, but place special emphasis on the aim of establishing rapport. The basic therapeutic tasks of listening, reflecting, and demonstrating genuineness and positive regard must not be given short shrift at this stage. While it is also useful to describe the cognitive model, it is important to minimize psychological jargon, and to stay as close as possible to ordinary language. This will help the wary and distrustful patient to view the therapist as being more of a "real person."

For example, the cognitive therapist would be ill-advised to speak in the following manner:

"We're going to be examining your thinking processes, to understand the kinds of cognitive distortions that lead you to engage in maladaptive behaviors such as drug abuse and antisocial activities."

Instead, a preferable alternative phrasing would be:

"Mr. X, I'd like to tell you a little bit about cognitive therapy, and I'd like you to feel free to ask me any questions you might have about what goes on here in treatment. We try to understand how you see things—your thoughts about yourself, about life, about using drugs, and about other things. The reason for this is that it's very important for me to understand where you're coming from and what you're going through. It's also important because you might learn some things about yourself that could help you turn your life around to be more the way you want it. What do you think of that?"

The therapist in the above example does not go into depth in describing cognitive therapy, but he sets some of the groundwork. It is more important that the therapist come across as being understanding and reasonable. If the patient remains in treatment for a sufficient period of time, there will be many opportunities to elaborate on the specifics of cognitive therapy, and to teach the patient the relevant cognitive and behavioral skills.

It is important that therapists communicate in as nonjudgmental a manner as they do with their non-substance-abusing patients. Most clinicians can sympathize with patients who are depressed or anxious but may have less tolerance for those who break the law and cause misery for their families because of their own substance abuse behaviors. Therefore, therapists need to monitor their thoughts and verbal behaviors so that they do not project an air of disdain or preachiness in the therapy session (we discuss this in more detail later in the chapter). The patient's drug abuse behaviors and cognitions need to be discussed as representing a problem, without implying an attack on the patient's morals or character.

Additionally, therapists can facilitate the development of rapport by focusing on other areas of their patients' distress as well. Since many of these patients are in treatment by virtue of having reached points of crisis in their lives (Kosten, Rounsaville, & Kleber, 1986; Sobell, Sobell, & Nirenberg, 1988), many of them have dual diagnoses (Castaneda et al., 1989; Evans & Sullivan, 1990; Nace et al., 1991; Rounsaville et al., 1991), thus making it appropriate to address such areas of concern as dysphoric mood, feelings of shame and low self-esteem, general difficulties in coping with life stressors, family problems, and the like. When therapists demonstrate that they are interested in the entirety of the patients' well-being, and are not simply seeking to stop their "bad" drug using, patients may begin to see their therapist as an ally. In this manner, therapists show that they are interested in getting to know the patient as a person, not simply as an addict. Therapists then gain a better chance at calling patients' attention to the fact that substance abuse is an important causal factor in their overall emotional, interpersonal, and physical malaise. This motivates patients to consider the cessation of substance abuse as a major ongoing goal of therapy.

Another useful rapport-building technique nicely doubles as a procedure to begin to educate patients about the cognitive model. Here, therapists freely ask their drug-abuse patients what they think about coming into therapy. Such questions can involve asking about patients' doubts and concerns, as well as their expectations, goals, and hopes for therapy. It is especially important to inquire about these thoughts during the initial therapeutic contact, to maximize the likelihood that the patient will return for a second session. Otherwise, the patient may harbor misgivings about ongoing sessions, and quietly exit therapy after one session without ever offering a clue that such intentions were present.

As illustrated earlier, these techniques serve two functions. First, they communicate a willingness to hear the patient's point of view, and show that the patient will have input into the treatment. Second, they allow the therapist to point out how certain thoughts (e.g., doubts about therapy) can lead to certain emotions (e.g., hopelessness and dysphoria) and behaviors (e.g., quitting therapy) that have a great impact on the patient. After discussing these doubts, the patient may have a more optimistic outlook on therapy. If the patient also feels better emotionally, the therapist can seize on this as a live example of cognitive therapy at work—positive thinking corresponds with positive mood. The following dialogue between patient (PT) and therapist (TH), based on one of our court-referred cases, illustrates this:

PT: (*interrupts the therapist to ask a terse question*) How many times do I have to come here [to therapy sessions]?

TH: Well, as I understand it, as often as you and I believe it makes sense that you come here. That might be once a week, perhaps more often, perhaps less, and we'll be meeting either until it's clear that you're no longer in need of regular sessions, or until the end of your probation period. Do you have some ideas in mind?

PT: Yeh, I have some ideas. (*long pause . . . patient frowns and has a scowling look*)

TH: I take it you're not too pleased about being here.

PT: You got that right.

TH: I'd like to hear you out if you're willing to tell me what's on your mind right now.

PT: What's to tell? I have to come here, and that's that. I ain't got no choice. So what else is new?

TH: Hmmm (*sympathetically*). You're pretty down and maybe pissed off that you have to come here. And it feels to you like it's something that was forced on you.

PT: Yeh.

TH: And that this isn't the only thing that's been forced on you?

PT: Yeh.

TH: I'd like to hear more about it.

PT: I'm just tired of the whole thing. (*long pause*)

TH: Go on. I'm listening.

PT: I did my time. Two years of my life. And now I'm supposed to be free, but no . . . I have to check in with my parole officer, and I have to give urines [toxicology screens each week], and I can't travel without permission, and I have to go see a head shrinker, and everything else.

TH: What is your opinion about all of this?

PT: It sucks.

TH: Well, I suppose that I wouldn't be too pleased myself if I were going through what you're going through right now. I don't think I'd take too kindly to having all these appointments.

PT: It's like, I'm always being checked up on. And being monitored. I'm sick of it already. It's as bad as when I was in jail.

TH: Are you saying that you view coming to therapy here as being "checked up on?"

PT: Yeh. (*sarcastically and incredulously*) Tell me you're not here to check up on me and report things to my PO about me.

TH: Well, you got part of it right, that's for sure. I am responsible for sending an attendance report to the parole office each month. I mean, after all, they are paying for your treatment and they want to see that you're getting something out of it and not just blowing it off. If you're not here, then it probably tells them that you're not getting any ongoing help. If you're not getting any ongoing help, then you don't stand as good a chance of remaining free of drugs, and you might violate parole and wind up in jail again. I don't think that they want you to have to go back to jail again, and neither do I.

PT: What's it to you?

TH: Well, I like to think I'm doing something worthwhile for people. I'd feel proud of myself and happy for you if our weekly meetings had something to do with getting this drug and prison monkey off your back once and for all so you can get back to living your own life again. My main goal is not just to check up on you.

PT: It's just such a hassle, you know.

TH: I know. [Therapist makes a conscious decision not to address this automatic thought at this time, but rather chooses to commiserate with the patient in order to build rapport]

PT: I guess I have to come here. But I don't have to like it.

TH: Well, that's true. You're the final judge on whether this whole therapy thing is worth anything to you. But I'd like to think that we could work together so that you can get something for your troubles. I'm not here to "shrink your head." I'm a psychologist. A therapist. I'm here to help you solve some problems. I can't do it alone, though. I need your assistance. I may be an "expert" in psychology, but you're the expert on you. I have to respect that.

PT: Well, yeh.

TH: What would you like to get out of therapy so that it's much more than just being monitored? Something for you.

Therapist and patient went on to talk at some length about the patient's goals for therapy, and the patient's mood brightened and her anger diminished. Before the end of the session, the therapist helped the patient to summarize the contents of the session, with special emphasis on an important point that paved the way to socialization into the cognitive model. The main point was that when the patient thought only about the down side of therapy, she felt sad and angry. However, when she opened up her mind to other possible uses of therapy, she acquired more information, thought of more useful ideas, and felt more hopeful. In short, she learned an important lesson about how untested thoughts could adversely affect her emotions, as well as her capacity for solving problems. She also learned that it was important to get all the facts before passing judgment on a situation (such as being in a therapist's office for the first time), especially when the situation seemed very negative to start with.

As highlighted by the preceding dialogue, it is useful to elicit the patient's negative thoughts about therapy. Therapists need to be able to hear the patient's complaints without feeling personally attacked. They may be tempted to engage in an argument with such a patient, and/or to dismiss the complaints as being pure folly. They need to resist such a temptation, lest the patients regard their expectations about the adversarial nature of therapy as confirmed. A sympathetic elicitation of the patient's thoughts, followed by sincere involvement by way of questioning and direct, honest, humble feedback, will be a boon to the establishing of rapport.

As patients attempt to engage in the process of treatment, therapists can help facilitate the establishment of rapport by giving positive verbal reinforcement for the patients' pro-therapy behaviors and attitudes. For example, therapists can provide encouragement and praise to patients for demonstrating good attendance, promptness, active participation in sessions, and cooperation with therapeutic homework assignments (e.g., writing down the disadvantages of using drugs each time the patient experiences a strong urge to go out to make a "score"). Such positive feedback from therapists helps patients to feel supported, to understand their role in therapy, and to decrease their anxieties and negative expectations about the process of working with mental health professionals.

BUILDING TRUST

Trust does not develop immediately. It cannot be asked for, and it cannot be artificially rushed. Only through the therapist's consistent professionalism, honesty, and well-meaning actions over a period of time can trust enter fully into the therapeutic relationship. It does no good for the therapist to say merely, "Don't worry, you can trust me." It is far more realistic to admit that there is little reason for the patient to trust the therapist in the beginning, but that "I hope that in time you will decide for yourself whether or not I can be believed and trusted."

Unfortunately, trust can be impaired or lost relatively quickly, and therefore it must be nurtured and managed in a delicate, painstaking fashion. In short, therapeutic trust with the substance-abusing population is difficult to establish, and may be more difficult to maintain. Furthermore, even if the patient learns to trust the therapist, there may be little reason for the therapist to trust the patient. Inaccurate and/or incomplete reporting by patients is a frequent phenomenon with this population, a situation to which the therapist must remain sensitive. Nevertheless, since the professional is held to a higher standard of behavior than is the patient, the therapist must be willing to continue benevolently to assist the substance-abusing patient, even if that patient has been untruthful. Later, we discuss ways in which the therapist can confront such dishonesty on the part of the patient, yet continue to strengthen the therapeutic relationship and work toward greater progress in treatment.

The following suggestions and illustrations are offered to assist the cognitive therapist in achieving and holding on to this most valuable therapeutic asset.

The basic elements of trust building are very simple and undramatic. They include behaviors that consistently demonstrate the therapist's genuine involvement in the therapeutic process, and commitment to being available to the patient. Such behaviors include (1) being available for therapy sessions on a regular basis, (2) being on time for sessions (even if the patient is not), (3) returning patient telephone calls in a prompt manner, (4) being available for emergency intervention (e.g., by giving the patient a telephone number where the therapist can be reached in case of the need for crisis intervention), (5) showing concern and being willing to try to contact the patient if he or she fails to keep an appointment, and (6) remaining in touch with the patient (and available for the resumption of outpatient cognitive therapy) if inpatient hospitalization, detoxification treatment, halfway house rehabilitation, or reincarceration takes place during the course of the therapeutic relationship.

Therapists foster trust when they assiduously avoid making disparaging comments about the patient, the patient's family members, other substance abusers with whom the therapist has had contact, or any socioeconomic, ethnic, or gender group. Even if the therapist makes the derogatory comment about someone else, the patient may think that this is how the therapist truly thinks of him or her when not working in the role of "therapist," and such a remark may foster the patient's possible belief that the therapist is insincere in his or her show of respect.

Trust is also built when therapists serve as role models who have "clean" lifestyles and attitudes. Offhanded comments by therapists about their own "partying" or "getting buzzed" clearly are contra-indicated. Such statements give drug-abusing patients a confusing mixed message. This message may lead the patient to perceive the therapist as a hypocrite who operates on a "Do as I say, not as I do" policy.

Related to this issue is the situation that arises when patients ask therapists about their own experiences with drug use. Certainly, thera-pists are under no obligation to answer this type of question. A typi-cal appropriate response would be, "I know you're curious about it, but I'm going to have to decline to answer your question. We really have to stick to talking about issues that are relevant to you."

At the same time, therapists may use their discretion in choos-ing whether to answer. A brief, honest reply may go a long way toward fostering the patient's sense of trust for the therapist. For example, the therapist might answer, "No, I've never used any drugs on more than a try-and-see basis, and even that was fifteen years ago. I was playing with fire, and I guess I'm lucky it never progressed. But I've seen enough misery in the lives of those who've gotten into more regular drug use to know that I'd be a damned fool to ever try any-thing again." Another honest answer could be, "No, I've never used drugs. I was always too afraid that I might like them. But really, we need to focus back on you because this is your session." Those thera-pists who have used drugs in the past may choose to be silent about this matter or may use the experience to make rare but relevant self-disclosures as a way of keeping a patient engaged in treatment or to drive home an important point. The goal here again is to nurture the therapeutic relationship, not to get sidetracked from the work of therapy.

SETTING LIMITS

While it is crucial that therapists strive to work in a collaborative fashion with their drug-abusing patients, they must take care not to become oversolicitous to the point that patients know they can take advantage of their therapist. Limits must be set (Moorey, 1989)—for example, that a therapy session will not be held if it is de-termined that the patient is in an inebriated or drug-intoxicated state.

Another such limit might be that the therapist will not condone "a little bit" of drug use.

Therapists can establish such ground rules without sabotaging the therapeutic relationship if they take care to maintain a respectful tone, and reiterate their commitment to act in ways that are in the best therapeutic interest of their patients (Newman, 1988, 1990). When one of our patients arrived drunk to a session, the following dialogue took place:

TH: Walt, pardon me for asking this . . . and if I'm mistaken please accept my apology . . . but have you had something to drink before coming to this session?

PT: I had a few. No big deal (*belches to be humorously obnoxious*).

TH: How many is "a few"?

PT: You know, a few.

TH: Walt, I think you're intoxicated.

PT: I'm fine. I can hold my beer pretty good.

TH: Walt, we've discussed this before. If you're in an altered state of mind . . . and believe me, drinking "a few" means that you're in an altered state of mind . . . there's no point in going through with this session. I have no reason to believe that you'll be able to pay serious enough attention to what we do here to warrant continuing with this session.

PT: Shit man, you're making a big deal out of nothing.

TH: Walt . . .

PT: I'm fine I tell you.

TH: Walt . . .

PT: I shouldn't have said anything.

TH: Walt . . . I'm glad you were up front with me. I respect you for it. I'm depending on you to be a man and tell me the real story to my face. It's just that we can't go through with this session. That was our agreement, and I think we should stick to our agreements.

PT: Shit, man.

TH: Did you drive here?

PT: No, I was beamed down (*sneers*).

TH: I have something important to ask you. I need to ask you to hang out in the waiting room for a couple hours until you're sober enough to drive safely.

PT: Doc, I don't got time for this shit. I got here fine, and I'll get home fine.

TH: Walt, you've worked too hard to get to this point to mess up now. If you get pulled over, or worse, you're risking going back to jail. I don't want to see that happen to you. What's a couple of hours to ensure your freedom? You can have my newspaper to keep you occupied for awhile.

The patient ultimately complied with this therapist's request. The limit was clearly set, but the tone of the communication was neither critical nor controlling. The therapist emphasized that he was looking out for the patient's welfare, and this had a lot to do with the patient's compliance and willingness to continue actively with cognitive therapy. When the therapist sets a limit, sticks to it, and does so in a respectful way, trust is fostered and the patient learns to have respect for the therapist as well.

Parenthetical to the above, it is necessary that the therapist be amenable to continuing with therapy once the patient is in compliance again after a slip (Mackay & Marlatt, 1991). Since many drug-abusing patients frequently test limits, no gains will be made if therapists are disinclined to go forward with therapy when their patients engage in defiant and/or manipulative behaviors. Therapists serve their drug-abusing patients best when they follow through on predetermined agreements on how to deal with counterproductive patient behavior but also show genuine support and encourage the patients to "get with the program" again.

The above vignette brings up the issue of the role of alcohol in the illicit drug-abusing patient's life and therapy. While we believe that it is theoretically possible for illicit-drug-abusing patients to continue to drink alcoholic beverages on a casual basis during treatment, in practice our experience tells us that the use of alcohol undermines their abstinence from drugs such as cocaine and heroin. One reason is that the use of alcohol lowers patients' inhibitions. Patients have reported that when they are drinking they are less likely to think about the compelling reasons for staying free of drugs. Even when they can stay focused on the disadvantages of drug use, patients report that they are less apt to care about the long-term consequences of their behavior than when they are sober. Thus, they are more likely to resume the use of harder substances. Further, when patients use alcohol as a "substitute" for drugs such as cocaine or heroine, their consumption quickly escalates to levels indicative of abuse and dependence. Therefore, we discourage the use of alcohol during patients' treatment and recovery from illicit drugs.

PROTECTING CONFIDENTIALITY

As alluded to previously, there are limitations to confidentiality. Therapists should spell this out to their patients from the very start. The following monologue may serve as a model:

"Mr. A, I want you to know that almost everything we discuss here will be kept just between you and me, unless you want me to talk to someone else about your situation or you otherwise give me permission. So, for the most part, things that you tell me here will be kept confidential. But I want to inform you that there are certain exceptions to this rule. If you tell me something that indicates that you or someone else is in danger, and you're not willing to help me fix the situation so that everyone is safe, then I am legally obligated to contact the authorities and anybody else who may be personally involved. This includes situations in which you intend to kill yourself or someone else, or where you are causing harm to a child. Another such situation would be where you have the AIDS virus, but you're not telling your sexual partners or making any attempts to protect them from infection. Please hear me out. I can promise you this: If it comes to pass that I have to break confidentiality in order to protect you or someone else, I will make every possible effort to let you know that I'm going to do this. I don't want to do things behind your back. That's not my style. I'd rather that you know exactly where I'm coming from. In fact, if the authorities have to be contacted, I'd be more than happy to stand by you while you make the phone call. If you cooperate in this way, and I support you, we can solve most any problem. What do you think about all that I've just said? Do you have any questions?"

(If the patient has been referred by a parole office district, the following can be added to the monologue):

"You should also know that I am obligated by law to let your parole officer know whether or not you are attending these therapy sessions, and to let him know if you are arriving on time. I don't have to tell him if you have started using drugs again, but he'll be asking you to submit to giving urines on a regular basis, so he'll have his own way of knowing whether you've started up again."

Patients will not be pleased to hear this, but they will appreciate the explanation and the warning. The alternative, namely, that the therapist necessarily breaks confidentiality without first alerting the patient to this possibility, will at the very least seriously undermine trust in the therapist.

MAINTAINING CREDIBILITY

Yet another way in which therapists can establish and maintain their credibility as trustworthy professionals is by being willing to admit that they do not know everything, and/or that they were wrong about something. To highlight this point, one of our patients asked his therapist if the therapist could use hypnosis to cure him of his crack addiction. The therapist admitted that he had no training in hypnosis, and therefore could not perform this technique. Instead, he explained a bit more about cognitive therapy and worked with the patient to formulate a goal list. In a later session, the patient stated that he knew that the therapist was "for real" because the therapist admitted that he did not know how to perform hypnosis. The patient added, "How did I know what you could do for me and what you couldn't? Now at least I know that if you say you can do something for me, you can actually do it—and if you can't, you tell me you can't. I wouldn't know what to believe if you always said you could help me with everything."

In another instance, the therapist was waiting for his patient to arrive for her session. After 20 minutes, the patient telephoned. Before the patient could explain herself, the therapist launched into a mini-lecture on the importance of attending therapy sessions on time. Just then, someone else got on the line. It was the patient's parole officer, who proceeded to explain to the therapist that he had been responsible for the patient's delay in leaving the parole office. Half an hour later, when the patient arrived for her session, the therapist immediately apologized for jumping to the conclusion (a cognitive error) that she was remiss in her obligation to attend therapy. He pledged that he would "get evidence" next time before passing judgment. He then asked the patient if she had any negative thoughts or feelings about this situation. She smiled and replied, "Not anymore."

In sum, humility, honesty, and aboveboard communication from the therapist will help to bring about the development of the all-important qualities of trust and rapport in the therapeutic relationship.

MAINTAINING A SPIRIT
OF COLLABORATION

When both the therapist and the patient are actively working together, rather than in opposition or in stagnant passivity, there is the greatest potential for therapeutic change. Cognitive therapy takes such a collaborative approach, whereby therapists communicate that they take their patients' points of view very seriously, downplay their own role as an "all-knowing" paragon of authority and power, and stress the importance of mutual work toward discovery and positive change (Beck et al., 1979).

In doing so, therapists do not have to take an overly lenient stance with regard to their patients' problematic drug use and drug-related behaviors, nor must they remain neutral regarding their opinions about drug abuse. Therapists can communicate a fundamental positive regard for their patients as individuals without condoning their abuse of substances. This separation of patients from their behavior may seem contrived to some degree, but it is just such a stance that may facilitate the spirit of the therapist and patient working as a team to fight the patient's drug abuse problems. In any event, the differences between the patient's personality when he or she is using drugs versus when he or she is free of drugs are typically so striking that it is not really difficult to mentally separate the patient from the abuse-related behaviors.

A key element of collaboration is compromise. Therapists must not allow themselves to be manipulated or conversely to become dictatorial in their dealings with their substance abuse patients. It is strongly advised that therapists take a firm stance, neither encouraging power struggles nor acquiescing fully to patients' threats and idle promises. Therapists best demonstrate both their strength of will and their character, as well their willingness to collaborate, by being *flexible*. On a small scale, this quality is demonstrated when therapists allow their patients some say in what gets discussed during the therapy hour. In a situation in which the therapist believes that the patient's chosen therapeutic agenda is too tangential to be valuable, the therapist would do well to agree to spend a limited amount of time on the patient's preferred topic, while noting for the record that other issues need to be discussed as well in order for treatment to have its strongest impact. Such a strategy fosters a positive working alliance.

On a larger scale, therapists may need to use diplomatic skill just to keep their patients from bolting from treatment. For example, a patient who loathed the fact that he was indeed in the role of a patient wanted to use therapy contacts as nothing more than "bitch sessions." In this manner, the patient could blame everyone else for his troubles and not have to face the fact that he himself had problems that needed attention. When the therapist highlighted this point, the patient threatened to discontinue treatment. After a long discussion (in which the therapist remained calm and carefully worded his comments), it was agreed that the even-numbered sessions would be reserved for complaining about others, but that the odd-numbered sessions would focus on the patient's problems with anger, depression, and drug abuse. For good measure, the therapist thanked the patient for being "so open minded and a good sport." Ironically, once the patient began to utilize the odd-numbered sessions to discuss his personal issues and drug abuse tendencies, he spontaneously began to use the even-numbered "bitch sessions" to do the same.

RESISTING COLLUSION WITH THE PATIENT

Many substance-abusing patients, on ascertaining that their therapists are supportive and genuinely trying to help, will try to take advantage of the situation. They do this by asking their therapists to single them out for special treatment, to conceal information from their parole officers, to ignore obvious trouble signs, and in general to assume the role of "enabler." Therapists then find themselves in the dilemma of trying to reassert the therapeutic ground rules without alienating their patients (cf. Newman, 1990). As difficult as this task might seem, it is essential if therapy is to continue in a fruitful direction. As we've mentioned previously, the therapeutic relationship can be preserved if the therapist communicates straightforward honesty and expresses a desire to continue to provide therapeutic assistance. One patient, "Charleen," called her therapist at home late at night, asking for the following "favor":

PT: I'm sorry to bother you so late, but I really need you to help me out.

TH: OK. What's going on?

PT: I'm on my way home from a [support group] meeting, and my boyfriend thinks I'm out messing around and getting high and he said he's going to kick me out if I stay out late again. Could you call him and let him know that I've been to a meeting and that everything's cool?

[Before saying anything in reply, a number of thoughts were already racing through the therapist's mind. For starters, he realized that he had no way of knowing whether or not what Charleen was saying was true. Second, he recognized that this request was an inappropriate use of therapeutic telephone privileges. He decided to engage the patient in further dialogue before passing judgment and before agreeing to do anything.]

TH: Charleen, you know that I want to help you out any way that I can, but I have to admit that I'm uncomfortable with how this all sounds.

PT: What do you mean? (*getting annoyed*)

TH: Well, you're asking me to comment on something I have no knowledge of. Now, if you had just been to my office and we had had a session, and you wanted me to call to let him know, then I would do it. But this is different. It would make much more sense for you to call your boyfriend yourself and let him know where you are, or just return home as usual. If I call, he's going to think that I'm giving him an alibi for you, and that will just raise his suspicions further. Have you thought this through?

PT: So what are you saying, that you're not going to help me out? Thank you very much, you're a great therapist (*angry, sarcastic tone*).

TH: Charleen, I'm more than happy to help you to *deal* with a problem or a situation, but I can't act to make it *go away* for you. There are certain things that you have to take responsibility for yourself. This is one of those things.

PT: So what am I supposed to do if my boyfriend throws me out?

TH: If that happens, call me again and we'll try to do some problem-solving. Can you call me from your mother's house if that happens?

PT: I don't want to go to my mother's house!

TH: You don't have to want to go there. I'm just asking if you can call me from there if you have to.

PT: Yeh. I guess.

TH: OK. Do you want to schedule an appointment for tomorrow so we can discuss this whole matter at greater length?

PT: I don't know (*disgusted tone*).

TH: Please level with me, Charleen. Have you been using [drugs]?

PT: No!

TH: Can I depend on you to stay away from drugs until tomorrow when we can get together and have a session?

PT: Yeh, yeh.

This dialogue illustrates the fact that therapists can offer appropriate therapeutic support without having to allow themselves to get sucked into playing the role of enabler. A certain degree of collaborative compromise was called for here. The therapist was unwilling to call the boyfriend for the patient, but he did express a willingness to receive another late-night telephone call in order to help the patient deal with a potential crisis. (Although therapists at the Center for Cognitive Therapy routinely provide patients with their home telephone numbers for use in emergency situations, we realize that some therapists may prefer instead to make use of an intermediary such as an answering service. In either case, we believe that it is necessary for patients to be able to make contact with their therapist after hours in the event of critical situations.)

APPEALING TO PATIENTS' POSITIVE SELF-ESTEEM

As many substance abusers evidence defiant attitudes and/or pathological levels of self-importance, it is often necessary for the therapist to appeal to patients' narcissism in order to elicit collaboration from them. This does not have to entail gross hyperbole on the part of the therapist. If fact, such an approach is contraindicated as the intelligent patient will rightly see it as an insincere, manipulative ploy. Rather, the therapist needs to focus on some of the patient's actual strengths and positive points, and express appreciation for these qualities. This approach serves to strengthen rapport and to elicit greater cooperation.

The following clinical vignette demonstrates an appeal to the patient's sense of entitlement in order to defuse his anger toward the therapist. The problem arose when the patient did not show up for his session, and instead called 5 hours later to say that he had gotten a flat tire on the way to the therapist's office. The dialogue (a condensed version of the actual interchange) proceeded in the following manner:

TH: Walt, we've talked about how important it is for you to get to these sessions on time, and to keep me informed of your whereabouts. The fact that you waited five hours to call me concerns me.

PT: (*Exasperated*) I was on the road. I couldn't get to a phone. I didn't have a spare tire so I had to wait to get help. There was no way I could call any sooner.

TH: Walt, ninety percent of me wants very much to believe you, but I have to be honest with you—ten percent of me has my doubts. I can't help but wonder whether your lateness in getting in touch with me is drug related.

[The patient responded very angrily, vilifying the therapist for being "such a hard-ass" and for insulting the patient by "calling me a liar." The therapist answered with a reply that was geared to use Walt's narcissism in the service of repairing the therapeutic relationship.]

TH: Walt, I'd like to believe everything you say to me. But you and I both know that you have a lot of skill and experience in covering your tracks. You could easily outsmart me if I'm not careful. If I just blindly believe everything you tell me, then I'm a fool, and frankly, I think you deserve better than to have a fool for a therapist.

This latter statement achieved its intended effect of disarming the patient's hostility long enough to get him to agree to come in for a session early the next day.

Later in treatment, the therapist and Walt were discussing Walt's unsafe sexual habits. Walt noted that he did use condoms when he had sex with prostitutes, but refused to wear one with his many "girl friends," stating facetiously that it was against his religion. Therapist and patient discussed these practices at length, trying to get a handle on the automatic thoughts and beliefs that led him to act so recklessly in this era of the AIDS epidemic. Additionally, the therapist attempted to focus Walt's attention on the dangers involved in his sexual behavior by noting the pros and cons of wearing condoms. Finally, when it seemed that these tactics were falling on deaf ears, the therapist resorted to making an appeal to Walt's intelligence by saying:

TH: The fact that you wear condoms with hookers is a smart move. I wouldn't expect anything less than a smart move where you're concerned. You're very good at taking care of number one. So it confuses me how you would stop short of doing the smart thing with your girl friends as well. It just doesn't seem like you, Walt. It's out of character for you to leave any loose ends like that [no pun intended]. You normally have all your bases covered [again, no pun intended].

This approach effectively pitted Walt's desire to be seen as an intelligent person against the "macho" rules that governed his unsafe sex practices. It allowed the therapist to be confrontive without damaging rapport or collaboration.

In other cases, we have helped bring our patients back into a collaborative mode by appealing to their sense of justice, their positive feelings for involved significant others, their survival skills, their integrity, their potential abilities to be positive role models for others, and other personal attributes.

MANAGING POWER STRUGGLES

In spite of the therapist's best efforts to maintain an ongoing positive therapeutic relationship with the drug-abusing patient, there will almost certainly be times when therapist and patient are at odds, and when negative feelings will be rather intense on one or both sides. However, this does not have to spell doom for the working alliance. We rely on the following guidelines for managing such power struggles:

1. Don't fight fire with fire.
2. Maintain honesty.
3. Remain focused on the goals of treatment.
4. Remain focused on the patient's redeeming qualities.
5. Disarm the patient with genuine humility and empathy.
6. Confront, but use diplomacy.

1. *Don't fight fire with fire.* When a patient becomes hostile, loud, intransigent, and/or verbally abusive, it does little good for the therapist to respond in kind. In fact, such a reaction on the part of the therapist could potentially lead to a dangerous escalation of the conflict. Instead, therapists must show confidence and conviction in their position in a matter-of-fact way. Concern and strong feelings can be expressed (e.g., "Ms. G, I urge you to reconsider your intentions in this matter. I am greatly concerned that you are headed for a big-time fall if you go ahead with your plans to attend that dealer's party!"); however, it is advisable that such sentiments be expressed in a way that communicates a genuine concern for the patient's well-being and best interests. A controlling or disrespectful response (e.g., "You're dead wrong! If you go to that party you're an idiot! I simply can't allow you to do it.") will undermine the therapeutic alliance and probably will not effectively control the patient's behavior anyway. Instead, the strategy advocated here is more akin to the philosophy espoused in Asian martial arts that states that a strong opponent must not be fought head on but rather through leaning back and allowing the adversary's misguided brute force to carry him past you, to stagger, and to fall.

2. *Maintain honesty.* During times of conflict with a drug-abusing patient, there is often a great temptation to try to appease the patient artificially through reassurances that are less than completely truthful (e.g., getting a patient "off your back" by telling him that it won't really matter too much if he continues to be late for therapy

sessions). Not only is it unwise to reinforce patients' maladaptive interpersonal behavior by capitulating to them, it also sets up the therapist to look like a liar if the therapist later reverses his/her position or otherwise reneges on the reassurances. Instead, the therapist must be willing to "take the heat," and not simply say things that the patient wants to hear in order avoid the unpleasantness of a power struggle.

3. *Remain focused on the goals of treatment.* When therapist and patient are at odds, it is extremely helpful if the therapist calls attention to mutually set goals. In effect, therapists can remind both themselves and their patients that a disagreement in one area does not alter the fact that there are fundamental areas of agreement and collaboration in other areas. One therapist diffused a heated exchange by telling his ex-football player patient, "We may not agree on whether we should run the ball, or pass, but we have to remember that we're on the same team and we both want to get into the end zone."

4. *Remain focused on the patient's redeeming qualities, as well as your own (as therapist).* Power struggles are often fueled in part by the therapist's cognitive biases. This happens when the therapist reacts to an aversive power struggle by focusing only on the patient's irritating qualities, and glossing over his/her strengths. Similarly, the therapist may lapse into dysfunctional self-blame (regarding the lack of the patient's therapeutic cooperation and progress), thus engendering more ill feelings. In such instances, it is extremely helpful for therapists to use cognitive therapy procedures on themselves in order to notice and modify the following types of automatic thoughts that might be exacerbating negative interactions with patients:

- "This patient is a loser. He'll never listen to me."
- "This patient is so dense. I'm going to have to beat this guy over the head with my point of view until he agrees with me."
- "Why can't I reach this patient? What am I doing wrong? I'm ready to give up on working with this patient."
- "Maybe I'm not cut out to work with such a patient. I don't like being reminded of my shortcomings, so this patient is really on my shit list."
- "You just can't compromise and be reasonable with these people. If you give them an inch, they take a light-year. Therefore, I will not budge from my position one iota."
- "Why did I ever take on the responsibility of treating this patient in the first place? I must have been an idiot. I almost wish this patient would get arrested so I can be rid of this case."

Obviously, the aforementioned automatic thoughts are very deleterious to the therapist, the patient, and the prospects for the continuation of treatment. Therapists would do well to focus on their own idiosyncratic automatic thoughts, to produce the kinds of rational responses that would diminish the anger, frustration, and exasperation that escalate power struggles and undermine problem solving and therapeutic collaboration (Weiner & Fox, 1982). Examples of such rational responses might be:

- "There have been a number of sessions in which the patient and I worked very well together. Those were very rewarding experiences that I must not forget.
- "This patient is not dumb. He's convinced he has his reasons for defying the therapeutic plan the way he's doing. Let me try to understand his resistant automatic thoughts and beliefs, rather than simply label him a troublemaker."
- "My worth as a therapist does not hinge on my patient believing everything I say, doing everything I suggest that she do, and staying free of drugs for the rest of her life. I'd like for her to be compliant and to make progress, but the fact that she sometimes thwarts this doesn't prove that she can't succeed in therapy with me, and it certainly doesn't prove that I should throw in the towel with all drug-abusing patients."
- "If I keep my cool, present my point of view resolutely, and also show that I'm willing to be flexible within reason, I'll probably get a lot more therapeutic mileage out of this conflict than I will if I become strident or stubborn."
- "This power struggle is a great opportunity to get at some really hot interpersonal cognitions!"

5. *Disarm the patient with genuine humility and empathy.* Frequently, drug-abusing patients will become angry if they perceive the therapist to be flaunting their authority over the patient or acting with a holier-than-thou air. This perception can lead the patient to fight against the therapist's position in order to reassert some measure of control. This implies that it is important for therapists to be aware of the possibility that the patient is viewing him or her in this negative way, and to respond with behavior that gives the patient evidence to the contrary. For example, one of our patients suffers from diabetes and frequently neglects his medical care as a sign of defiance, much in the same way that others might choose to go on a hunger strike. Ray and his therapist often engaged in power struggles over whether

or not Ray should consult his medical doctor. Finally, after a great deal of heated disagreement, the therapist resorted to a more humble, empathic approach:

"Ray, I'm not trying to give you a hard time. Who am I to tell you how you should run your life? I'm just worried about you, man. I get this mental picture of you in a diabetic coma and it alarms me. I don't want this to happen you. I want to keep working with you and I want to see your life become happier and healthier again, but instead I worry that when you walk out that door I'm not going to see you anymore because you're going to wind up dead. I guess that's why I come on so strong about going to see your doctor. Do you see where I'm coming from, Ray?"

6. *Confront, but use diplomacy.* As mentioned earlier, therapists must be prepared to confront their drug-abusing patients when they break therapeutic ground rules (Frances & Miller, 1991), but a tone of respect and concern must prevail (Newman, 1988). A particularly effective method of subtle confrontation involves the therapist's use of the patient's own words in order to make a point. For example, a patient may say in a given session, "I know I have to stay on top of myself—I can't let down my guard when things are going well because that's when I always get stupid and think I can go back to using again." Later, this same patient may betray his own words by asking for a discontinuation of treatment because "everything's cool in my life now," a statement that the therapist evaluates to be a gross oversimplification and distortion. Rather than telling the patient that he's fooling himself and then hounding him into staying in therapy, the therapist can use the patient's earlier statement as evidence against his current position:

"I'm a little confused right now. You're telling me that everything's cool right now and that you can leave therapy. But you told me something—and I wrote it down here because I was so impressed with what you said—that it would be times just like now that you would have to stay on top of yourself, because you know that you're prone to relapsing when you think everything is going great and you let your guard down. Now, I took what you had to say very seriously, and I thought you really knew the story. It seems that what you said would apply to this situation we're in right now. What do you think?"

The above example also highlights *the importance of the therapist's documenting important patient statements for future use in session.*

Confrontation is often called for when the therapist suspects that the patient is lying (about his/her whereabouts during a missed therapy session, about level of abstinence, etc.). Here, it is useful for the therapist to develop a repertoire of carefully worded statements that "nicely" say the equivalent of "I think you're lying." Such statements include but are not limited to:

- "I don't get the feeling you're being completely straight with me right now."
- "I'm going to ask you the same question again. This time please level with me. Whatever the story is, I'll try to help you in any way that I can."
- "Are you sure you're telling me the whole story here? It sounds like there's some stuff you're leaving out."
- "I get the feeling that you're struggling to try to tell me something, but you're not sure you can get the words out. Take your time—I'll listen to whatever news you have for me."
- "Are you being honest with yourself here?"
- "I hope you're not fooling yourself right now."
- "Usually the things you say make a lot of sense, so I'm a little confused right now because I have to admit that what you're saying to me at this moment doesn't make sense to me."
- "Are you willing to prove what you're saying? I'd like you to show me up by proving it. But if you can't, I'm not sure I can completely buy what you're telling me."
- "You know, this is one of those instances where your intelligence works against you. The fact that you're so smart means that you're capable of bullshitting me and making it sound golden. Now I know that you're smart, and that means that I have to wonder whether you're telling me the truth, especially at times like these when your excuses and alibis are extremely convincing and clever."

SUMMARY

This chapter has emphasized the vital importance of establishing a positive therapeutic relationship with the drug-abusing patient. Along the way, we have noted the difficulties that are entailed in this task, and have proposed methods by which to actively nurture and maintain a functional working alliance. We have illustrated ways that therapists can engender a sense of rapport, trust, and collaboration with their drug-abusing patients, without having to collude with their patients' dysfunctional beliefs and behaviors. Finally, we have emphasized the role of confrontation in the therapeutic relationship, and demonstrated that this need not lead to the therapist and patient becoming adversaries. In fact, an honest, humble, direct approach can allow the therapist to use the therapist-patient interactions to make significant headway in treatment.

CHAPTER **5**

Formulation of the Case

A good case formulation helps the therapist to understand the complexity of the substance abuser. By weaving together the patient's history, constellation of beliefs and rules, coping strategies, vulnerable situations, automatic thoughts and images, and maladaptive behaviors, the therapist has a better understanding of how patients become drug dependent. The case formulation also helps to answer many of the following questions:

1. Why did the patient start using drugs?
2. How did using drugs lead to abuse and dependency?
3. Why has the patient not been able to stop on his/her own?
4. How did key beliefs develop?
5. How did the patient function prior to using drugs?
6. What interpretations can we make about high-risk circumstances as they relate to using drugs?

A well-formulated case helps to give direction to the session (Persons, 1989). The therapist is guided to ask important relevant questions and to develop strategies and interventions that are most likely to succeed. Without a case formulation, the therapist is proceeding like a ship without a rudder, drifting aimlessly through the session.

CASE FORMULATION

The essential components of a case conceptualization are as follows:

1. Relevant childhood data
2. Current life problems
3. Core beliefs or schemas
4. Conditional assumptions/beliefs/rules
5. Compensatory strategies
6. Vulnerable situations
7. Automatic thoughts and beliefs (especially *drug related*)
8. Emotions
9. Behaviors
10. Integration of the above data

Relevant childhood data are those early experiences that contributed to the development and the maintenance of core beliefs. These experiences are not necessarily traumatic but are early messages that children receive about themselves that help to form the foundation for their positive and negative views of themselves. For example, a patient might come from a family where one member is an alcoholic and unpredictable. The message that the patient might receive is that "alcohol is a way to cope" and "people are unpredictable." Some patients come from homes where they are often put down and their acceptance is dependent on "perfect behavior." These patients might develop the core belief "I'm unwanted," "I'm unlovable," or "I'm bad."

Current life problems comprise the full spectrum of difficulties that drug-abusing patients experience in their lives as they enter treatment—problems that transcend the simple abuse of mind-altering substances, that will need additional attention in treatment (cf. Sobell et al., 1988). These problems commonly include relationship difficulties, unemployment, health problems, legal trouble, low motivation, unstable living arrangements, hopelessness, and others. As therapists conceptualize these difficulties, they attempt to determine which of the patients' problems contribute to the *onset* of the substance abuse, which problems are *sequelae* of the drugs, and which are *both* causal and consequential factors. Therapy with substance abusers is incomplete without a treatment plan to address the kinds of life problems mentioned above.

Core beliefs or schemas are the most central and important beliefs that reflect how patients view themselves. We have found that these beliefs generally fall into two categories: (1) "I am unlovable" or (2) "I am helpless." It is important to note that core beliefs might not necessarily be manifested by these exact words, but there can be derivatives or correlates of the core belief. For example, "I am helpless" might be expressed in such terms as "I am inadequate," "I am powerless," "I am trapped," "I am inferior," "I am ineffective," "I am incompetent," "I am weak," or "I am vulnerable." The belief that "I am unlovable" might be expressed as "I am unattractive," "I am undesirable," "I am rejected," "I am unwanted," "I am uncared for," or "I am bad."

Conditional assumptions/beliefs/rules help patients to cope (for better or worse) with their core beliefs. These assumptions can be in a positive or negative form. A conditional positive assumption might be the following: "If I do everything perfectly, then I will be wanted and accepted by others." The negative counterpart to this assumption might be, "I am unlovable if I am not accepted by everyone."

Compensatory strategies are those behaviors that also help patients to cope with their core beliefs. On the surface, compensatory strategies seem to work. However, the problem with many compensatory strategies is that they are often compulsive, inflexible, inappropriate, energy depleting, and not balanced by adaptive strategies. In addition, these compensatory strategies often still do not prevent the patient from having hidden doubts, secret fears, and negative self-concepts. A typical compensatory strategy for substance abusers is the use of drugs in order to feel more confident or feel better about themselves. However, it should be noted that the use of drugs is not limited to being a compensatory strategy. People use drugs for many reasons. However, we have found that in the drug-dependent patient, drug use can clearly be demonstrated as one of several coping strategies to "remedy" the sense of helplessness or hopelessness.

Vulnerable situations are best described as those problematic circumstances in which core beliefs and drug-related beliefs become activated. An example of this is the cocaine addict who has been abstinent for several months and is faced with the situation of going into a neighborhood where he has previously purchased cocaine. He has an image of the last time he used, which is followed by strong urges and cravings. This, in turn, activates a drug-related belief such as "The urges and cravings make me use."

Automatic thoughts stem from the activation of core beliefs, conditional beliefs, and drug-related beliefs. Some typical automatic thoughts of substance abusers are: "I can't stand the urges and cravings," "Just a little bit won't hurt," and "Go for it. You deserve it. You've worked hard all week."

These automatic thoughts often potentiate patients' urges and cravings to use drugs and/or alcohol, and provide them with impetus to enact plans to procure the drugs (Beck, Wright, & Newman, 1992).

Emotions are usually associated with particular automatic thoughts or beliefs. Patients who abuse drugs often are unaware of the cognitive processing that precedes a particular emotion, such as anger, anxiety, or sadness. However, through therapy, patients can be taught to be more aware of the thinking process that is associated with their emotional life.

The patient's *behaviors* are the end products of the vulnerable situations, and the activation of beliefs, automatic thoughts, and emotions. Common dysfunctional behaviors include actively seeking drugs, using drugs, engaging in irresponsible activities (e.g., unprotected sex), abusive interpersonal confrontations, avoidance of self-help activities, and others.

The *integration* of the above data is the most challenging and most important step in the ongoing process of conceptualizing the patient's life and problems. Here, therapists piece together all the information into a "story of the patient's life" that provides plausible explanations for the patient's difficulties and suggests treatment recommendations that may break into the patient's self-defeating patterns and vicious cycles.

For example, the therapist may posit the following:

"The patient was subject to a frequent barrage of harsh disapproval in childhood, and came to believe that he was inadequate and unlovable. These core beliefs have been carried into adulthood, where the patient experiences chronic discomfort in social situations where he believes that he will not measure up. The patient took to using cocaine in the belief that it would make him feel confident enough to make positive impressions on others. Unfortunately, this dysfunctional compensatory strategy has led to compulsive use of cocaine, leading further to a depletion of his money and endangering his marriage. These life problems have fed back into the patient's cycle of anxiety, sadness, low self-worth, and renewed belief that the only way to be accepted is to become outgoing through the use of cocaine. As a result, his drug, financial, and marital problems have worsened, and his sense of helplessness and hopelessness have increased."

CASE STUDY

The following case illustrates in more detail the ten essential components of a case formulation. The patient (described in the integrative example above), David, is a 40-year-old white male. He has been married for eight years and has one child. His complaints at intake evaluation included high anxiety and a long history of alcohol and cocaine abuse. He reported recently feeling more anxious in social situations, and he feared that if his anxiety got worse he might have a relapse and start using cocaine and alcohol. In other areas of his life, he was working and received a good salary; however, he was $40,000 in debt as a result of his cocaine "habit." His marriage was "on the rocks," and he also suspected that his wife was an alcoholic.

Upon completion of his intake evaluation, David met the DSM-III-R criteria for polysubstance use, with cocaine as his preferred drug, social phobia, and generalized anxiety disorder. The social phobia was the area on which David wanted to work first. David felt an urgency in this regard because it was the holiday season and he had several business obligations that required his attendance at social functions such as dinner–dances and parties. David felt that if he did not learn to cope with his anxiety in these situations, he would lose control and start using cocaine again.

David grew up in a household where his father was seen as a workaholic and someone who "drank too much." David stated that his mother was nurturing but somewhat timid around her husband. In school, David did not do well. He received mostly C's and D's and only stayed in college for one year. David first began drinking at about age 9. Because of his father's business, the family was involved in many social activities and David would often go around drinking out of the glasses of some of the guests. By age 13, David already had experimented with alcohol, marijuana, speed, and diet pills.

As a child David was often humiliated and degraded by his father, usually at social events, after his father had been drinking heavily. On one occasion after his father called him "stupid," he ran outside and sat under a tree and felt humiliated, worthless, and helpless. On another occasion, he ran out onto a pier and sat there feeling ashamed and helpless. These were significant childhood events for David, and they served as the foundation for some of his core beliefs and compensatory strategies. His typical style was to run away and avoid unpleasant situations. Later in life, David realized that alcohol and drugs helped him to cope with unpleasant emotions. Since drugs and alcohol worked so well, David did not develop many other strategies for coping with unpleasant emotions.

Under *relevant childhood data,* we can see that there were several incidents when David was shamed by his father. These incidents helped to form his core belief, "I am unloved, unwanted." He later developed a conditional assumption for coping, "If I do everything perfectly, then people will like me." David had several compensatory strategies, such as always to strive to do things perfectly or to avoid doing things that were unpleasant. Other strategies included avoiding showing others how he really felt, and using alcohol and drugs. After using cocaine, David felt especially confident that he could do "everything perfectly," which in turn led him to believe that he was loved and wanted by others.

A *vulnerable situation* occurred when David was invited to a dinner party at a friend's house. Prior to going to the friend's house, David was acutely aware of the fact that he was becoming anxious and nervous. He was also aware of the fact that his automatic thoughts centered on such ideas as "I'll screw up," and "They will see me trembling," and he imagined himself being "overcome with anxiety" and eventually running out of the house. This, in turn, led to taking a drink and snorting a line of coke before going to the party.

From this example, the clinician can see the relationship between the development of David's *core belief*, his *conditional assumptions*, and his *compensatory strategies*, as well as their cumulative impact on a *vulnerable situation*—being invited to a dinner party at his friend's house (see Figure 5.1). Once again, we need to remember that these compensatory strategies tend to be rather compulsive, inflexible, inappropriate at times, energy depleting, and not balanced by other adaptive strategies. In addition, in spite of the compensatory strategies, the patient still tends to have hidden doubts and secret fears about coping.

GATHERING DATA FOR CASE FORMULATION

The Case Summary and Cognitive Conceptualization Worksheet is an excellent form for compiling data that will be used in the case formulation. This worksheet is divided into eight main sections:

  I. Demographic Information
  II. Diagnosis
  III. Inventory Scores
  IV. Presenting Problem and Current Functioning
  V. Developmental Profile
  VI. Cognitive Profile
  VII. Integration and Conceptualization of Cognitive and Development Profiles
  VIII. Implications for Therapy

The *demographic information* section is where the therapist collects such information as the patient's age, sex, race, religion, employment

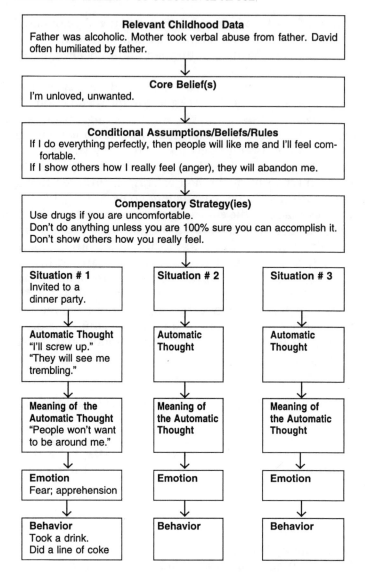

FIGURE 5.1. Cognitive conceptualization diagram developed by Judith S. Beck. From J. S. Beck (in press). Copyright Guilford Press. Reprinted by permission.

status, marital status, and other pertinent identifying characteristics. This is standard information that would be a part of any psychological evaluation.

In the *diagnosis* section, it is advantageous to formulate a diagnosis on all five axes of DSM-III-R. Clinical syndromes are designated on Axis I. On Axis II, developmental disorders and personality disorders are noted. Physical disorders and conditions pertinent to the patient's psychological difficulties are presented on Axis III. Severity of psychosocial stressors is identified on Axis IV. The level of severity of psychosocial stressors ranges from code 1 (none) to code 6 (catastrophic), such as the death of a child, the suicide of a spouse, or a devastating natural disaster. Axis V can be determined from the Global Assessment of Functioning Scale, which has a code number descending from 90 to 1, with 90 signifying abstinence and ideal coping, and progressively lower numbers indicating an increasing severity of drug use or deficits in coping and functioning. All the data on the five axes will have an impact on the clinician's understanding of the patient, and in the subsequent designing of the treatment plan.

Inventory scores, such as the Beck Depression Inventory, Beck Anxiety Inventory, and Beck Hopelessness Scale (discussed later), are listed in this section. Intake scores plus scores from the first six sessions are reported. There is also an extra column in order to note the scores of the most recent session. These inventory scores are extremely important because the therapist can quickly see general trends and patterns—changes for the better or for the worse.

The *presenting problem and current functioning* section describes the patient's current difficulties and focuses on such areas as employment, concurrent psychiatric disorders, nature of drug use, criminal activity, interpersonal problems, and other data. This is a cross-sectional analysis of the patient's current functioning.

The *developmental profile* examines the patient's social history, educational history, medical history, psychiatric history, and vocational history. In addition, relationships with parents, siblings, peers, authority figures, and significant others over the life span are also noted. It is also important to ascertain any significant events or traumas in the patient's formative years or recent past. This longitudinal analysis is akin to paging through a family photo album. The therapist can see the patient in different stages of development. This retrospective analysis also includes an evaluation of the patient's introduction to psychoactive substances and how the problem became a full-blown addiction.

The *cognitive profile* section addresses the manner in which the patients process information. The patients' typical problem situations are noted, and the corresponding automatic thoughts, feelings, and behaviors in these situations are outlined. In addition, possible core beliefs, conditional beliefs, and drug-related beliefs are described in this section.

The integration of cognitive and developmental profiles takes into consideration the patient's self-concept and concept of others. It also focuses on the interaction of life events with cognitive vulnerabilities, as well as compensatory and coping strategies. An important part of this section is a description of how self-concept and concept of others might have played roles in the onset and progression of substance abuse. This section is illustrated by the case of Mike, a 31-year-old cocaine addict. The patient lives with his parents in a rundown neighborhood where there is high unemployment and high crime rates. He grew up around drugs and alcohol, and his mother and all his siblings have had problems with drugs and alcohol. Mike is now serving five years probation for insurance fraud.

The patient's work history is poor. After dropping out of high school, Mike found only unskilled labor jobs, and he is currently unemployed. There is lots of dealing in his neighborhood; Mike has sold drugs in the past and knows there is lots of fast money in dealing. Mike sees himself as a loner and does not have any real friends. His problematic beliefs are "I'm no better than the rest of my family," "I'll never get a job," "I can't get away from it (drugs)," "Dealing is the only way out of here (urban ghetto)," and "Using is the only way to cure the boredom."

His circumstances and beliefs have led to the following behavioral patterns: brief periods of abstinence from drug and alcohol followed by solitary use of alcohol with Valium, which, in turn, leads to intermittent use of crack cocaine, and then to daily use of crack cocaine.

Mike's case shows many of the cognitive factors (among other factors) that can influence drug use (see Figure 5.2).

The section on *implications for therapy* examines some of the following areas:

1. The patient's initial "aptitude" for cognitive interventions;
2. The patient's personality characteristics, such as "sociotropic" or "autonomous";
3. The patient's motivations, goals, and expectations for therapy;
4. The therapist's goals; and
5. Anticipated difficulties in treating the patient.

In this section, the clinician hypothesizes how psychologically minded the patient is. For example, is the patient aware of the nature and severity of his or her problems, and does he or she have the ability

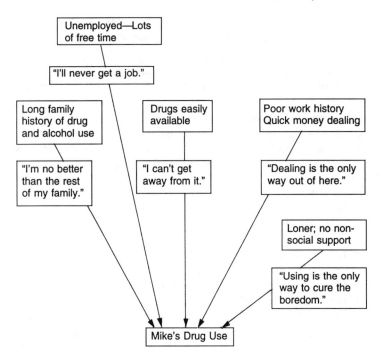

FIGURE 5.2. Beliefs and other factors contributing to Mike's drug use.

to self-monitor automatic thoughts? The patient's capacity for access-
ing automatic thoughts and beliefs certainly has important implications for the pace of treatment. In addition, personality characteristics—for example, sociotropic or autonomous—can provide the
therapist with some indication as to the conditions under which the
patient might relapse, for example, the sociotropic person in situations in which there is social pressure, and the autonomous individual
when blocked from reaching his/her achievement goals. The patient's
motivation, goals, and expectations for therapy are noted and discussed on the conceptualization form. Also noted are the therapist's
goals for treatment, and how compatible these are with the patient's
goals. Finally, it is also useful to anticipate difficulties that might arise
during the course of therapy that might warrant special attention. For
example, if the patient has a history of periodic homelessness, this
will need to be addressed early in treatment lest the patient suddenly
"disappear" from treatment and be unreachable by mail or telephone.
    A case study illustration of the Cognitive Conceptualization Work-
sheet (for patient "D.D.") follows.

CASE SUMMARY AND COGNITIVE
CONCEPTUALIZATION WORKSHEET

Dr. R.	D.D.	1/10/92	6
Therapist' Name	Patient's Initials	Date	Session #

I. Demographic Information
Ms. D is a 38-year-old, white, single female who is currently unemployed. She lives alone and has recently broken up with her boyfriend. She was in school but stopped going to class this month.

II. Diagnoses
Axis I:	Cocaine abuse
	Alcohol abuse
	Major depression, recurrent
Axis II:	Avoidant personality disorder
	Histrionic personality disorder
Axis III:	No physical illness reported
Axis IV:	Code 2 (Mild)—Not attending her college classes
Axis V:	GAF Code 60—Moderate depressive symptoms; not functioning well in school; difficulties eating, sleeping, and concentrating

III. Inventory Scores

	Intake	Sess. # 1	Sess. # 2	Sess. # 3	Sess. # 4	Sess. # 5	Sess. # 6	Latest Sess.
BDI	25	26	20	21	17	17	16	16
BAI	2	1	1	12	11	12	13	13
BHS	11	11	12	12	12	10	7	7

Other

General Trend of Scores: BDI and BHS scores are improving; however, her BAI scores have worsened over the past six sessions. (Higher scores indicate greater symptomatology.)

IV. Presenting Problem and Current Functioning
There were three presenting problems: (1) history of alcohol and cocaine use (though she reported that she had not used in the past 30 days), (2) moderate number of depressive symptoms and related fear that the symptoms would get worse, and (3) worry and fear that she might start using drugs and alcohol, progressing toward total relapse.

(continued)

V. Developmental Profile

A. History (family, social, educational, medical, psychiatric, vocational)

The patient was born on the East Coast and spent most of her life in an urban setting. Her father had numerous businesses and her mother was a homemaker. When D was 13, her mother and father divorced. The patient liked elementary school but was anxious. She "hated" high school. D went through inpatient detox in 1985, and previously suffered from major depression in 1987.

B. Relationships (parents, siblings, peers, authority figures, significant others)

The patient described her father as a loving, dedicated man. She stated that he was a heavy drinker—unpredictable when he was drunk. Her mother was the "perfect mother," always there for the family. D was the oldest of five children. She stated her relationship with all of them was "great."

C. Significant events and traumas

The patient described three significant events: (1) her parents' divorce, (2) her unhappiness throughout high school, and (3) her realization in 1985 that she had a drug and alcohol problem.

VI. Cognitive Profile

A. The cognitive model as applied to this patient

1. Typical current problems/problematic situations:
   Situations that can lead to her taking drugs:
   (a) When she is around former drug friends.
   (b) When there is a breakup in a significant relationship.
   (c) When bored and alone.
2. Typical ATs, affect, and behaviors in these situations:
   Automatic Thoughts:
   "They still use."
   "I'll never find someone who really cares."
   "I can't stand the boredom."
   Affect:
   Angry
   Depressed
   Hopeless
   Behavior:
   Uses alcohol first, then cocaine

B. Core beliefs (e.g., "I am unlovable")

"I am unlovable."
"I am undesirable."
"I am powerless."
"I am weak."

(continued)

C. Conditional beliefs (e.g., "If I fail, I am worthless")
   "If I do what is expected of me, then people will accept me."
   "If I do things perfectly, then I feel competent."
D. Rules (shoulds/musts applied to self/others)
   "I must be accepted by others or I'm worthless."
   "I must be emotionally in charge or there is something wrong with me."

VII. **Integration and Conceptualization of Cognitive and Developmental Profiles**
   A. **Formulation of self-concept and concepts of others**
   The patient believed she had to do the "right" thing as a child or her father would push her away.
   The patient could not always please her father predictably because his drinking led to erratic and "fickle" treatment of his children.
   Father left mother without any explanation; led to D's belief that men are not to be trusted.
   B. **Interaction of life events and cognitive vulnerabilities**

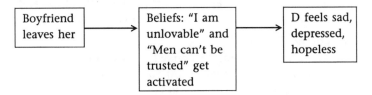

   C. **Compensatory and coping strategies**
   Avoids doing things that she feels she cannot do perfectly.
   Tendency to use drugs and alcohol when she is upset.
   D. **Development and maintenance of current disorder**
   Low frustration tolerance for anxiety, boredom, and depression.
   Drug-related beliefs such as "Cocaine is the only way to relieve the boredom."

VIII. **Implications for Therapy**
   A. **Aptitude for cognitive interventions (rate low, medium, or high, and add comments, if applicable):**
   1. Psychological mindedness: very good
   2. Objectivity: good
   3. Self-awareness: very good
   4. Comprehension of cognitive model: very good
   5. Accessibility and flexibility of automatic thoughts and beliefs: very good
   6. General adaptiveness: very good
   7. Humor: Excellent

(continued)

B. **Personality characteristics: sociotropic vs. autonomous**
   Sociotropic: Strong need for attachment to others.
   Achievement needs are far less pronounced.

C. **Patient's motivation, goals, and expectations for therapy**
   Strong motivation to stop using drugs and alcohol.
   Other goals are realistic (i.e., would like to finish college).

D. **Therapist's goals**
   1. Teach patient to monitor, examine, and respond to negative automatic thoughts.
   2. Help her to acquire skills for coping with drug and alcohol urges and cravings.
   3. Improve D's problem-solving skills.

E. **Predicted difficulties in therapy**
   1. Lapse could turn into a relapse if patient does not contact the therapist as soon as possible, which she might not do if she feels ashamed of her behavior and expects the therapist to criticize her.
   2. Patient will tend to minimize her problems (e.g., as she did when she described her relationships with family members in glowing terms in spite of serious conflicts).
   3. Patient still maintains contact with drug friends who may try to sabotage her abstinence goals.

ADDITIONAL DATA FOR THE CASE CONCEPTUALIZATION

In addition to the clinical interview, self-report inventories provide data that are important in the conceptualization of the case. The following is a list of such questionnaires and scales.

1. Beck Depression Inventory
2. Beck Anxiety Inventory
3. Beck Hopelessness Scale
4. Dysfunctional Attitude Scale
5. Beliefs about Substance Use Scale
6. Relapse Prediction Scale
7. Craving Beliefs Questionnaire
8. Sociotropy–Autonomy Scale

Beck Depression Inventory

The Beck Depression Inventory (BDI) (Beck, Ward, Mendelson, Mock, & Erbaugh, 1961) is a self-report scale composed of 21 items, each comprising four statements reflecting gradations in the intensity of a particular depressive symptom. The respondent chooses the statement that best corresponds to the way he or she has felt for the past week. The scale is intended for use within psychiatric populations as a measure of the symptom severity of depressed mood and as a screening instrument for use with nonpsychiatric populations.

Beck Anxiety Inventory

The Beck Anxiety Inventory (BAI) (Beck, Epstein, Brown, & Steer, 1988) is a 21-item, self-report instrument designed to measure the severity of anxious symptoms. The BAI overlaps only minimally with the BDI and other measures of depression while measuring anxiety.

Beck Hopelessness Scale

The Beck Hopelessness Scale (BHS) was developed by Beck, Weissman, Lester, and Trexler (1974) to measure negative expectancy regarding the future. The BHS is composed of 20 true–false items assessing the expectation that one will not be able to overcome an unpleasant life situation or attain the things that one values in life. The BHS has demonstrated predictive validity for completed suicide (Beck, Steer, Kovacs, & Garrison, 1985).

Dysfunctional Attitude Scale

The Dysfunctional Attitude Scale (DAS) (Weissman & Beck, 1978) is a self-report scale composed of 100 items. It was developed to assess underlying assumptions and beliefs that constitute schemas by which individuals construe their life experiences.

✓ Beliefs about Substance Use

The Beliefs About Substance Use inventory is a self-report scale composed of 20 items that can be scored on a range from 1 to 7. A "1" indicates that the person totally disagrees with the statement. A score of "7" means that the person totally agrees with the statement. This scale measures many of the commonly held beliefs about drug use (see Appendix 1, page 311).

Relapse Prediction Scale

The Relapse Prediction Scale (RPS) is a 50 item self-report scale. Each item is composed of situations that typically are reported to trigger urges for cocaine or crack. Each situation is rated on two dimensions: "Strength of Urges" and "Likelihood of Using," with all situations being rated on a 0–5 scale (0 = none to 5 = very high) (See Appendix 1, page 313).

Craving Beliefs Questionnaire

The Craving Beliefs Questionnaire (CBQ) is a self-report scale that measures beliefs about the craving phenomenon as it pertains to cocaine and crack. Each of 28 items is rated on a 1–7 scale (e.g., 1 = totally disagree and 7 = totally agree) (See Appendix 1, page 312).

Sociotropy–Autonomy Scale

The Sociotropy–Autonomy Scale (Beck, Epstein, & Harrison, 1983) is a measure of two broad personality dimensions that are associated with depression (Beck, 1967). One is "sociotropy," which refers to the degree of importance a person places on interpersonal affiliation in order to be happy. The second is "autonomy," referring to the degree to which a person believes he or she must achieve and attain success in order to be happy.

Each of the 60 questions asks the respondent to rate the percentage of time that a statement applies to himself or herself. Half of the questions indicate a sociotropic personality style, and the other half indicate an autonomous personality style. One example of a sociotropic item is, "I find it difficult to say no to people." There are five possible responses—this applies to me (1) 0%, (2) 25%, (3) 50%, (4) 75%, (5) 100% of the time. Sociotropy and autonomy subscores are summed separately; therefore, a person may be high on both scales or low on both scales.

SUMMARY

The purpose of this chapter has been to provide the therapist with a comprehensive methodology for achieving a sound case formulation.

We began with a rationale supporting the importance of a good case formulation, and suggested key questions for the clinician to ask when treating substance abuse patients. Next, we introduced what we consider the ten essential components of the formulation: (1) relevant childhood data, (2) current life problems, (3) core beliefs, (4) conditional assumptions/beliefs/rules, (5) compensatory strategies, (6) vulnerable situations, (7) ATs, (8) emotions, (9) behaviors, and (10) integration of the data. Each component was described in detail and pertinent examples presented, followed by an illustrative case study.

Next, we reviewed methods for gathering and organizing data for the case formulation. We introduced the Cognitive Conceptualization Worksheet, provided an explanation of its use, and noted examples to aid in the understanding of the use of this form. This chapter concluded with a description of eight self-report inventories used in producing information toward a sound case formulation.

CHAPTER **6**

Structure of the Therapy Session

T he structure of the therapy session is one of the more noticeable and essential characteristics of cognitive therapy. Structure is important for the following reasons: (1) Within a typical 50-minute session, substance abusers often present a large amount of material to discuss, either longstanding or acute crises, yet there is a limited amount of time. Structuring the session provides the opportunity to *make maximum use of time.* Patient and therapist collaborate to most effectively handle problems in the time allowed. (2) Structure assists in *focusing* on the most important current problems. (3) Learning new skills, such as better problem solving, requires hard work. Structuring the therapy session sets the tone for a *working atmosphere.* (4) Structured sessions fight against therapy drift, whereby continuity from session to session is lost. Knowing the elements of the structured session facilitates adherence to the cognitive model and minimizes the chances that drift will occur.

This chapter focuses on eight important elements of the structure of a session:

1. Setting the agenda
2. Mood check
3. Bridge from last session
4. Discussion of today's agenda items
5. Socratic questioning
6. Capsule summaries
7. Homework assignments
8. Feedback in the therapy session

SETTING THE AGENDA

Time is precious. Setting an agenda helps to make efficient use of time and provides a focus for the therapy session. It also teaches patients to set priorities, usually a skill deficiency in impulsive drug-addicted individuals. Because they spend a considerable amount of time seeking, using, or recovering from their drug use, patients often spend little time focusing on solving the other problems that are plaguing their lives.

Setting agendas has a positive effect on the therapeutic alliance as well. It reinforces the collaborative agreement between patient and therapist as each party has an opportunity to contribute to the process of therapy. It allows patient and therapist to target specific goals (see Chapter 8, this volume) for the session and to discuss the appropriateness of focusing on specific topics. It also sets the stage for modeling better ways of resolving conflicts, for example, when the patient's agenda item seems incompatible with what the therapist wants to discuss. This is illustrated in the case in which the patient says, "I want to give you all the details . . . I just want to get it off my chest . . . It makes me feel better." In order to preserve collaboration, the therapist might reach an agreement with such a patient that a certain portion of the session can be used to "let off steam" but may also suggest that other topics will also need to be covered, such as ambivalence about abstinence, continued drug use, and triggers to using.

Some patients have a low tolerance for anxiety and therefore avoid bringing up topics that provoke discomfort. When therapists provide a rationale for putting such topics on the agenda in spite of the discomfort the topics evoke, they help to avoid power struggles between themselves and their patients. Therapists also make good, collaborative use of the agenda by demonstrating empathy for their patients' reluctance to discuss certain hot topics, such as their spouses' substance abuse problems.

At times, therapists need to be flexible in setting agendas. Sometimes patients come to a session in crisis, such as after being fired from a job or being left by a spouse. These types of problems may require immediate attention, superseding ongoing issues. Likewise, a lapse or relapse should be dealt with immediately because patients who have used often feel hopeless about their ability to stay off drugs, and thus are at increased risk for a full relapse. This in turn often leads to feeling hopeless about therapy and may precipitate a premature flight from treatment.

A key point to remember is the importance of the therapist's not being rigid or dictatorial in setting and following agendas. For example, when it becomes clear that a high-priority agenda item will require most of the session to addresss adequately, the therapist needs to be willing to shelve less important topics. Also, therapists can modify agendas by periodically checking the number of agenda items to be covered and the amount of time left in the therapy session. If there is insufficient time, patient and therapist then collaborate on deciding which agenda items might need to be postponed.

The following is a transcript of the beginning of a therapy session in which the therapist and patient are setting an agenda collaboratively. In reading this transcript, keep in mind that the therapist is working with the patient to set an appropriate agenda with a specific target problem, to keep the agenda suitable for the amount of time available in the therapy session, and to prioritize the topics.

TH: Well, what are we going to focus on today?

PT: Some things, but you know . . . my burden now . . . my thing is that I need a job.

TH: That is something important to put on the agenda for today. Are there other things that we need to talk about? For example, your current frequency of drug use?

PT: No, I'm doing all right as far as my drug things are concerned.

TH: How much of anything have you used since the last time I saw you?

PT: Nothing.

TH: Nothing?

PT: Nothing. I go to my meetings now.

TH: No drinking? No alcohol?

PT: Nothing.

TH: OK.

PT: When I wake up in the mornings now, I really don't have that craving for drugs. Do you know what I mean? So, now I have to just put this energy into getting up in the morning and getting out and getting a job. That's a real problem; let's make sure we get to that.

TH: OK. What I will do is write on the board a list of things that we need to cover. We might not be able to get to everything today. First we have "finding a job"—difficulty getting up in the morning to go looking for one. The next thing I was going to put there had to do with "cravings." So, at some time today, I would like to talk with you about what happened that led to your last slip. The whole point of doing this is for you to get more familiar with what happened so you can recognize when you are feeling bad, what that usually leads to, and to try to come up with some ways to keep it from going all the way down to your using again. To the alcohol, then to the coke, then to the heroin. Oh, we also need to go over the homework from last week.

PT: Finding a job is the most important.

TH: OK. Maybe we can start with that. Is there anything else you want us to focus on?

PT: No, this is good.

As this brief transcript illustrates, the therapist set the stage for focusing on two primary goals for treatment: reducing drug use, "What happened that led to your slip?" and doing problem solving, "Finding a job . . . difficulty getting up." The therapist asked two of three important questions that should be asked at every session: (1) Have you used since the last session? (2) Have you had any urges/cravings to use? and (3) Are there any situations coming up before our next session where you might be at risk to use? (This third question was not asked by the therapist.)

MOOD CHECK

Since depression, anxiety, and hopelessness are internal stimuli that have the potential to trigger continued use and/or relapse, it is important to monitor these (and other) states. Therapists should pay special attention to feelings of hopelessness as it has been shown that a chronic, marked negative view of the future is one of the best predictors of suicide (Beck, Steer, et al., 1985).

It is desirable to have the patient complete the BDI, BAI, and BHS at every session (see Chapter 5, this volume, for descriptions of these instruments). Scores and their meanings should be discussed with the patient, especially if there are substantial changes in scores. Sometimes there can be a change in mood as measured by these instruments, but the patient seems unaware of the change. Therefore, the therapist should ask the patient if he or she is aware of changes in his or her mood. The therapist might say, "Your score on the BDI is higher this week, which may indicate that you have been feeling more depressed. Do you agree with that?"

Important points to remember are (1) mood is an important variable with regard to drug use and relapse, (2) hopelessness is one of the best predictors of suicide, (3) mood levels should be measured at each session, and (4) therapists should discuss scores obtained from the BDI, BAI, and BHS with their patients.

BRIDGE FROM LAST SESSION

Drug and alcohol abusers often have chaotic lives; therefore it is easy for therapists to get drawn into a pattern of jumping from one topic to another in a disjointed fashion. Therapists should think carefully as to how they will stay focused and *maintain continuity across therapy sessions*. They should ask themselves, "How do the present agenda items relate to what was discussed in the previous session, and how do these items relate to the overall goals of treatment?"

The therapist also reviews the patient's feedback about the previous session. There are two ways to accomplish this. First, the therapist asks the patient if there is any unfinished business from the most recent session, including any negative reactions he or she might have had. Second, the therapist may reflect on the Patient's Report of Therapy Session (see Appendix 5, page 324), which patients are asked to complete after each session. Usually this is brief; however, some responses might require considerably more attention and time to address. For example, one patient reported after the last session that he did not *expect* to make any progress in that session, that he did not *in fact* make any progress, and that he did not expect to make progress in *future* sessions. The therapist, recognizing that this feedback indicated that the patient held very negative views about therapy, suggested that this be discussed at some length in the current session. To get a sense of the patient's world, it is helpful to review briefly the patient's life during the past week. Therapists can use activity schedules to structure this review. Therapists must encourage their patients to keep this review as brief as possible, so that it does not deteriorate into idle chit-chat about the patient's general goings-on that takes up valuable time in the session.

DISCUSSION OF TODAY'S AGENDA ITEMS

When therapists and patients proceed to discuss the agreed-on agenda items for the session, they must bear in mind the following points. First, it is important to prioritize the list of topics. It is not always possible to discuss every item within the time constraints of a given session. Some topics will need to be shelved until the following session. Therefore, it makes the most sense to determine which topic or topics are essential to discuss in the present session, and to discuss these topics first. By doing so, therapists can avert unfortunate problems such as an entire session being used to discuss a patient's complaints about his car troubles, only to find out as the sessions ends that the patient went on a drinking binge after his wife walked out on him. Clearly, this latter topic needed to be discussed first and foremost, not just for 2 minutes at the tail end of the session.

Second, therapists must be alert to patients' tendencies to stray from agenda items and to go off on irrelevant tangents. A polite but prompt statement, such as "I don't mean to interrupt, but I think we should refocus on the topic we started talking about," usually is sufficient. At times, when patients seem to "stray" to even more important issues (e.g., a discussion of the patient's marriage leads into hints that the patient is contemplating suicide), it is advisable for therapists to switch gears to accommodate and follow up on these important topics by revising the agenda. In general, *topics such as the patient's active drug use, suicidality, or hopelessness about therapy will supersede most other agenda items.*

Third, therapists need to be somewhat conscious of time in the session so that the various topics are covered in sufficient breadth and depth, and so that transitions from one agenda item to the next can be made in a timely manner. At times, therapists may choose to interject the following question in order to facilitate this process: "We're about halfway through the session, and we have a decision to make. Should we keep talking about our current topic a while longer, or would it make sense to wrap this up and go on to our next item?" This is a collaborative, flexible way to stay focused on meaningful therapeutic material, and to be as efficient as possible in making the best use of valuable therapy time.

Fourth, therapists need not be stymied by patients who say "I don't know" when asked what topics should be discussed as part of the agenda. (In fact, *good cognitive therapists almost never take "I don't know" for an answer.* They persist nicely, find alternative ways to ask the question, or ask the patient to deliberate further.) Instead, therapists can explain that one of the patient's responsibilities in therapy is to think about what he or she would like to talk about in session. At first, the therapist may assist the patient by *suggesting* some agenda items, asking, "Which of these is most important to you?" The therapist may also ask, "What has been on your mind lately? What's on your mind right now?" Later, if the patient continues to be unwilling or unable to generate topics for discussion, *this problem in and of itself can become an important agenda item.* For example, the therapist may say, "Let's discuss your difficulty in thinking of things to talk about in session. Let's try to understand where the problem is, and how to overcome it." In doing so, the therapist avoids falling into the trap of accepting the patient's helplessness or resistance as an unchangeable fact. In addition, the patient learns that saying "I don't know" will not be reinforced, and that this strategy will fail as an intended means of escape from the work of therapy.

SOCRATIC QUESTIONING

Overholser (1987, 1988) defines Socratic questioning as a method of intervening that encourages the patient to contemplate, evaluate, and synthesize diverse sources of information. This type of questioning, also referred to as "guided discovery," is utilized over the entire span of the session.

In contrast to questions typically designed for the therapist to gather information regarding the frequency, intensity, and duration of the substance abuse problem, Socratic questioning is used to bring information into the awareness of the *patient.* Therefore, Socratic questions are designed to promote insight and better rational decision-making. Questions should be phrased in such a way that they stimulate thought and increase awareness, rather than requiring a correct answer. The proper choice, phrasing, and ordering of questions has a strong impact on the organization of thought in the patient. Further, we have found that most of our drug-abusing patients respond more favorably to exploratory questioning than to didactic "lecturing."

Socratic questioning is a powerful technique to use while discussing the various agenda items. Therapist asks questions in such a way as to help patients to examine their thinking, to reflect on erroneous conclusions, and, at times, to come up with better solutions to problems. This often leads to patients' questioning, and thereby gaining greater objectivity from, their own thoughts, motives, and behaviors. Also, Socratic questioning establishes a nonjudgmental atmosphere and thus facilitates collaboration between patients and therapists. This can help patients come to their own conclusions about the seriousness of their drug abuse problem.

As a rule of thumb, therapists should start utilizing Socratic questioning from the beginning of treatment. This helps to orient patients to an active thinking mode. If therapists find that Socratic questioning appears to be overwhelming patients more than helping, then the therapists may choose to be more direct, such as pointing out inconsistencies and errors in thinking and asking if the patients agree with and follow this logic.

While it is important to use questioning to explore problems and to help patients draw their own conclusions, there should be a balance between questioning and other more direct modes of intervention, such as reflection, clarification, giving feedback, and educating the patient. The following dialogue illustrates such a balance, with the therapist starting with some basic assessment questions:

TH: Charleen, have you used any drugs or alcohol this week?

PT: No, none. It's been over a month now.

TH: What about your pain medication from the dentist?

PT: What about it?

TH: Well, I have a number of questions. First, are you taking the amount that you're supposed to take, and not more than that? Are you taking it when you're supposed to take it, and not more often than that?

PT: I'm doing just what I'm supposed to do, so don't worry.

TH: Do you know why I'm asking? Do you know why it matters?

PT: Yeh, because you told me that pain medication is like a drug . . .

TH: Not *like* a drug. It *is* a drug. It's a mild narcotic.

PT: And I could get addicted to it.

TH: Right. And do you know why I'm concerned about the *amount* and the *frequency* with which you're taking it?

PT: No.

TH: Think about it for a minute. Why do you think we should be concerned about it?

PT: I don't know.

TH: Well, I realize that you might not know *exactly* why, but could you try to guess some possible reasons. I'll be happy to tell you my reasons after you give me *your* theory.

Note that the therapist is asking a number of open-ended questions in the hope that the patient will begin to do some active thinking in the session. The fact that the patient does not respond to the latter question does not deter the therapist. Instead, he finds a tactful, collaborative way to encourage the patient to apply some cognitive effort. Later, he plans to "reward" the patient for her effort by giving her some additional information in order to educate her about the dangers of pain medications in the hands of a recovering addict. First, however, he continues with some Socratic questioning.

PT: I guess if I took more than I'm supposed to, I could get addicted faster.

TH: That's right. What else?

PT: I could get high on the pain medication and lose control and go out and use other drugs.

TH: Absolutely right. Excellent answer. See, you *do* understand. Anything else you can think of?

PT: No. Not really.

TH: Well, consider this. What would happen if you ran out of the pain medication before you were supposed to run out?

PT: I'd have to get more.

TH: Yes, but if the dentist knows that you're supposed to still have some medication left, and you're already asking for more, what would happen?

PT: He might say no.

TH: What might you do then?

PT: I might have to find some other way to kill the pain.

TH: Such as?

PT: Such as whiskey. (*laughs*)

TH: Why would that be a problem?

PT: Because then I would blow my streak of staying off stuff I shouldn't take.

TH: And would you just drink whiskey?

PT: I might also use crack if I had the chance.

TH: Right. Now, you've worked very hard to get to this point. It would be a crying shame if you set yourself back by taking too much pain medication.

PT: I agree.

TH: So, Charleen, have you been taking the medication as prescribed?

PT: Yes, but I still have pain, so I've been taking the Advils and the Tylenols too.

At this point, the therapist is satisfied that the patient has arrived at her own conclusion that she could be at risk for a lapse or a full-blown relapse if she misuses her prescribed medications in any way.

At the same time, he has just heard something a bit disturbing; therefore he will ask for clarification before proceeding with some non-Socratic, didactic education.

TH: Uh oh. You're taking more medications? How much?

PT: (*Getting a little annoyed*) Until I feel better, that's how much!

TH: Do you read the instructions before taking the over-the-counter medications?

PT: No, I just take it until I feel better.

TH: Charleen, please bear with me for a few minutes. I can tell you're getting a little ticked off right now, and I don't mean to get you angry but this is important. Can you hear me out?

PT: Do I have a choice?

TH: Well, yes. You could ignore me if you wanted to, but I'm hoping you'll give me a chance to make my point before you decide whether to disregard it or not.

PT: Go ahead.

TH: Thanks, I appreciate your being a good sport. Charleen, there are good reasons why medications have instructions. If people ignore the instructions, they can overdose. Or, they can cause something called "interactions" with other drugs. In your case, the over-the-counter medications could combine with the dentist's medication to create an effect in your body that's equal to many, many, many medications, which could be dangerous. Also—and I'm not sure that you knew this—every time a person takes a pain medication he lowers his body's own natural ability to kill pain. So, if you take too much of *anything*, it can suppress your ability to feel well after you stop taking the medication. You see, if the medication runs out, and you've suppressed your body's own natural abilities to kill pain, you're going to go into withdrawal and be in a lot of discomfort. Then, you won't be able to get a refill of the dentist's medication and you'll probably think that you have no choice but to drink whiskey or get some crack. That's why it's so important for you to take *only what is prescribed, and nothing more, not even over-the-counter stuff.* Do you get my point?

PT: You mean if I take these medications, my body will never be able to kill pain by itself?

TH: Not "never." It will just be suppressed for a few days. That's the withdrawal phase, just like for any drugs. But can you hold off on using drugs for a few days when you're in pain?

PT: No way.

TH: That's my point. If you go on the way you're going on right now, you'll be in danger of using alcohol and crack, especially when you run out of the prescription.

PT: I see. What should I do?

TH: That's an excellent question. Can I turn it back to you? What do you think you should do?

Now, the therapist shifts back into the mode of Socratic questioning.

PT: I guess I have to stop taking the Advils and the Tylenols.

TH: And how about the dentist's medication?

PT: I guess I have to make sure I read the instructions.

TH: But what if you do exactly what you're supposed to do, and you're still in pain?

PT: I don't know.

TH: What do you think I would do in your situation?

PT: You would call the dentist.

TH: I might do that, yes. What else?

PT: You would try distracting yourself with activities, right?

TH: Correct! Could you try that?

PT: I could try.

TH: What kinds of things could you do?

The therapist continues to ask open-ended questions so that Charleen can generate her own interventions, the likes of which she is more likely to follow between sessions than those interventions simply directed toward her. Thus, the dialogue has demonstrated that a mixture of interventions, including education, clarification, and Socratic questioning, can help patients to do meaningful work in session, and to elicit the maximum amount of information and cooperation.

CAPSULE SUMMARIES

Capsule summaries are an important part of the learning process in therapy sessions. As a general rule, therapists and patients should summarize what has been discussed in a session a minimum of three times. This provides opportunities to adjust agendas and to maintain the focus of the therapy session. The first capsule summary typically is done after the agenda has been established, the second one approximately halfway through the therapy session, and last, toward the conclusion of the therapy session.

The first summary helps patients make a connection between the agenda of the present session and the long-term goals of therapy. The following represents a typical first capsule summary:

TH: OK, let's summarize what we are going to focus on today. One thing is the situation when you had the strong urge to pick up on some crack. Second is your situation at work. You are anxious about the fact that you might be laid off. Was there anything I missed?

PT: No, that's it.

TH: Both of these issues fit very nicely with your long-term goals of treatment, one being coping with urges to use crack, finding other methods for coping with anxiety, and, last, your concerns about employment and saving money. Do you see how they connect?

PT: Yeh, it all makes sense.

The second summary helps the therapist to collect his own thoughts, to decide what to do next (such as advancing to the next item on the agenda), to convey understanding of the patient and provide an opportunity to correct any misunderstanding, and to make the therapy process more understandable to the patient.

Initially in treatment the final summary is done by the therapist. However, as therapy progresses the therapist should move very quickly to get the patient to do end-of-session summaries. When patients summarize, it gives them responsibility for processing the session, and it lets therapists check on patients' understanding of what went on in the session. Further, patients improve their retention for the contents of the session when they actively review what has been discussed.

HOMEWORK ASSIGNMENTS

The homework assignment is a collaborative enterprise generated and agreed on by the therapist and patient as a team. Its two main functions are to serve as a bridge between sessions, ensuring that the patient continues to work on his or her problems, and to provide an opportunity for the patient to collect information to test erroneous beliefs and to try new behaviors (Blackburn & Davidson, 1990).

Patients are encouraged to view homework as an integral and vital component of treatment (Burns & Auerbach, 1992; Burns & Nolen-Hoeksema, 1991; Persons, Burns, & Perloff, 1988). Since the therapy session is time-limited, normally less than an hour, homework assignments become extremely important as they offer patients ongoing opportunities to practice various skills that they have been taught in the therapy session.

It is best to assign homeworks that draw from the therapy session, as homework is most effective when it is a logical extension of the therapy session (Newman, 1993). This can be done by reviewing what has happened in the therapy session and then focusing on how these points or lessons can be continued and reinforced outside treatment. Ideally, such assignments ultimately lead to the continued use of new skills, even after the termination of formal treatment.

It is generally advisable to review the previous week's homework as an early agenda item in each therapy session. By doing so, therapists convey to patients that homework is an important part of the therapy process (Burns & Auerbach, 1992). Also, by reviewing homework from previous sessions, therapists can correct patients' mistakes early in treatment—for example, in completing a Daily Thought Record (DTR) (see Chapter 9, this volume). By making sure that the homework assignment is reviewed, therapists can make certain that patients are practicing new cognitive and behavioral skills correctly.

Therapists who neglect to review the homework in each session create three problems. First, the patients usually begin to think that the homework is not important and, therefore, that treatment is something done to them rather than something they actively work on even in the absence of the therapist. Second, the therapists miss opportunities to correct mistakes such as the patients' inadequately responding rationally to their automatic thoughts. Third, the therapists lose the chance to draw helpful lessons from the homework and to reinforce these lessons.

The therapist can minimize patient noncompliance by being sure to explain the rationale for the assignment and by discussing with the patient any possible or expected difficulties (Newman, 1993). For example, the therapist might ask: "What are some things that could happen that might get in the way of completing the assignment?" and/or "What are the odds of your completing the assignment?" In addition, if the therapist has some doubt about the patient's understanding of the task, he or she should, if possible, rehearse the assignment before the patient leaves the session.

If a homework assignment is not carried out, therapists should address this issue. One method is to use the "Possible Reasons for Not

Doing Self-Help Assignment" Checklist (see Appendix 6, page 327). This checklist helps to identify those reasons why patients often do not do homework assignments. The therapist can pull out a copy of this list and ask the patient to select those items that apply to his/her noncompliance. The following are some examples of items on this checklist: "I don't have enough time, I'm too busy," "I feel helpless and I don't really believe that I can do anything that I choose to do," and "It seems that nothing can help me so there is no point in trying."

These beliefs become new targets for examination and testing. In summary, the homework assignment functions as a bridge between therapy sessions and provides an opportunity to test beliefs and practice skills learned in the session. The task should be a logical extension of the session and be relevant to the goals of therapy. The therapist can minimize noncompliance by giving rationales for assignments and discussing possible difficulties with the patient. To facilitate patients' understanding, homework assignments can be rehearsed in session. Therapists should explain the importance of homework, and are advised to review assignments at each session. Incomplete assignments should be discussed as an agenda item in the session. The reasons that patients cite for not doing the homework can be ascertained through questioning or a checklist, and these reasons are treated as beliefs to be tested.

FEEDBACK IN THE THERAPY SESSION

Therapists and patients regularly exchange feedback during therapy sessions. Throughout the session, the therapist asks questions to be sure that the patient understands what the therapist has said and where the therapist is heading. For example, the therapist might ask, "Can you tell me what point I'm trying to make with these questions?" Sometimes patients misunderstand what therapists are trying to accomplish. Asking questions at these points gives patient and therapist an opportunity to clarify miscommunications in the therapy session. At the end of the session, the therapist should try to get feedback from the patient regarding (1) what was learned in the session, (2) how the patient felt during the therapy session, and (3) how the patient feels about the therapy in general.

For example, the therapist might ask the following questions: "What did you get out of today's session?" "Was there anything that I said or did that rubbed you the wrong way during today's session?" "Do you feel we are accomplishing something useful?"

Other ways of eliciting feedback include responding to nonverbal behavior in the therapy session. For example, if the therapist notices that the patient is frowning, the therapist might say, "I noticed you just had a frown on your face. What thoughts were going through your mind right then?" This will often result in eliciting valuable feedback.

The key points to remember are that the therapist should endeavor to become adept at eliciting and responding to verbal and nonverbal feedback throughout the therapy session, that the therapist should regularly check for the patient's understanding of what is going on in the therapy session, and that key points should be summarized periodically throughout the therapy session. This, in turn, helps to build a strong collaborative relationship.

SUMMARY

In this chapter the importance of session structure and its eight components are discussed. Setting agendas helps to make maximum use of time, keeps the sessions focused, sets the tone for a working atmosphere, and counters therapist drift. Repeated mood checks identify changes in mood that might lead to relapse. Bridging sessions provides continuity across sessions and keeps therapy sessions focused on goals of treatment. In discussing the list of agenda items, therapists help their patients to prioritize the list, to stay focused on important material, to make the most efficient use of time, and to contribute actively to the discussion. Also, therapists use skillful Socratic questioning as often as possible, which helps patients make their own discoveries. Capsule summaries should occur at least three times in a session. The importance of homework must be conveyed to the patient, and the appropriate steps for minimizing noncompliance should be taken. Therapists provide and elicit feedback to clear up possible misunderstanding and/or misinterpretation of what is happening in the session.

CHAPTER *7*

Educating Patients in the Cognitive Model

$\mathbf{A}$s the cognitive therapy of substance abuse is a collaborative enterprise between therapist and patient, it is essential that patients gain a conceptual grasp of the key components in the model, such as understanding the associations and causal relationships between cognition, affect, behavior, craving, and using. Patients need to learn about the phenomenon of automatic thoughts and the key elements for testing hypotheses.

Some therapists start educating drug abuse patients in the treatment model before they themselves have gained an adequate understanding about their patients' formulations of the various problems. In doing so, therapists may miss an opportunity to foster an atmosphere of teamwork that is so important to nurture early in treatment. Asking patients for *their* views helps to nurture the collaboration. In some cases, patients are quite aware of the specifics of their problems; they just feel stuck and are not sure what steps they need to take to arrive at functional solutions. While gathering the patients' formulations, therapists can begin to educate patients in the cognitive therapy model by focusing on the *beliefs* that are inherent in their interpretations of their drug problems.

ELICIT PATIENTS' FORMULATIONS OF THE PROBLEM

Substance abuse patients generally have explanations for their drug problems, such as "I have a high-stress job," "Today everybody uses drugs," "It's this marriage; if she would only change," and so on. By beginning to explore these "reasons," the therapist starts to understand the patient's "internal reality" and to establish a collaborative set for therapy.

Therapists ask patients how they believe their drug problem developed, and how they would explain their current difficulties with work, relationships, the law, and other important life areas. In addition, therapists inquire about what the patients think they must do to solve their drug problem. Similarly, clinicians ask why patients believe that they have not been willing or able to solve their drug and general life problems on their own to this point.

Although patients may present what appear to be understandable reasons for their drug abuse, they usually have some degree of doubt (as do their skeptical therapists!). How much they believe their own explanation can be assessed by asking them to rate it on a scale of 0 to 100, with 0 meaning they do not believe it at all and 100 meaning they believe it completely. This subtle tactic begins to teach patients that their beliefs are not the same as facts and will be subject to evaluation.

For example, one patient explained to the therapist during the initial therapy session that he believed his alcohol and cocaine use were the direct result of where he lived. He stated that the conditions were miserable: "There's high unemployment, poor housing, and drugs all over the place." He believed that anyone with these types of hardships would also be drinking and using cocaine. When the therapist asked how much he believed in his own explanation, the patient replied "85%." The patient stated that there were indeed some people in the area who did not use drugs, but they were "religious." However, on closer review, the patient noted that there were two members of his own family who were using neither drugs nor alcohol—his sister and father.

The patient was given an assignment to list all of the people on his street that he believed used and those who he believed did not use. Although there were a large number of users, a clear majority of people on his street did not use drugs or abuse alcohol. The patient was quite surprised with these findings. Therapist and patient then agreed that looking at other explanations for his cocaine and alcohol abuse would be worth pursuing.

DEMONSTRATE THE RELATIONSHIP BETWEEN SITUATIONS, COGNITIONS, AFFECT, CRAVING, BEHAVIOR, AND DRUG USE

The following is an example of a didactic presentation:

"An automatic thought is a spontaneous thought or picture in your mind. Right now you might not pay much attention to these thoughts or pictures or make any connection between them and how you feel, but they do in fact affect your emotions and cravings for drugs. Automatic thoughts can be related to past, present, or future events, such as 'I knew I should not have gone in that bar,' 'I can't stand this craving,' and 'Oh hell, I'm never going to kick this problem.' Furthermore, these thoughts seem completely believable when they occur; therefore, they are accepted as fact without question. Further, they seem to make sense in spite of evidence to the contrary."

A powerful method for teaching patients how to recognize automatic thoughts is to have them relate their ongoing thoughts live in the therapy sessions. Therapists might say, "I want you to remember when you were in the waiting room just prior to this session. How were you feeling?" Patients sometimes will respond by saying "anxious," "nervous," "unsure of myself," "bored," "angry," and other emotions. Therapists can then ask, "*What was going through your mind right then as you were sitting out there?*" Some typical responses are, "I hope no one sees me here," "I wonder what this is going to be like," "Is the therapist going to like me?" "Am I going to be able to do this?" "What is this therapy all about?" "What am I doing here?" "I won't be able to stop using," and "I don't need to see a shrink." Patients then are told that these are examples of automatic thoughts and that they have direct bearing on the aforementioned emotions. For homework, patients may be instructed to self-monitor some of their automatic thoughts between therapy sessions. They are asked, for example, to write down their thoughts while feeling depressed, bored, anxious, angry, and especially when having cravings or urges to use drugs.

The next phase entails demonstrating the relationship between situations, emotions, cognitions, behaviors, and cravings. This may be accomplished by using examples patients bring to the therapy sessions. Therapists use the patients' examples to show how the patients' thoughts played a role in their negative feelings, their urges to use drugs, and their resultant drug-related actions.

For example, "Walter" stated that he was extremely angry because the therapist had implied that the patient's failure to attend a recent therapy session was drug-related. He added, "I was so pissed off that I thought about going out and getting bombed." The therapist, rather than becoming defensive, seized this opportunity to teach Walter about the connections between situations, thoughts, emotions, and drug urges. Specifically, he helped Walter to realize that his thoughts about "getting bombed" did *not* arise spontaneously, nor did his urges to use result purely from having a chemical addiction. Rather, Walter's thought that the therapist distrusted him triggered an angry reaction (a thought led to an emotion), and the anger in turn sparked thoughts about reasserting control in the therapeutic relationship through using drugs (an emotion led to a drug-related belief), and this finally stimulated an urge to use (a drug-related belief led to a drug urge). Thus, a potentially destructive interaction between patient and therapist was turned into an opportunity to learn about the cognitive model of drug abuse.

As patients become more skillful at making their own connections between situations, affect, cognitions, and craving, the therapist can begin to discuss with them the concept of beliefs.

The therapist explains that the way we interpret events is largely determined by our belief systems. Beliefs tend to lie in a dormant state out of awareness until they are activated by specific situations. Patients who have difficulty understanding the notion of beliefs within a drug use context may be given the following nonclinical example:

"A person has the belief that 'all people are created equal.' This is a belief that usually is dormant; it is not a statement that he goes through life thinking to himself. However, under certain circumstances, this belief is activated, such as when the person sees an injustice occur (e.g., someone who is guilty of a serious crime is set free because he is wealthy and influential). In these examples, the belief 'all people are created equal' is activated because circumstances occur that have to do with the belief. This, in turn, leads to a series of automatic thoughts, such as 'This shouldn't happen,' 'This is unfair,' and 'Why is this happening?' At this point, when the belief is triggered, the automatic thoughts are brought to awareness for that person and he becomes righteously angry."

Therapists explain that while the above belief is adaptive, many drug-related beliefs are *not*, and the thoughts and feelings they lead to may make matters worse by triggering drug cravings and urges. Dysfunctional beliefs lead people to misinterpret situations, to overgeneralize, to exaggerate, to see things in all-or-none terms, and to engage in other errors of thinking. Drug-abusing patients often make the mistake of assuming that their dysfunctional beliefs are valid and, therefore, that their interpretations are correct. One way to illustrate the notion of accurate/inaccurate beliefs is to remind patients of the story of Christopher Columbus. At one time, many people in the Western world held the belief that the world was flat. However, this did not make it so. It took a bold expedition to test the accuracy of this belief. One might say that when Columbus proved that the world was not flat, many people updated their information or belief about the surface of the world. However, there were still a few skeptics who held on rigidly to the idea that the world was flat. In the same way, people may believe that drugs are the only way to feel good, even though drugs have time and time again been proven to cause more misery than joy.

As pointed out earlier (Chapter 2, this volume), addictive beliefs are an essential component in the sequence leading to compulsive using. Patients often start off with the belief that their drug of choice is not harmful. They may also have the belief that they function better with other people when under the influence of drugs such as cocaine. This belief can lie dormant until the patient faces a situation such as a social event. Being informed of an upcoming party may activate this belief and thus lead to craving, followed by certain automatic thoughts that give permission to use the cocaine. This in turn leads to a series of habitual behaviors that facilitate finding the cocaine.

Patients also have beliefs that develop over time. For example, a patient may start off with the belief that it is OK to use cocaine, that "it's not addictive." He may also entertain th belief that using cocaine makes him more sociable. However, over time, he might also develop a new set of beliefs regarding the cocaine, such as "I can't be social without it" and "I must have the cocaine in order to function." In this scenario the patient has moved from being a recreational user to substance dependence.

In educating drug-abusing patients about the cognitive therapy model, it is helpful to teach them to identify drug-related beliefs. As stated earlier, drug-related beliefs can take different forms. They may be (1) beliefs about the drug itself, such as "Cocaine is not addictive," (2) beliefs about what is expected from the drug, such as "Coke will help to chill me out," and (3) permission-giving beliefs, such as "I deserve to feel good."

Mr. C., a 34-year-old polysubstance abuser, had the initial belief that he could not become addicted to using cocaine. He started off using cocaine socially—"only" at parties. Later he developed the belief that he could work better using cocaine. This, in turn, led to his use of cocaine at work when he was under pressure to meet deadlines. He had the illusion that he was much more productive at work when using coke. However, he overlooked the large amount of money he was spending on cocaine. Furthermore, he was not as productive because he began to miss days at work after cocaine binges. Later, when he tried to stop and he began to experience strong urges and cravings, Mr. C.'s beliefs centered on the cravings themselves. Some of these were, "I can't stand the craving," "These feelings won't go away," and "The urges make me use."

In order to assist therapists in the process of identifying patients' beliefs about drugs, we have developed the Beliefs About Substance Use questionnaire (see Appendix 1, page 311). This questionnaire, clinically generated, lists 29 common beliefs that patients report about substance use. We have found that patients who are otherwise un-skilled in reporting their thoughts can *recognize* beliefs that they main-tain regarding drug use when they utilize this inventory. A noteworthy feature of the Beliefs About Substance Use questionnaire is that it allows patients to endorse beliefs that are contradictory to one another. This can be important in helping patients understand that they may hold conflicting beliefs about their drug-taking behavior. Thus, both their ambivalence and the dysfunctional nature of their thinking styles may be highlighted.

Another useful method for identifying beliefs is via inductive questioning (also known as the "downward arrow technique"; cf. Burns, 1980). The substance-abusing patient first recognizes an auto-matic thought; then the patient and therapist attempt to understand underlying meanings of the thoughts.

This technique is illustrated by the following example: Mr. C. reported that during the week he was feeling extremely angry and anxious. The therapist then asked the patient to describe the specific situation. Mr. C. reported that while at a party, he had seen other people using and also saw some of his drug buddies, and he started having urges to use.

TH: What thoughts were going through your mind right then?

PT: It's not fair; they can use and I can't.

TH: Let's presume for the moment this thought is accurate. What about it is important—what does it *mean* to you?

PT: I'll never be able to use again.

TH: And if you'll never be able to use again, what will be the sig-nificance of *that*?

PT: I'll always have these urges and feel anxious.

TH: And what are the implications for your life?

PT: There's no escape. I'm trapped and helpless.

As one can see, an important core belief ultimately was uncov-ered through using the downward arrow technique (see Figure 7.1), and the patient came to understand the role of beliefs in his prob-lems a bit more clearly.

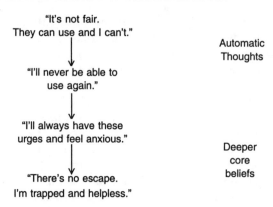

FIGURE 7.1. The downward arrow technique.

THE "CRAVING SCENARIO"

Therapists can teach their patients a great deal about the patients' substance abuse as seen within a cognitive therapy perspective by diagramming a "craving scenario." Essentially, this entails spelling out the cognitive model of substance abuse in the form of a flow chart, complete with examples that pertain directly to the patient's subjective experiences with drugs.

For example, Ms. L. reported a cocaine lapse to her therapist, who proceeded to map out the patient's "craving scenario" (see Figure 7.2), which highlighted the sequence of events and beliefs that led up to the actual episode of drug use.

PROBLEMS IN EDUCATING PATIENTS IN THE COGNITIVE MODEL

Sometimes patients initially fail to identify their automatic thoughts. They report, "I don't have any thoughts." In order to overcome this problem, therapists may wait for the patients to demonstrate affective shifts in the therapy session and then ask, "What is going through your mind right now?" When aroused in this manner, patients often have access to their thoughts. Patients are also asked, "If you don't have any thoughts, can you report what you are feeling?" Oftentimes, they report feelings in the form of cognitions; for example, "I feel like I don't want to be here today." Initially, therapists may choose to accept these responses as feelings, but, at a later point, it will be important to educate patients to make a distinction between cognitions, such as "I don't feel like being here today," and feelings, such as anxiety, anger, sadness, shame, and guilt.

Some patients have difficulty labeling the particular feelings that they are experiencing. They say such things as "I feel like shit" or "I feel awful." One method to help patients label feelings is to encourage them to use the simplest terms possible in describing their feelings, for example, mad, sad, or glad. Also, if a patient says, "I'm upset," the therapist could ask, "And *where in your body* do you experience this feeling of being upset?" The patients may then report some type of physiological indicator such as tightness in the stomach, tightness in the chest, stiff neck, and so on. Patients can be taught to use these bodily sensation cues to ask themselves the important question: "What's going through my mind right now?" With repetition, patients eventually come to understand that it is important to notice and to modify their thoughts and beliefs.

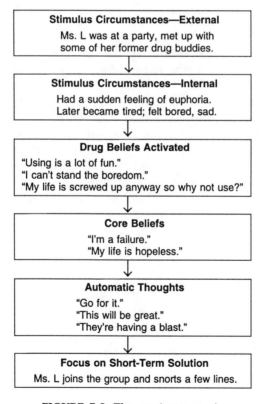

FIGURE 7.2. The craving scenario.

SUMMARY

An important part of the early stages of therapy involves educating patients about the cognitive model of drug addiction and its treatment. Most fundamental to this process is the therapist's explication of the causal and correlational connections between stimulus situations, thoughts, beliefs, emotions, drug urges, and drug taking.

Therapists can achieve this important goal by highlighting naturally occurring sequences of events in the patients' lives, as well as in session. In this manner, patients learn that therapy entails much more than simply venting about problems and/or being persuaded to give up their drug use. Rather, patients learn that their drug problems involve an understandable series of external and internal events that, left undiscovered and unmanaged, "automatically" lead to drug use. They learn that these same events, once understood, offer a number of choice points for patients to minimize the chance that they will experience opportunities, urges, and actions that will perpetuate drug use. Most important in this process is the patients' understanding that their automatic thoughts, triggered by core beliefs and beliefs about drugs, play an important role in their addiction. As a result, they learn that by modifying these thoughts and beliefs, they assist themselves in the process of recovery.

The "craving scenario" is one useful method for illustrating the series of external and internal events outlined above. Another useful tool is questionnaires, such as the Beliefs About Substance Use inventory, which helps patients to recognize some of the implicit beliefs that fuel their drug use. In addition, skillful questioning by therapists can help patients to illuminate the central role that their thinking plays in any situation that is pertinent to their risk for using drugs. Ultimately, the patients themselves become adept at modifying their thinking styles, a vital therapeutic step.

CHAPTER 8

Setting Goals

There is an old saying that maintains, "If you don't know where you're going, you won't know when you get there." This statement rings especially true for therapy with addicted individuals. In this chapter, we examine the reasons it is important to establish goals for therapy.

Setting goals creates a therapy map that helps to give a sense of direction to patients and therapists. Generally, patients enter treatment wanting to feel better—to get rid of the depression, anxiety, panic, and other negative affect states. When the patient and therapist agree on a set of goals, they collaboratively focus on change in the patients' behavior, for example, being abstinent from cocaine and finding better ways of solving real-life problems. In the absence of clearly defined goals, therapy sessions often appear fragmented or disjointed. In one case, a patient came in with a long history of cocaine use. However, her presenting problem was wanting to "feel better" about herself. Through careful questioning, the therapist was able to conclude that this might be achieved by her going back to school, finishing school, and pursuing a career. Since her use of cocaine was interfering with these goals to a large degree, the therapist assumed that one of her goals was to become totally abstinent. It was not until they were halfway through the first therapy session that it became apparent that the patient planned to continue her cocaine use, "but only on the weekends," and wanted to work only on the goal of going back to school. She saw no contradiction between these goals.

Formulating goals tends to make explicit what patients can expect from treatment. Sometimes patients' expectations of therapy are unrealistic. By initially discussing the expected outcome of therapy and defining it in concrete behavioral terms, patients know where therapy is headed and, through understanding the cognitive therapy model, have an idea as to how the goals will be obtained. In sum, as alluded to at the beginning of the chapter, patients will know where they are going and how they are going to get there.

Focusing on the expected outcome of therapy tends to make patients feel hopeful about the possibility of change. Many substance abusers have made numerous unsuccessful attempts in the past to stop on their own and feel hopeless about kicking their habit. Clear goals direct their attention to the possibilities for change. For example, "Jake" entered treatment and, at the very first therapy session, stated that he could not imagine himself being off of cocaine, even though he had recently finished a detoxification program and had not used cocaine for several weeks. It was a difficult (but not impossible) task to get this patient to focus on the possibility of change and to try to imagine himself being cocaine free and coping with many of the other concerns that he brought into therapy—excessive debt and family discord.

Setting goals helps to prevent therapy drift. Many substance abusers enter therapy only after accumulating many problems such as the loss of a job, marital problems, poor health, depression, and anxiety. With so many presenting concerns, it is quite easy to shift haphazardly from one topic to another in each session. Knowing specifically the long-term goals of therapy and the priority order in which they will be addressed helps to prevent drift from taking place. The therapist and patient can focus on one or two of the most immediate and pressing problems, yet still fully realize that there are additional issues that will be dealt with as therapy progresses.

Specific goals tend to act as anchors and thus make it more obvious to the therapist when therapy has taken a turn in a new direction. For example, consider the case of a patient who came into treatment for help with his anxiety about abstinence from cocaine. He had not used cocaine for over a year, but in the past few weeks he noticed that he was becoming more and more anxious about the possibility of using again. The initial goal in therapy was to help the patient develop better ways of coping with his anxiety about some of the urges and cravings that were reappearing. Although this was the primary focus of therapy, it became obvious after several sessions (when the patient was less anxious about relapse) that he was also experiencing severe marital discord. He disclosed that his wife was also abusing diet pills and alcohol and that this was causing a great deal of strife between them. Knowing the original goal of therapy, which was to help him deal with the anxiety about a possible relapse, the therapist and patient were able to see that focusing on marital concerns was going to be a change in the original treatment plan. It would have been very easy to drift automatically into working on the marital discord *at the expense* of a discussion about managing anxiety and cravings for drugs. Instead, patient and therapist put both topics on the therapeutic agenda, allotted a certain proportion of session time for each, and decided that future sessions would explore the *causal connection* between his renewed drug cravings and his wife's substance abuse.

The setting of mutually established goals reinforces the therapeutic alliance and the spirit of collaboration between patient and therapist. It also gives the patient a sense of active participation in his or her treatment. This is especially important for substance abusers who often see their lives in disarray and feel out of control and at the mercy of their dependency. Collaboratively setting goals aids in fostering the patient's sense of efficacy and confidence to overcome drug dependence and other problems. For example, a young cocaine addict reported the following after a goal-setting session: For the first time since he had tried stopping on his own he had some sense of control over his life and it was clear what he wanted to get from therapy—to learn techniques for coping with cravings and to learn better ways of finding a job. He felt as if he was part of the therapeutic process, and that therapy was not something that was "being done" to him.

To define positive therapeutic outcomes in concrete terms is an important part of the structure of the cognitive therapy session. Goal setting, along with other elements of the structure of the therapy session, such as agenda setting, helps to avert the common trap whereby each session is reduced to a series of crisis interventions. Therefore, patient and therapist gain a sense of the long-term goals of therapy along with the short-term goals of the session at hand.

Understanding the goals of therapy also is important for *evaluating therapeutic progress and outcome.* Oftentimes, patients become discouraged in treatment because of a lack of progress or setbacks, such as lapses in drug use. This, in turn, often stimulates black-and-white thinking about therapy: "Therapy is not working *at all.*" By referring back to the original goals of treatment, and by reviewing the patient's progress throughout, the therapist can undermine some of the patient's hopelessness about treatment.

For example, one patient and his therapist had documented the following goals at the beginning of treatment: to abstain from cocaine and alcohol, to gain more confidence in social situations, and to obtain and maintain a steady job. Over a period of about 6 months, the patient did remain abstinent from cocaine and alcohol. However, he was unable to obtain any type of employment. This was very discouraging for the patient and he began reporting negative automatic thoughts about the therapy. The therapist then was able to point out that, although he had not found employment, the patient was feeling much better and had a strong sense of pride about being able to stay away from drugs and alcohol. Thus, an important goal of treatment was being met. In addition, the therapist questioned the patient about the specifics of the original goal of employment. In order to achieve this goal, the patient and therapist had agreed on the short-term goal of developing job-seeking skills, such as how to conduct himself at an interview, where to look for a job, and how to prepare a resumé. Indeed, the patient had made gains in these areas. After their discussion, the patient was able to see the progress he had made and was able to challenge his negatively biased thinking about the therapeutic "failure" of not finding a job. The patient felt a bit more hopeful about therapy and more motivated to continue in treatment.

Conversely, a patient who is discouraged because she has not completely quit her smoking and drinking may be cheered somewhat on realizing that some of her more general goals for therapy are being met, thus giving her momentum to tackle further her alcohol and nicotine addictions. This brings up an important point; namely, that goals for therapy do *not* simply entail cessation of problematic drug use. Criteria for success in therapy must be assessed across a number of important life concerns, including family relationships, social functioning, and work productivity, to name but a few (Covi et al., 1990; McLellan et al., 1992).

There are numerous issues that can be brought up and discussed in any one particular session. With clear, concrete goals, the therapist and patient can make maximum use of the therapy time, and can address problems in an organized and systematic fashion.

GENERAL RULES FOR SETTING GOALS

Therapists should collaborate with their patients in establishing goals for treatment. When patients enter treatment they frequently are ambivalent about abstinence from drugs and alcohol (Carroll, Rounsaville, & Keller, 1991; Havassy et al., 1991; Miller & Rollnick, 1991). It is inadvisable for therapists simply to proclaim that their patients must strive for abstinence as a condition of being in treatment. Instead, it is important for the therapist to explore collaboratively with the patient the benefits of total abstinence from drugs such as cocaine. The act of collaboration will help the patient to feel that he or she truly is a part of the process of change.

In setting goals, therapists try to highlight the relationship between abstinence and problem-solving. For example, therapists discuss with patients how being drug free can contribute to keeping a job and to having better relationships and more money for other things such as clothes, vacations, and a car. Nevertheless, it must be explained that while abstinence increases the chances of obtaining the desired outcome, it does not *guarantee* it. As a case in point, Ms. F. presented as her primary goal the wish to stop using crack. The therapist then asked her what the benefits of not using crack would be. She stated that by not using she would be able to save money, that she would be able to pay her bills, and also that she would feel like going to work each day. The therapist then summarized, "Being drug-free is your primary goal and other goals will be to save money, to be able to pay your bills, and to be able to keep your job. It is important to note that abstinence alone will not insure achieving these other goals. It will *help* you to be in a better position to learn how to get what you want in these other areas of your life. Perhaps we'll work on these skills as well."

Goals are best stated in concrete, specific terms. Often, at the beginning of therapy, patients present vague, nonspecific goals for treatment, such as "I just want to get my life in order," "I just want to be my old self again," or "I just want this anxiety to go away." Therapists assist patients in defining treatment goals in more circumscribed behavioral terms, such as finding a job; staying away from people, places, and things associated with drugs; being able to go out and have a good time without using drugs; or reestablishing a broken relationship. For example, Mr. R., a 42-year-old cocaine addict, stated that he wanted "his world to stop falling apart." In order to concretize the goals, the therapist asked what he would like to be doing differently at the end of treatment. Mr. R. then presented more focused objectives: "First of all, I would like to get a chance to see my children more often. I'm separated from my wife right now and she doesn't allow me to see the kids. I would like to stop using coke. I want to get involved with the church again. I used to be really into it. I would like to have a regular job. I'm tired of doing odd jobs. I want more excitement in my life. I'm bored most of the time except when using drugs." The therapist facilitated this process by periodically asking, "And what else would you like to be doing differently?" As a result, Mr. R.'s goals were translated from a vague statement of his "world to stop falling apart" to much more concrete, behavioral, measurable events. The therapist summarized Mr. R.'s goals as follows:

1. See children more often.
2. Stop using coke.

3. Get involved with the church.
4. Have a regular job.
5. Have more excitement, but stay drug free.

Once the patient's goals are concretized, the therapist can start to think of the necessary operations to achieve them, and the criteria on which to assess treatment outcome. An example of goal attainment was Mr. R.'s finding a permanent job with a construction company. Another goal was reached when, after getting a job, his wife allowed him to see the children each weekend. Further, through urine testing, the therapist was able to establish that Mr. R. was not using cocaine. Finally, therapist and patient worked on developing sources of *nondrug* positive reinforcement, such as hobbies and physical recreation (cf. Stitzer, Grabowski, & Henningfield, 1984).

Having these specific goals in the forefront helped to keep the therapist and patient from drifting in each therapy session. Also, having these goals written down at the beginning of treatment proved to be a powerful motivator for Mr. R., as the patient was able to compare his situation at the beginning of treatment with his functioning at later stages in treatment, and thereby to recognize his progress in therapy.

In setting goals, it is important to remember the following:

1. Be collaborative in setting goals.
2. Establish goals in positive terms as they relate to abstinence.
3. Be concrete and define goals in measurable behavioral terms.

STANDARD GOALS OF TREATMENT

Two standard goals of treatment are (1) to reduce drug dependency, with the cornerstone being to help the patient develop techniques for coping with urges and cravings, and (2) to help patients learn more adaptive methods for coping with life problems.

When substance abusers enter therapy, they often are ambivalent about their desire to stop using. Increasing their motivation to reduce drug dependency becomes an important early focus in therapy. In the first phase of treatment, it is imperative to facilitate the patient's understanding of the various advantages and disadvantages of using or not using drugs and alcohol. The following is a transcript of a therapist discussing with his patient the advantages and disadvantages of using cocaine.

TH: One thing that we said that we would go through are the advantages and disadvantages of using drugs. What are some of the advantages to using cocaine? Why is it good to use?

PT: It ain't good. It ain't good but it makes me feel good.

⁻TH: OK. It makes you feel good.

PT: Yeah, that's an advantage of it. It makes me feel good for awhile.

TH: What is another advantage?

PT: I see everybody else doing it, so I want to do it too.

TH: So, are you saying that it makes you fit in?

PT: Yeah, it makes me fit in the crowd. When I see somebody else doing it, I want to be part of the crowd. People to talk to when I'm doing it. It seems like I have friends, but they are not friends, you know.

TH: OK, so you have more friends, but they are not real friends. Maybe we can consider this as a *disadvantage* to using? What do you think?

PT: Yeah. It seems like you have more, but you don't really have no friends.

TH: OK. Now let's focus on certain advantages for *not* using. Why is it good *not* to use cocaine?

PT: You save money.

TH: "You save money." (*Therapist writes this down*)

PT: You can think clearly. Your brain ain't all messed up. You can think clearly. You can function better and work.

TH: Some people say that they can function better at work when they have cocaine. What do you think about that?

PT: Oh, I can't. It just makes me want to take days off. I don't feel like working.

TH: So another advantage to not using is that you feel like going to work?

PT: Yeah, I can go to work. I can work. I can maintain my bills. Yeah, because when I used I was taking days off. You just don't have the motivation to do nothing but smoke.

TH: So, some advantages for not using is that you can save money, think more clearly, feel like going to work, and pay your bills on time.

PT: Yeah, and I feel better about me.

TH: Are you saying that sometimes when you don't use coke you feel better about yourself? In other words, you feel proud of yourself when not using? Is that right?

PT: Yeah, that's the feeling I'm talking about. Yeah, and when I use, later I feel depressed and guilty that I gave in.

TH: Well, yeah. That's something we can look at. Something we will put under the category of disadvantages for using and, that is, we could say that after using cocaine—how would you say it? You feel bad about yourself?

PT: Yeah. You feel real bad about yourself for picking up. Then it's like you are on a merry-go-round again. You just want to keep on using once you start.

TH: Now, can you think of any other advantages for not using? Any good reason for not using?

PT: My kids, my family, I have more time for them.

TH: Good. OK, let's switch tracks now. Let's look at the disadvantages for not using it. In other words, right now you are not using it. Are there any problems when you are not using coke? What's the cost of not using?

PT: 'Cause I'm not using it?

TH: Yeah, you are not using it. Do any thoughts go through your mind?

PT: A little voice saying, "Go ahead, one time ain't going to hurt" [a permission-giving belief].

TH: One time won't hurt?

PT: Yeah, I can handle it. One time ain't going to hurt you.

TH: Yeah, that thought crosses your mind often?

PT: Yeah, sometimes the thought does come, "Yeah, go ahead and take one. It ain't going to hurt you."

TH: So what is the price you pay for not using?

PT: The only one I can think of is this voice saying, "OK you can go try." This urge to use.

TH: So, are you saying that the disadvantage when you are not using is that sometimes you are troubled by these thoughts telling you to use?

PT: Yeah, just go ahead and use, just once.

TH: OK. I get your drift now.

PT: Saying, "Go ahead, it's good to use it." It makes me uncomfortable. I start getting that urge again.

TH: So, in other words, when you are not using coke, the thought makes you uncomfortable and you start getting the urge to use. Having these urges can certainly be the price you pay for not using, and these urges certainly are uncomfortable. Now what are the disadvantages for using?

PT: For picking up? I spent my money on it. It is something I don't want to do. And then I say, "All right then, you already did it. You might as well continue" [permission-giving belief; abstinence violation effect].

TH: So the disadvantage is that once you start using it, you give yourself permission to keep using it and later you feel bad about yourself?

PT: Right, I give myself permission to keep on using it and feel depressed and guilty later. I let myself down. And then I use all of that money. It's an awful lot of money used. And also I've gotten into legal trouble for using it. That's certainly a disadvantage. And also my life is a lie. I end up lying to some of my best friends.

TH: OK. These things that we just went over—the advantages of using, the advantages of not using, the disadvantages of using, and the disadvantages of not using—are some things that I think we need to review in therapy over and over again. First, let's write them down on some index cards for you to carry around with you as reminders.

In this example, one sees that by reviewing the advantages for using and the advantages for not using cocaine, the therapist has elucidated some important goals for treatment. For example, under the "advantages for not using" category, there are some concrete, positive goals to be obtained: having more money, being able to think more clearly, being able to pay bills, and so on. However, there is another set of goals (that is a bit less obvious) that was highlighted as a result of discussing the "advantages for using"; that is, the patient viewed the cocaine as making her feel good, fitting in with the crowd, and having more friends. A set of goals can be derived from these statements, with the therapist saying, "If we could work on helping you to feel good, to be able to fit in with the crowd, and being able to have friends, but *without* using cocaine, would these be important goals for us to try to achieve in therapy?" By using this strategy, the therapist focuses on the positive aspects of abstaining from cocaine and presents the goals in a positive manner, while still empathizing with the patient's desire for the drug. This is important since some patients view abstinence from drugs as a form of deprivation in the sense that it is something that is taken away from them (Jennings, 1991). The therapist collaboratively helps the patient to reframe the goal in a more positive way. Therefore, the patient can work on attaining the perceived positive aspects of using cocaine but without incurring the disadvantages involved in actually using the drug.

As previously mentioned, the two standard long-term goals of treatment are the reduction of cocaine dependency and the learning of more adaptive methods for coping with real-life problems. Regarding the latter goal, substance abusers tend to have poor problem-solving skills. They tend to blame others for their problems, to be impulsive in making decisions, to ruminate about their problems without actively taking steps to solve them, and to withdraw and avoid instead of thinking about their problems and coming up with practical solutions.

This withdrawal and avoidance often is achieved through the use of drugs. For example, one patient blamed his current situation—being unemployed and being on parole—on society. He claimed that given his current situation, anyone would be using cocaine. For example, even after he had been off of cocaine for awhile, he impulsively decided that he would make some extra money by "bagging cocaine." He also tended to ruminate about his problems and to spend a great deal of time fantasizing about how he would get out of his current dismal situation—unemployed and living with his parents. Yet, when questioned by the therapist, the patient was able to see that he was taking no active steps to solve this problem. In addition, he tended to withdraw from others and his problems by daydreaming and by using alcohol and cocaine.

The therapist was able to help this patient with his problem-solving strategies first by encouraging him to define his problems in clear, specific terms; for example, he was unable to find a job because he was not actively looking for a job and, in addition, the patient had poor job-hunting skills. The therapist also helped the patient identify errors in his thinking that interfered with looking for solutions. For example, the patient was under the assumption that since he was on parole, no one would hire him. The reality, though, is that there are firms that hire people who are on parole, and many parolees are able to find jobs in spite of their criminal records. In addition, this patient valued his autonomy and therefore had a great deal of difficulty reaching out to others. He believed that it was a sign of weakness to do so when it was really in his best interest to make maximum use of the social support systems in his area, such as public assistance, food stamps, support group meetings, and therapy.

ADDRESSING THE PATIENT'S AMBIVALENCE DIRECTLY

As noted earlier, many patients are ambivalent about being in therapy and about giving up their drug use. These mixed feelings and attitudes can be addressed as part of the early process of establishing therapeutic goals, as illustrated by the following dialogue:

TH: One thing that we said we would do today is continue working on goals. I would like to start with that. Is that OK with you?

PT: Yeah, I guess so.

TH: At the last session you seemed a bit uncertain about totally giving up cocaine.

PT: Yeah. And I'm still not sure. Sometimes it seems like a good idea but then I feel like it would sure be nice to pick up every now and then. You know what I mean? Sort of control my use like when I first started.

TH: So sometimes you think that you want to go for total abstinence then at other times you feel you still want to use but be able to control it.

PT: Yeah.

TH: OK, what do you think would happen if you tried to stop completely?

PT: I'm not sure . . . it would be hard . . . I would miss it.

TH: It would be hard and you would feel a sense of loss . . . (*patient nods in agreement*) . . . that would be the down side, but what about the up side? Are there any benefits to stopping totally?

PT: I think I would feel better about myself.

TH: So you would feel better about yourself. How is that?

PT: I feel terrible about how far down I have fallen the past year. I've tried to quit several times . . . and each time I fail . . . maybe if I could stop this I could feel good about myself, the way I used to.

TH: That would certainly be a benefit. Remember in the last session we talked about some specific advantages for not using. Maybe this would be a good time to take another look at that list and also to talk about how hard it is to give up cocaine and that you will miss it. Does that sound OK to you?

PT: OK.

Often patients feel overwhelmed because, through errors in their thinking, they exaggerate their difficulties and minimize the possibility of corrective action. This, in turn, leads them to believe that there are no solutions and that drug use provides their only respite. In response, the therapist can help the patient to reframe his or her problems in a more hopeful way. Reframing involves getting the patient to collect objective data about situations, to generate alternative ways of looking at the situation, and to begin to brainstorm solutions. The process of searching for an alternative in order to combat the patient's hopelessness is illustrated by the following:

TH: Let's discuss this problem of your girlfriend calling you when she is high.

PT: No need to talk about that . . . there's nothing I can do about it . . . she's my son's mother.

TH: So there is nothing that can be done about it . . . sounds like you feel it's pretty hopeless.

PT: You're right.

TH: Can you tell me more about what happens? . . . I'll jot down some of the details of this problem.

PT: She goes out and gets ripped on crack. Then when she is crashing, she calls me . . . she's crying . . . complaining . . . wants me to come over and that's what I usually do, you know. . . .

TH: She gets high, calls you, crying and complaining, she asks you to come over and you do?

PT: Yeah.

TH: How do you end up feeling?

PT: Like hell . . . I get angry with her . . . I can't stand to see her that way . . . I feel sorry for her, kind of sad.

TH: What thoughts go through your mind?

PT: Here we go again . . . I'm tired of this . . . she lied again [girlfriend told patient several times she would stop using and get help] . . . when I get real angry I want to just go out and get drunk . . . get high thinking about coke . . . sometimes I do just that, you know, just chill out.

TH: So, she calls, you get angry, feel sad, you go over to her house, you want to get high to deal with the anger and sadness?

PT: That's exactly it.

TH: You said earlier there is nothing you can do about it. What would you *like* to see happen?

PT: For her to stop calling me when she's high or crashing.

TH: Let's think about this for a few minutes. Her calling you, unless you take your phone out, is for the most part out of your control. I was wondering, are there things that are still within your control?

PT: I don't have to talk with her . . . I don't have to go over.

TH: True. But, what would it mean if you didn't talk with her and you didn't go over?

PT: She's the mother of my son . . . it would mean that I'm not helping her.

TH: So you believe, at this point, that by talking to her and going over you are helping her? Is that really true?

PT: Not really. I keep doing the same thing over and over again . . . she still doesn't stop and she won't get any help.

TH: So, maybe an alternative way of looking at this is that it's best if you decide to steer clear of her when she's using. You believe you are helping her by talking to her and going over to her place. But, when you look back, you are really not helping her situation and you set yourself up possibly to use cocaine to deal with the anger.

PT: That's right.

TH: Would your not talking to her and not going to her house be part of a solution to this?

PT: True.

TH: I believe that when she calls, this incorrect belief within you gets activated, fired up, and you behave as if it were true.

PT: That's right. It's only afterwards that I see I'm not really helping and it's the same thing over and over again.

TH: I think this gives us something to work on to help you solve this problem. First thing we'll do is to help you deal with her calling and the second is to explore *other* things you might do to help her.

SUMMARY

This chapter examined some reasons why it is important to establish goals for therapy: (1) to foster a sense of direction, (2) to help patients feel more hopeful, (3) to prevent therapist drift, (4) to reinforce collaboration, and (5) to evaluate therapeutic progress and outcome. The following general rules for setting goals also were covered: (1) be collaborative, (2) highlight the relationship between abstinence and problem solving in positive terms, and (3) state goals in concrete, specific terms. We discussed in detail two standard goals of treatment: to reduce drug dependency, and to learn better problem-solving skills, as well as presented methods of addressing the patient's ambivalence and negativity about getting help.

CHAPTER 9

Techniques of Cognitive Therapy

For optimal results, the vicious cycles associated with substance abuse are best addressed with a combination of cognitive and behavioral techniques. Cognitive techniques address drug-related beliefs and automatic thoughts that contribute to urges and cravings, while behavioral techniques focus on the actions that causally interact with cognitive processes. Behavioral techniques help the patient test the accuracy of drug-related beliefs that trigger and perpetuate drug use, and are also used for teaching the patients skills (e.g., assertiveness and relaxation) in order to deal with high-risk situations, urges, and cravings. In this chapter we describe some of the most common, widely used techniques of cognitive therapy. Although some of these techniques are adapted for specific use with substance abusers, most are applicable to patients across the diagnostic spectrum.

BASIC PRINCIPLES

The Therapeutic Relationship

The efficacy of cognitive and behavioral techniques is dependent, to a large degree, on the relationship between therapist and patient. Beck et al. (1979) explain that the relationship requires therapist warmth, accurate empathy, and genuineness. Without these, the therapy becomes "gimmick oriented."

The Cognitive Case Conceptualization

Effective treatment requires a comprehensive and accurate cognitive case conceptualization. The case conceptualization

(Chapter 5, this volume) is defined as the collection, synthesis, and integration of data about the patient so that testable hypotheses about the etiology and treatment of the patients' various maladaptive beliefs and other symptoms can be formulated and tested. These data include demographic information, presenting problem, DSM-III-R diagnosis, developmental profile, and cognitive profile of the patient. Without an adequate case conceptualization, the choice of specific techniques may be arbitrary and even inappropriate for a particular patient. This is seen in the case of a patient who uses cocaine ostensibly in order to give him more "energy" to work late hours at the office. Such a patient would *not* be receptive to the therapist's blind application of relaxation techniques.

The Socratic Method

In cognitive therapy, effective interaction between therapist and patient is best accomplished by frequent use of the Socratic method (i.e., guided discovery). Through the Socratic method, patients are guided through a process of discovering their distorted patterns of thinking and behaving. Despite the fact that cognitive therapy involves learning new beliefs and behaviors, these are not taught through lectures or preaching. Instead, the cognitive therapist uses probing questions, reflections, summaries, and hypotheses to elicit, examine, and test patients' basic beliefs and automatic thoughts.

Overholser (1987) provides an excellent description of the Socratic method. He explains that "the Socratic method of interviewing encourages the client to contemplate, evaluate, and synthesize diverse sources of information . . ." (p. 258). This process, when done properly, should reduce "subjective distress" and reduce "acute symptomatology." Overholser further explains that Socratic questioning promotes insight and rational decision-making by making the patient aware of important information. Most important, this process shapes thinking through active questioning and selective reflecting. The goal of the Socratic method is for the patient to learn to think independently (i.e., autonomously) and rationally.

Homework Assignments

To a large degree, success in therapy is facilitated by the completion of formal (assigned) and informal (spontaneous) homework assignments (Burns & Auerbach, 1992; Persons et al., 1988). Formal homework assignments involve the practice of cognitive and behavioral techniques between sessions, where change is most important. For optimal compliance with homework, assignments should be jointly formulated whenever possible. Further, the therapist should check to see if the patient understands the specifics of the assignment and its rationale, perhaps by practicing in advance in the session. The therapist and patient can put their heads together to anticipate potential barriers to completing assignments, and backup plans can be formulated for times when homework cannot be completed (e.g., the patient is instructed to list the automatic thoughts that inhibited facing the issues inherent in the assignment). Homework compliance will be further reinforced if the therapist regularly checks on the status of previous homework assignments at each session.

COGNITIVE TECHNIQUES

Advantages–Disadvantages Analysis

The person who uses drugs typically maintains beliefs that minimize the disadvantages and maximize the advantages of doing so. Hence, the advantages–disadvantages (A–D) analysis is an extremely useful cognitive therapy technique. In the A–D analysis, the patient is guided through the process of listing and reevaluating the advantages and disadvantages of drug use. Typically, a four-cell matrix is drawn for patients and they are asked to fill each cell with the consequences of using versus not using drugs.

An illustration of the A–D analysis is provided here. "Jill" is a 34-year-old woman who was seen in therapy for her cocaine addiction. As she had had an extended abstinence from cocaine, she expressed an interest in cigarette smoking cessation. Jill explained that she did not know if she "really" wanted to quit. The therapist engaged the patient in the A–D analysis as follows (the matrix they completed is presented in Figure 9.1:

TH: You say you're not sure whether you really want to quit.

PT: Yes, that's right.

TH: OK, let's look at the potential advantages and disadvantages of quitting smoking. I will draw a window like this (*draws matrix*) so that we can keep track of your thoughts.

PT: All right.

TH: On the vertical axis we write "advantages" here and "disadvantages" here. On the horizontal axis we write "quitting" versus "not quitting."

PT: OK.

	Quitting Smoking	Not Quitting
Advantages	• breathe easier • smell better • live longer • save money	• continued stress relief • avoid withdrawal • less hassle
Disadvantages	• withdrawal symptoms • no way to deal with stress and boredom • giving up a "friend"	• self-esteem will eventually suffer from not taking control • probably die from smoking • still have this dirty, disgusting, nasty habit

FIGURE 9.1. Advantages–disadvantages analysis.

TH: Now what are the advantages of quitting?

PT: I will breathe easier.

TH: What else?

PT: I will smell better.

TH: What else?

PT: I will live longer.

TH: What else?

PT: Aren't these *enough* reasons to quit?

TH: They might be, but let's try to exhaust the possibilities for each cell of the matrix before we stop.

PT: OK, then there is the money.

TH: You will save money. Any more?

PT: I can't think of any.

TH: OK. What about the advantages of smoking?

PT: I can't think of any right now.

TH: You must see advantages of smoking or else you wouldn't be a smoker today.

PT: Well, I guess I can. Smoking seems to relieve my stress at times.

TH: What else?

[This discussion continued until all cells of the A–D analysis were full.]

When the A–D analysis is successful, the patient should have a more accurate, objective, balanced view of substance use than previously held. As stated earlier, those who abuse drugs otherwise tend to minimize their drug-related problems and maximize (i.e., romanticize) the benefits of drug use.

Identifying and Modifying Drug-Related Beliefs

In previous chapters, the cognitive therapy model of substance abuse has been presented. It has been explained that the patient who abuses substances is likely to have such drug-related beliefs as the following:

"I work hard. I deserve to party."

"Smoking relaxes me."

"Drugs make me more creative."

"I have a successful career, so I can't possibly have a drinking problem."

"My life's a mess anyway, so drugs couldn't make it worse."

"If I stop using, I'll get depressed."

Individuals who abuse drugs are typically not attentive to their drug-related beliefs, often viewing their drug use as a function of extrinsic factors. For example, they attribute cigarette smoking to "stress" rather than to their attitudes about smoking. Therefore, it is essential to help patients monitor and identify their beliefs about drugs and drug use.

In cognitive therapy the drug user is taught about these beliefs as they apply to his or her drug-use patterns. Specifically, the therapist explains and illustrates the "cognitive model of substance abuse" (see Figure 3.5, page 47) to the patient, and together they fill in each box of the flow chart with examples of basic beliefs, automatic thoughts, feelings, and behaviors that are pertinent to the patient's life. For example, consider the case of "Mack," who reported to his therapist, "I went on a binge on Saturday night." The following dialogue ensued.

TH: Tell me about your binge.

PT: What's there to tell? I just felt pretty good and I decided to drink.

TH: Let's look at the cognitive model together. [The therapist took out a printed copy of the cognitive model of substance abuse and showed it to the patient.] So the initial stimulus was internal; you "felt pretty good."

PT: Yeh.

TH: In response to feeling good, what was going through your head that contributed to your drinking?

PT: I guess I was thinking "Gee, a drink would make me feel even better."

TH: And what automatic thought went through your mind?

PT: "What the hell! I might as well."

TH: And by that time you were beginning to crave?

PT: Big time!

When patients are systematically taught to monitor their basic drug-related beliefs and automatic thoughts, and when these cognitive processes are shown to be related to their subsequent drug use, patients tend to report an increased understanding of why they use, and a better sense about how better *not* to use.

Downward Arrow Technique

It is common for drug-using patients to have catastrophic (all-or-none or overgeneralized) thoughts not only about their substance use but about themselves, their life, and their future (the cognitive triad; Beck, 1976). Such thoughts might include the following:

"My life is going to crumble."

"I'll fall apart if I can't get my fix."

"I can't do anything right."

"Nobody gives a damn about me."

"I am totally out of control."

The downward arrow technique is quite useful for addressing such beliefs as these. Many patients are unable to articulate these underlying beliefs until they have been asked to consider the personal *meaning* that their more manifest thoughts have for them. Therefore, when patients exhibit strong negative emotions that seem to be far more intense than their automatic thoughts alone would cause, therapists can ask patients to probe a bit deeper by asking successive variations of the question "What does that *mean* to you?" Oftentimes, the end result of the question is the elicitation of an underlying or core belief. The following is an illustration:

TH: Phil, you seem to be having a very strong reaction against the idea of trying to steer clear of drinking alcohol at your upcoming office party. *What is your concern about being sober at the party?*

PT: I wouldn't be any fun at parties if I didn't drink.

TH: And if you weren't fun at parties, *what would the implications be?*

PT: People wouldn't hang around me.

TH: And if people didn't hang around you, *what would that mean?*

PT: It would mean they didn't like me.

TH: And assuming that all of the above is true, *what would the consequences be?*

PT: It might mean that my career would suffer since I am a salesman, and I depend on people liking me for me to succeed.

TH: And if your career suffered, *what would the ultimate consequences be?*

PT: I could lose my house and my family and everything I've worked for!

TH: And all this would happen because you weren't drinking alcohol at social events?

PT: Well, when you put it that way, I guess it's pretty unlikely.

TH: I agree, but do you see how a chain of progressively more problematic beliefs leads you to assume that catastrophe would result if you followed through with the assignment of being "dry" at the party?

PT: Yes, I never realized that before. It *does* seem like it's do or die, but maybe it isn't.

TH: We'll have to stay alert to similar chains of beliefs. For now, let's write down what we've just learned on paper [See Figure 9.2.]

The downward arrow technique (so-called because of the way it is illustrated on paper, with each successive belief pointing an arrow downward to the next underlying belief) is effective because it helps a patient to "decatastrophize" (i.e., to reevaluate and modify catastrophic thoughts). In the above example, the downward arrow technique helped Phil to articulate the catastrophic thought that he would lose his career, family, and house if he stopped drinking. On doing so, Phil was able to see the distortion in his thinking. As a result, he

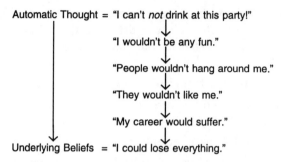

Automatic Thought = "I can't *not* drink at this party!"

"I wouldn't be any fun."

"People wouldn't hang around me."

"They wouldn't like me."

"My career would suffer."

Underlying Beliefs = "I could lose everything."

FIGURE 9.2. Downward arrow illustration.

was in a better position to modify this thought. In fact, the irony of Phil's catastrophic thinking truly came to light when he did an A–D analysis and determined that he could "lose everything" if he *did not* stop drinking.

Reattribution of Responsibility

Those who use drugs will often attribute their use to extrinsic factors. For example, the alcoholic may attribute drinking to a bad marriage, a stressful job, and drinking buddies exerting pressure to be "one of the guys." The therapist can help individuals to reattribute responsibility for their drug use to themselves so that they may take initiative to modify drug-using behaviors. Reattribution of responsibility requires the skillful application of the Socratic method, so that patients do not feel that their therapists are being judgmental or accusatory. The following is an example of this process:

TH: You say that you've been drinking again. What are your thoughts about why this is happening?

PT: Well, my wife has really been hassling me lately. I might be able to stay sober if she would get off my back once in a while.

TH: So you see your wife as causing your drinking?

PT: In a way, yes . . . but it's not that simple.

TH: OK. Tell me more about some of the complexities involved here. Exactly what role does your *wife* play, and what role *your* beliefs and actions play.

PT: She criticizes me, and I start thinking that I can't get any peace and that I'm trapped.

TH: And then?

PT: And then I think that my only escape in life is to get bombed and forget about my miserable marriage.

TH: So when you focus on the misery in your marriage, you determine that there is only one remedy—to drink until you go "blotto." Am I on target?

PT: Yes.

TH: Would it be fair to say that you *decide* to drink, rather than choosing some other way of resolving your problems with her?

PT: Yes. I guess it's my decision, but it's easier to blame her. (*chuckles*)

TH: It may be easier to blame her, but does that help you to reach your goal of dealing with your problem with alcohol?

PT: No.

TH: What *would* help?

PT: If I take charge of my own life and my own decisions, regardless of how pissed off I am at my wife.

TH: Not easy, I admit, but a worthy goal.

In this example, the patient's focus shifted from external to internal factors. Initially, he blamed his wife for his drinking. At the end of this dialogue he had begun to see that he had some responsibility for his drinking. As a result, he may begin to take some responsible actions toward changing his drinking.

Daily Thought Record

The Daily Thought Record (DTR) is a fundamental strategy in cognitive therapy, which has been useful in the treatment of depression, anxiety, and other problematic mood states (Beck et al., 1979; Burns, 1980). The standard DTR is a five-column form that is completed by the patient (see Figure 9.3).

Those who abuse substances tend to do so as a result of their beliefs (often maladaptive) about drugs. For example, the alcohol abuser, prior to going to the corner tavern, may have the belief "I *need* a drink." By using the DTR, the patient is able to examine this belief and consider its validity in a more systematic, objective fashion. In addition, the DTR provides a time lag after the initial urge during which the patient may choose not to drink (or use other drugs), and may experience a natural diminution of the craving. Additionally, the DTR provides a method for coping with negative mood states so that they are not as likely to trigger drug use.

Consider the case of Mack, who reported that he was most tempted to drink when alone on weekends. For homework his therapist asked him to complete a DTR based on the experience of being alone on a Saturday night (see Figure 9.3). Mack initially described himself as being lonely and angry as a result of not having a date. He rated these emotions as quite high: 80 and 75, respectively. These feelings were based on his beliefs: "No one cares about me" and "It's unbearable to be alone." Using the DTR as a guide, Mack's therapist helped him to consider alternative rational responses, such as "My friends and family care about me" and "I CAN bear to be alone." As a result of doing so, Mack reported feeling sufficient relief that he held off on having a drink. This result boosted his sense of self-efficacy markedly.

A useful method for teaching patients to generate objective rational responses involves the application of a series of open-ended questions (see the bottom of Figure 9.3). These questions include the following:

1. What concrete, factual evidence supports or refutes my automatic thoughts and beliefs?
2. Are there other ways I could view this situation? Is there a blessing in disguise here?
3. What is the *worst* thing that could happen? What is the *best* thing? What is most likely to *realistically* happen?
4. What constructive *action* can I take to *deal* with the situation?
5. What are the pros and cons of my changing the way I view this situation?
6. What helpful advice would I give my best friend if he/she were in this situation?

Any or all of these questions can help stimulate patients to think of rational responses. We have found that the regular application of these questions makes for an excellent ongoing homework assignment and helps patients learn to use DTRs to their maximum benefit.

Imagery

Imagery techniques can be used with drug users to help them visualize "self-control" and avoid drug use. Imagery can be a useful technique for focusing patients on drug-related beliefs and automatic thoughts, or distracting them from their cravings and urges.

Directions: When you notice your mood getting worse, ask yourself, "What's going through my mind right now?" and as soon as possible jot down the thought or mental image in the Automatic Thought column.

DATE/TIME	SITUATION Describe: 1. Actual event leading to unpleasant emotion, or 2. Stream of thoughts, daydreams or recollection, leading to unpleasant emotion, or 3. Distressing physical sensations	AUTOMATIC THOUGHT(S) 1. Write automatic thought(s) preceded emotion(s) 2. Rate belief in automatic 0–100%.	EMOTION(S) 1. Specify sad, anxious/angry etc. 2. Rate degree of emotion 0–100%	RATIONAL RESPONSE 1. Write rational response automatic thought(s) 2. Rate belief in rational 0–100%.	OUTCOME 1. Re-rate belief in automatic thought(s) 0–100%. 2. Specify and rate subsequent emotions 0–100%

Questions to help formulate the rational response: (1) What is the evidence that the automatic thought is true? Not true? (2) Is there an alternative explanation? (3) What's the *worst* that could happen?Could I live through it? What's the *best* that could happen? What's the *most realistic* outcome? (4) What should I do about it? (5) What's the effect of my believing the automatic thought? What could be the effect of changing my thinking? (6) If _____ was in this situation and had this thought, what would I tell him/her?

(friend's name)

FIGURE 9.3. Daily Thought Record (blank).

It can also serve as a method for *changing* drug-related beliefs and thoughts. Examples of imagery used in this fashion include imagining assertive, direct methods for "saying no" to others who offer drugs; imagining positive, enjoyable activities as alternatives to drug use; and imagining a healthy, productive life as a result of freedom from drugs. The following example demonstrates the use of imagery in smoking cessation.

PT: I don't know how I'll survive without my first cigarette of the day.

TH: What are your thoughts just before you smoke that cigarette?

PT: I usually don't think. I just go to my pack, take one out, and light up.

TH: Perhaps your thoughts are so automatic that you don't pay attention to them. I'd like to help you recall thoughts that lead to smoking that first cigarette of the day. Close your eyes for a moment and imagine what happens when you first wake up in the morning. What do you see? Smell? Hear? How do you feel? Now, what thoughts are going through your mind? What are you telling yourself?

PT: Well, first I'm just kind of groggy. When my mind starts to clear, I lie in bed thinking about what I have to do that day. I feel myself getting a little nervous and I think "Oh just relax. Go to the kitchen for a cup of coffee and a cigarette."

TH: What happens next?

PT: Well, to be honest, I usually go the bathroom first, but after that, I go to the kitchen and have a cigarette and coffee.

TH: As you head to the kitchen can you recall what you are thinking?

PT: Sure! I am thinking about the lift I'll soon get from the cigarettes and coffee.

TH: So you think "I'm going to get a lift from that first cigarette. Quick, go smoke!" What do you feel with that image and what happens next?

PT: I feel an urge to smoke and I indulge myself.

TH: OK, let's try something. The images of smoking and drinking coffee are quite positive. Can you replace these with an alternative image of what could happen in the morning?

PT: I guess so. Last time I quit smoking I would wake up and go jogging.

TH: What were your thoughts prior to going jogging?

PT: They were sort of like the smoking thoughts, but instead I thought that the *run* would give me a lift.

TH: OK, let's try to imagine jogging in the morning. What do you see? Smell? Hear? Feel? Make it as attractive and tempting as possible.

PT: I see the soft light of the morning sun as it shines on the trees, the house, and the landscape. The morning air smells fresh and clean. I hear lots of birds chirping because it's early morning. I feel healthy and alive.

TH: What happens when you produce that new image?

PT: I lose some of my interest in the cigarette.

TH: Great! So now you have an alternative image to the smoking image when you wake up in the morning. Can you try to voluntarily "call up" this image to your awareness in the morning?

PT: I'll try.

TH: Let's also make sure your family physician agrees that it is safe for you to take up a regimen of jogging again before you start, OK?

BEHAVIORAL TECHNIQUES

Activity Monitoring and Scheduling

Patients who abuse drugs tend to engage in activities and behaviors that support their drug abuse and may concurrently fail to take part in activities that promote prosocial life goals, such as work, hobbies, community service, and stable relationships. Activity monitoring and scheduling can be useful basic strategies for understanding and modifying drug-related behaviors and for increasing productive behaviors.

The process of activity monitoring and scheduling is simple and straightforward. The patient receives a blank grid (the Daily Activity Schedule) which contains the 7 days of the week divided into 1-hour blocks (see Figure 9.4). For a period of 1 week the patient records daily activities and the degree to which he or she felt a sense of pleasure or mastery from participating in each activity. Pleasure and mastery, recorded on a scale from zero (none) to ten (extreme), provide an indication of the patient's mood and the level of reward or satisfaction derived from each activity.

The Daily Activity Schedule can be used for at least three pur-

NOTE: Grade Activities M for Mastery and P for Pleasure 0–10

	M	T	W	Th	F	S	Su
MORNING 6–7							
7–8							
8–9							
9–10							
10–11							
11–12							
12–1							
AFTERNOON 1–2							
2–3							
3–4							
4–5							
5–6							
6–7							
EVENING 7–8							
8–9							
9–10							
10–11							
11–12							
12–6							

REMARKS:

FIGURE 9.4. Daily Activity Schedule (blank).

poses. First, it serves as a journal of present activities. By reviewing a completed schedule, therapist and patient gain a baseline understanding of the patient's activities and how they relate to drug use. Second, the Daily Activity Schedule can serve as a prospective guide for future activities. That is, patient and therapist can use a blank form to schedule alternative activities that are less conducive to drug use. Furthermore, to the degree that the patient lacks satisfaction and a sense of accomplishment in life, the therapist may choose to examine the patient's core beliefs about his or her lovability and adequacy, respectively. And finally, the Daily Activity Schedule can be used to evaluate the extent to which the patient has been following his or her proposed schedule successfully. That is, after a weekly plan has been completed, patients may take home a blank form to monitor actual behaviors. Frequently, a failure to follow through with planned activities comes about as a result of drug-related behaviors, along with their concomitant beliefs, such as "I can't do anything right" or "I never reach my goals." When this happens, therapists must remain upbeat, helping patients to see that useful information has been obtained, and that goals can still be achieved in spite of early setbacks.

When patients succeed in planning and completing nondrug activities that give them satisfaction and build their self-efficacy, they begin to view themselves as less helpless, less out of control, and less dependent on chemical "fixes."

Behavioral Experiments

Behavioral experiments are used to test the validity of patients' drug-related beliefs and core beliefs. For example, consider the patient who believes "I would lose all my friends if I didn't smoke pot." A behavioral experiment might involve having this patient participate in "usual activities" with friends, without using marijuana. (The patient would be encouraged to fully participate in all non-drug-related activities.) Thus, the "independent variable" in this behavioral experiment would be the patient's use of marijuana. The "dependent variable" would be maintenance of friendships. The patient would be encouraged to avoid any "extraneous variance" by maintaining consistency in all other aspects of his or her behavior. Regardless of the results of this experiment, the patient is likely to learn some important lessons. Specifically, if he loses friends, he will be encouraged by the therapist to examine the meaning of his pre-abstinence friendships. If he maintains his friendships, he will, it is hoped, modify his original distorted belief: "I will lose all my friends if I don't smoke marijuana."

Another form of behavioral experimentation is the *"as if"* technique. Using this technique, the therapist encourages the patient to act as if a desired behavior or set of circumstances were true for him. For example, the patient who wishes to quit smoking might spend a week acting "as if" he were a nonsmoker. For example, he might ask others not to smoke around him, he might exercise, or he might sit in the nonsmoking sections of restaurants. Such activities are designed to modify the patient's drug-related beliefs as well as behaviors.

Behavioral Rehearsal (Role Play and Reverse Role Play)

Many patients with substance abuse problems have concurrent problems with interpersonal communication (e.g., assertiveness, self-disclosure, and active listening) (Platt & Hermalin, 1989). As a result, they often feel frustrated and overwhelmed in interpersonal situations, resulting in a vulnerability to drug use. Hence, the therapist may initiate role-playing to teach the patient effective interpersonal skills. The following is an example:

PT: I feel like getting wasted every time my wife nags me.

TH: What do you mean when you say she "nags" you?

PT: I mean when she asks me to do more than my share of the work.

TH: What do you do when you think she's nagging?

PT: Well, typically I go to another room or I just leave. That's when I'm most likely to drink.

TH: So you withdraw.

PT: Yeh.

TH: How else could you handle the situation?

PT: I have no idea.

TH: OK, let's try some different options. I will play the role of your wife, and I would like you to discuss your feelings with me as honestly as possible, without attacking or being aggressive.

PT: I don't understand. What should I do?

TH: Simply pretend that I am your wife and practice talking to me in a constructive fashion about my nagging.

PT: OK, who starts?

TH: I will. (*acting as patient's wife, sounding annoyed at patient*) I want you to take care of the yard this weekend. It's been three weeks since you promised to plant grass and soon it will be too late to even try. I'm sick and tired of waiting for you to do things around here! (*silence; patient looks puzzled*) [The therapist momentarily stopped role play to encourage patient.] Now you respond to me as your wife.

PT: Man, that sounded too much like her!

TH: OK, now talk to me as you would to her.

PT: (*Another pause, then role play continues*) Mary, I'm pretty sick of you nagging me!

TH: It's the only way anything gets done around here!

PT: I do a lot around here! (*in raised voice*) You're so busy complaining that you never notice!

TH: [Again, role play stopped. Therapist talked to patient.] Now, let's look at what has happened. What are your thoughts about this role play?

It became apparent that this patient lacked effective conflict resolution skills. Thus, the therapist must begin by teaching the behavioral skills of active listening, assertiveness (vs. aggressiveness), and compromise. The teaching process involves some didactic training, along with frequent role-playing, to learn and practice more effective interpersonal behaviors.

One way to gain a reluctant patient's active participation in role playing is to volunteer to take the *patient's* role while the patient portrays the "problematic other" (e.g., an employer, a spouse, or an old drug associate who is trying to convince the patient to get high). In this manner, the patient can show the therapist just how difficult the situation is to manage, while the therapist can model some responses that the patient might not have thought of before.

A more demanding variation of this procedure has been described by Moorey (1989), who suggests that drug abusers can learn to empathize with important people in their lives by role-playing the part of a significant other who has been hurt by the patients' drug use. This exercise also serves to highlight the destruction that the drug abuse has wrought on the patients' personal lives.

On the plus side, repeated role playing helps patients develop new, mature, effective repertoires of social behavior in a safe environment where errors can be corrected without actual consequences.

Relaxation Training

There is often a component of anxiety to drug use (see Chapter 15, this volume). For example, cigarette smokers and heavy alcohol users often report that they smoke or drink to relax. Hence, drug use may be a form of self-medication for people who have difficulty relaxing (Castaneda et al., 1989; Khantzian, 1985). Even cocaine users, who consume cocaine for its stimulating effects, may feel anxious or tense in anticipation of using, especially if there is some delay between the time they crave and when they actually use.

Thus, relaxation training may be a useful technique in that it provides the patient with a safe (drug-free) method of relaxing. Second, it provides the patient with a time lag after the initial craving experience, during which the craving may subside (Carroll, Rounsaville, & Keller, 1991; Horvath, 1988). Ultimately, relaxation training may be useful in building the patient's new belief that he or she is in control of and responsible for his or her coping responses (see Chapter 15, this volume, for additional information).

Graded Task Assignments

Quite often patients must make dramatic behavioral changes in order to facilitate a drug-free (or drug-reduced) life. For example, the patient whose only friends are other crack users will have to restructure his or her social life almost entirely in order to minimize the chances of relapse. Common sense and experience tell us that this is no easy task. Hence, the patient is encouraged to engage in *approximations* of the desired behaviors in order to *build* toward the end goals. For example, the patient who needs to modify her friendships might be encouraged to begin by spending drug-free time with a non-drug-using acquaintance (e.g., a new friend from a support group meeting), such as going to lunch or to a movie. On successful completion of this exercise, the patient would choose another (more challenging) assignment until he or she had built up a new drug-free network of cohorts.

Problem Solving

Drug users who frequently demonstrate impulsivity often are very poor problem solvers. In fact, in advanced stages of drug abuse, many patients either ignore their problems (denial, avoidance) and/or respond to their problems by anesthetizing themselves with drugs. For those patients with a long history of drug use, it is strikingly apparent that they have precious little accumulated experience in recognizing and solving life's problems constructively.

For example, one of our drug-abusing patients was troubled by her husband's ongoing drug abuse. One day she found a stash of his crack cocaine. Rather than confront him with this finding, or flush the drugs down the toilet, she smoked every cap until the stash was used up. When she reported this to her therapist, he shook his head in disbelief and asked her what her rationale was for such a self-defeating act. She replied, "I didn't want him to use, so I figured if I smoked it all, he wouldn't be able to use." The therapist noted that this was an example of a "permission-giving" belief, and that it reflected a failure to think the problem through carefully (to say the least). Another patient reported a scheduling conflict between his therapy sessions and his job. His immediate response was to quit the job, rather than wait a week to work out a new schedule with the therapist.

The upshot of these illustrations is that drug-abusing patients must be taught the principles of problem-solving (Nezu, Nezu, & Perri, 1989). The steps of problem solving include the following:

1. Defining the problem in clear specific terms
2. Brainstorming a number of possible solutions
3. Examining the pros and cons of each brainstormed solution (for the present, for the future, and for significant others as well)
4. Choosing the best hypothesized solution
5. Implementing the behavior after some planning, preparation, and practice
6. Evaluating the outcome and assessing for more problems to solve

This is a long, gradual process that is fraught with frustration along the way. Therapists must remain supportive, patient, and encouraging if patients are to persevere in learning these skills.

Exercise

Most substance abuse is incompatible with physical health and sustained exercise. For example, cigarette smoking and regular aerobic exercise (e.g., jogging) would seem to be incongruous. Hence, regular aerobic activity is likely to heighten a person's awareness of the disadvantages of substance use and the advantages of quitting.

The therapist may encourage the patient to engage in physical exercise as part of the treatment program (of course, only with a physician's medical approval). Such activity may help the patient to redefine him- or herself as a healthy, physically fit person. This image should cause cognitive dissonance for the patient and may motivate him or her to modify the pattern of substance abuse.

[A notable exception to the above involves athletes who abuse anabolic steroids, thinking that it is *very* much compatible with athletic achievement. In such cases, therapists would *not* want to focus on exercise as an intervention. Instead, anger control, interpersonal conflict resolution, and focusing on the unappealing side effects of steroids (e.g., balding, acne, reduced sexual responsivity, and myriad serious medical consequences) should be the central focus.]

Stimulus Control

At first glance it would seem that an effective strategy for reducing substance abuse would be to eliminate all stimuli that trigger drug use. However, it quickly becomes apparent that doing so is not practically possible: all people will have episodes of feeling sad, lonely, anxious, bored, frustrated, and other internal sources of high risk. Ex-smokers inevitably find themselves in places where others are smoking, alcohol-dependent individuals eventually face enticing advertisements, and many users of illicit drugs have to come in contact with relatives who abuse such drugs.

In order to minimize contact with drug triggers, patients are encouraged to identify those stimuli (internal and external) that put them at high risk for the activation of drug-related beliefs that trigger drug use (Carroll, Rounsaville, & Keller, 1991). For example, some people are vulnerable to negative moods (boredom, anxiety, sadness, etc.) while others are vulnerable to positive moods (joy, happiness, excitement, etc.). Still others are vulnerable to extrinsic cues (meals, other users, time of day, geographic location, etc.). Patients are encouraged to *plan ways* to avoid these cues whenever possible. However, more importantly, patients are encouraged to prepare methods for dealing with these cues when the cues are encountered (see Chapter 10, this volume).

COMMON OBSTACLES IN TREATMENT

When a patient does not appear to be responding favorably to cognitive therapy, it is possible that there is a problem in the therapeutic relationship. The patient who does not trust the therapist or feel comfortable in therapy is likely to be guarded in sessions; therefore, he or she might avoid important self-disclosures for fear of judgment or retribution. Without these admissions it is unlikely that the patient will objectively examine or acknowledge biased thinking patterns. Such examination is central to the success of cognitive therapy, and can be fostered via an accepting, warm, collaborative therapeutic approach.

When the therapeutic relationship is judged to be sound, but the techniques appear to be ineffective, it is important to review the case conceptualization for missed diagnoses, overlooked beliefs, and important unassessed historical events. For example, many substance-abusing patients have a coexisting personality disorder (borderline, antisocial, avoidant personality disorders, etc.). These patients require careful attention simultaneously to their chronic maladaptive personality (i.e., belief) patterns and to their substance abuse problems. Patients may also have problems with anxiety and depression, and they may be attempting to treat these problems with psychoactive substances (i.e., to self-medicate). Therapists must keep in mind that such a patient's "resistance" to treatment simply may reflect an unspoken fear that without drugs his or her anxieties or dysphoria will become overwhelming. Also, taking an updated review of the patient's history can stimulate a breakthrough in treatment. For example, one therapist did not realize until many months into treatment that his patient had gone through humiliating failure experiences in grade school and that memories of this had led the patient to resist anything called "homework," for fear that it would make him look stupid. Once this was understood, the therapist was able to help the patient to generate rational responses to combat these negative expectations and fears.

The topic of homework is important enough to merit its own separate discussion. Patient nonparticipation in homework assignments can hinder the therapeutic learning process. It is tempting in any medical or psychological intervention to simply tell the patient to "go home and do. . . ." However, for homework to be maximally effective it should have certain qualities. First, it should be collaboratively determined. Second, the therapist should check for the patient's understanding of the exact nature of the assignment, as well as the patient's understanding of the underlying rationale for the assignment. Third, the therapist and patient should consider any potential barriers to completing homework assignments and prepare contingency plans. Finally, the patient should have an opportunity to practice the homework with the therapist in order to test his or her understanding of and ability to do the assignment.

A final problem in applying the techniques of cognitive therapy to substance abuse might be in the therapist's therapeutic style. It is essential that the therapist stimulate the patient's thinking process with sensitively worded open-ended questions, rather than by lecturing or preaching to the patient. When the cognitive therapy techniques described here are presented in a dictatorial fashion, the therapist's words are likely to "go in one ear and out the other." Generous application of the Socratic method often is an antidote to this problem.

SUMMARY

In this chapter, we presented many of the most widely used techniques of the cognitive therapy of substance abuse. Most of the techniques that have been successfully applied in the treatment of other psychiatric syndromes are useful in the treatment of substance abuse. It is important that these techniques be applied with careful attention paid to the therapeutic relationship, the patient's individual case conceptualization, the patient's application of these techniques in the form of homework assignments, and the therapist's use of open-ended questioning.

The techniques that we described do not represent an exhaustive list. In fact, we encourage therapists to make use of their creativity and their patients' unique individual needs and strengths to devise new variations of cognitive therapy techniques and assignments. As long as the technique serves a logical purpose, fits within the case conceptualization, adheres to ethical guidelines, and focuses on changes in *beliefs* as well as drug-related *behaviors* per se, there is no limit to what may be applied successfully.

CHAPTER **10**

Dealing with Craving/Urges

Because of their resurgence during and after treatment, uncontrolled cravings and urges to use are major factors contributing to treatment dropout and often lead to relapse even after long periods of abstinence. Teaching patients to cope with craving is therefore one of the most important goals of treatment (Annis, 1986; Carroll, Rounsaville, & Keller, 1991; Childress et al., 1990; Covi et al., 1990; Horvath, 1988, in press; Shulman, 1989; Tiffany, 1990; Washton, 1988). The therapist initially assesses the patient's idiosyncratic perception of craving. Then, over the course of treatment, the therapist helps the patient to understand the various factors that contribute to craving, to reframe the experience, and to develop better ways to deal with this problem.

Horvath (1988) has distinguished the phenomenon of cravings from urges, describing the former as the subjective sense (e.g., physical arousal, emotional arousal, "need," and "desire") of wishing to attain the psychological state induced by drugs. In contrast, urges are described as the behavioral impulse to seek and use the drugs. Although these are useful theoretical distinctions, in practice we have used the terms "cravings" and "urges" interchangeably, as we will in the remainder of this chapter.

TYPES OF CRAVING

We have identified four major types of craving, each with its own unique characteristics (although there is some overlap from one type to another).

1. *Response to withdrawal symptoms.* Heavy users of drugs such as cocaine and heroin often come to experience a diminishing sense of gratification from the use of the drug, but an increasing sense of internal discomfort on cessation of the use of the drug. In such cases, the craving takes on the form of a "need to feel well again." This is especially true for the heroin user who experiences severe, flu-like symptoms during withdrawal, and the cocaine user who becomes deeply depressed during a "crash." Therapists who treat patients who are going through this type of craving will need to be empathic to the patients' acute sense of pain and suffering as a result of abstinence. It is most important to inform such patients that this discomfort is temporary (although in extreme cases medical supervision may be necessary).

2. *Response to lack of pleasure.* Another type of craving involves patients' attempts to improve their moods in the quickest and most extreme way possible. This phenomenon is most likely to occur when patients are bored, are unskilled in finding prosocial means of enjoyment, and wish to "self-medicate" (Castaneda et al., 1989; Khantzian, 1988) in order to blot out unpleasant thoughts or feelings. Here, therapists must be aware that the therapy sessions themselves may be sufficiently upsetting to patients that they may experience a craving for drugs in order to forget their troubles. Therefore, therapists are advised to assess their patients' moods and degrees of craving at the end of particularly stressful (i.e., productive and meaningful) sessions.

3. *"Conditioned" response to drug cues.* This type of craving requires no particular dysphoric mood, stressor, or hedonic urge on the part of the patient. Patients who have abused drugs have learned to associate many otherwise neutral stimuli (a particular street corner, a given person, a telephone number, a certain time of day, etc.) with the acute gratification obtained from the use of drugs. These neutral stimuli therefore become "charged" with meaning and can induce automatic cravings even in the absence of stressors. Therapists must help their patients to become aware of, and cope with, the cravings that arise simply as a result of their association with these everyday stimuli.

4. *Response to hedonic desires.* Patients sometimes experience the onset of drug cravings when they wish to enhance a positive experience. For example, some patients have made a habit of combining drugs and sex as a way to magnify the sexual experience. Others, for example, seek drugs as a way to make their social interactions more "enjoyable and spontaneous." Unfortunately, the high that is achieved by such practices is difficult to match (in the short term) in a drug-free life. Therefore, these are particularly difficult types of cravings to combat in therapy. Therapists have the most leverage when patients'

drug use has progressed to such a degree that their life problems have overwhelmed their isolated moments of drug-induced hedonic joy. Under these conditions, patients typically are more willing to work to find other means of achieving gratification in life. Still, there will be an ongoing battle with these cravings whenever the patient experiences a natural good mood.

CRAVINGS: UNDERSTANDING THE PATIENT'S EXPERIENCE

A therapist can begin to understand the patient's craving experience first by identifying automatic thoughts (ATs) associated with the experience. Cravings can be triggered in the therapist's office by having patients simply describe the last time they used drugs. Induced imagery is a more powerful method for evoking these cravings. As a word of caution, it is important that the patient understand the rationale for this induction, namely, to learn to identify and cope with cravings and cues to craving. Also, therapists must be prepared to help reduce the strong feelings of craving prior to the end of a session (Childress et al., 1990). If not, patients may leave the therapy session highly aroused and without the skills necessary to cope with their cravings. Thus, a lapse may ensue. Craving induction techniques should *not* be implemented until *after* patients have had practice with general cognitive therapy skills and coping techniques (see Chapter 9, this volume).

In a typical craving induction, patients are asked to imagine the last time they used cocaine, and then to describe the image. They are instructed to give as much detail as possible. The aim is to have patients relive the experience as vividly as possible, and therefore gain access to the "hot" cognitions that accompany the craving.

A typical way to introduce a craving experience is the following: "Jim, today I want to try to understand your experience of craving so that I can help you to develop better strategies for coping. Therefore, I'm going to ask you to do a short exercise with me."

"I want you to think back to the last time that you used cocaine [or another drug relevant to the patient's problem]. [Wait a minute or two for the patient to get into the image.] Now I want you to think about the events that led up to your using. I would like you to try to picture it in your mind, describe the setting, tell me the sequence of events, and relate what you are feeling. As soon as you notice that you are beginning to have a craving, please indicate this by lifting your hand." (*Patient indicates he's having an image*) "Describe what you are feeling and what thoughts are going through your mind just now."

Therapists should ask patients to compare how similar the cravings experienced in the office are to those they experienced outside. In addition, patients can be asked to come up with their own methods to help induce the craving. For example, some cocaine abusers report that one of the strongest cues for craving is remembering a particular sex partner that they had while using cocaine. The thought of that person and the image of having sex serve as powerful cues for eliciting strong desires to use cocaine.

COPING WITH CRAVINGS

Patients can be helped to *reduce* the aroused cravings by a number of techniques, including (1) distraction, (2) flashcards, (3) imagery, (4) rational responding to urge-related automatic thoughts, (5) activity scheduling, and (6) relaxation training. These techniques should be demonstrated and taught early in treatment. To develop a durable strategy for handling cravings, of course, patients must also learn to deal with the dysfunctional beliefs that facilitate using.

Distraction Techniques

The key goal of distraction techniques is to get patients to change their focus of attention from internal (e.g., automatic thoughts, memories, physical sensations) to external. Although some of these techniques seem quite simple, they do help to diminish strong cravings.

The following are brief descriptions of commonly used distraction techniques:

1. Instruct patients to concentrate their attention on describing their surroundings, such as cars, people, trees, and storefronts. Initially, patients can practice in the office. The more that they can focus and give details about these external events, the more likely they are to focus less on the internal cravings.

2. Use talking to distract. This can involve starting a conversation with a friend, a relative, a support group sponsor, or the therapist.

3. Patients can remove themselves from the cue-laden environment. They can take a brisk walk, visit a friend, or go for a drive. One of our patients found the public library an excellent place to escape in order to reduce cravings.

4. Perform household chores as a positive distraction. If patients are at home and they notice these cravings and urges, something as simple as beginning to clean the house can distract them from the craving. In addition, this goal-directed activity also helps increase their self-esteem because they have accomplished something useful. (As a caveat, this activity may be ill-advised if drugs and paraphernalia are scattered in hiding places throughout the house.)

5. Encourage patients to recite a favorite poem or prayer. For some patients, it is more helpful actually to write down the poem or prayer on a piece of paper.

6. Suggest that patients spend time involved in games, such as cards, video games, board games, and puzzles. These activities can be quite challenging and therefore require focused concentration. Further, patients can do some of these activities even if they are alone.

Flashcards

When cravings are strong, patients seem to lose the ability to reason objectively. Generating coping statements can be helpful in getting patients through this critical period. The usefulness of coping statements can be enhanced by asking patients to write these statements on flashcards (e.g., 3" × 5" index cards). Some examples include a flashcard with the list of advantages for not using drugs and a list of things that could be bought with the money intended for cocaine.

The following are examples of statements that one patient wrote on his flashcards:

1. You feel more sane when you don't use.
2. Things are going great with my wife; keep it that way!
3. You look good physically; keep it that way!
4. Get the hell out of this situation *now!*

Imagery Techniques

These techniques include (1) image refocusing, (2) negative image replacement, (3) positive image replacement, (4) image rehearsal, and (5) image mastery.

Refocusing is essentially a distraction technique. Patients direct their attention away from internal cravings by imagining external events. Refocusing can begin first by saying "Stop!" In order to accentuate this thought-stopping technique, patients may interject a visual image of a stop sign, a police officer, or a brick wall, to name a few.

They then begin to describe to themselves what they see going on around them.

For example, one patient was at a picnic where many people were drinking and having a good time. He began to have spontaneous memories of the last time he used cocaine, which led to a desire to use in the present. He said "Stop" to himself, pictured a stop sign, and then began focusing his attention on the people around him who were not drinking. He identified them by name, what they were wearing, and what they were doing. In doing so, he was able to focus his attention away from the cocaine memories and he experienced subsequent reduction in the craving.

Another imagery technique is negative image replacement. Oftentimes during the first few weeks of abstinence, patients report picturing themselves using, sometimes even having dreams about using. In these images they see the use of drugs as a method for coping with their current distress, and the image takes on a positive glow. In response, it is helpful for patients to substitute a *negative* image regarding the many unfortunate consequences of taking the drug, such as feeling helpless and hopeless (especially after a period of abstinence) or losing money, jobs, and relationships. For example, one patient, while at a nightclub, became quite angry that he could no longer drink alcohol. He saw other people around him drinking and this brought back nostalgic memories of some of his drug and alcohol days. In response, he replaced the image with one pertaining to the unpleasant physical experiences that he would have when he crashed the day after using alcohol and cocaine. This image was strong enough to dissuade him from taking the first drink.

Positive image replacement is a related technique to help cope with cravings and urges. For example, one patient experienced very strong negative images about his current situation, that almost his entire family was strung out on drugs. His father was about to lose the house where the patient was living. Consequently, the patient had images of losing his children, having to put them in a foster home, and having to live in a shelter. At that moment, in his sense of hopelessness, the patient began to have thoughts of giving up his abstinence from cocaine. However, he instead referred to a flashcard that described a positive scene. He imagined himself being back at work again, being in his own home, and able to take care of his children. Also, a concomitant of this positive image was the self-satisfaction that he would have after a long day of working. This technique diminished his hopelessness somewhat and, along with it, his craving.

Imagery rehearsals should be used to prepare patients when it is known that they are going to be in cue-laden situations. One patient, who had been abstinent from cocaine and alcohol for about one year, planned to go to a formal banquet where alcohol would be served. In the image rehearsal the therapist asked the patient to imagine going to the banquet and saying, "No thanks, I'll have a club soda," when he was offered a drink. The therapist told the patient to repeat the image several times and monitor his thoughts and feelings associated with the imagery rehearsal. The patient initially was quite anxious while doing this, but later developed a sense of mastery or confidence in being able to go to the banquet and still deal with alcohol being served all around him.

Some patients fear that while experiencing very strong cravings and urges to use drugs they will not be able to tolerate the negative feelings that they are experiencing without giving in to the urge to use (Horvath, 1988; Washton, 1988). We have found that it is helpful to teach these patients mastery imaging, seeing themselves as a very strong and powerful person who is overcoming cravings and urges. One patient who was an intravenous cocaine user reported having repeated images of what he described as "the cocaine lady." In this image, he would be have the sensation of strong cravings for cocaine as he would picture a beautiful woman who was going to offer him cocaine. The patient was taught by his therapist to change the image so that he would have more control. A metaphor that was used was that of a director of a play; that is, the cocaine lady was one character in the play and the patient was the director, able to decide what she would look like and how she would act. He subsequently redirected the image so that "the cocaine lady" was a grotesque-looking person who was very small, while the patient was a heavyweight boxer able to fight off the urges that he was experiencing.

Rational Responding to Urge-Related Automatic Thoughts

Therapists start by training patients to self-monitor automatic thoughts when they are having unpleasant emotions such as anger, anxiety, sadness, or boredom. Later, the patients are instructed how to assess their automatic thoughts while experiencing cravings and urges.

It is helpful to have patients carry a "therapy notepad" and a pen in order to write down these thoughts. Patients are told that anytime they experience strong cravings or unpleasant emotions, they should ask themselves *"What thoughts are going through my mind right now?"* They are also instructed to note any physiological distress and then to ask themselves, "What am I feeling?" and "What thoughts are going through my mind?" They then write down the answers and bring their notepads to the next therapy sessions.

The Daily Thought Record (DTR) is used to help patients examine negative automatic thoughts and to generate adaptive responses. DTRs can be completed before, during, and after episodes of craving. The use of DTRs can demonstrate to patients that they are not helpless in the face of their cravings/urges, and a review of old DTRs can serve as a reminder of this key fact.

Figure 10.1 depicts "Jim's" DTR. As can be seen under the Situation column, Jim was sitting at home. He had recently had an accident at a construction site, resulting in a broken hand and wrist. Under the heading "situation" he wrote: "Sitting at home, my hand is broken, and I can't go to work. There is plenty of money in my pocket." Also, he started thinking about some of his old drug buddies and the last time that he used cocaine. Jim was also aware of having a strong craving for cocaine. He rated at 95% the amount of boredom and anxiety that he was experiencing—an indication of strong negative feelings. Some of the automatic thoughts he identified were "There is nothing to do" and "I can't stand this boredom."

In examining their automatic thoughts, patients ask themselves five basic questions (see Chapter 9, this volume). The first question is "What is the evidence for and against my automatic thoughts?" The second question is "Are there other ways of looking at this situation?" The third question is "If it is true, what are the realistic consequences?" The fourth question is "What are the drawbacks to my continuing to dwell on these thoughts?" The final question asks, "What constructive action can I take to solve this problem?"

Jim began examining the automatic thought, "There is nothing to do," by asking himself, "What's the evidence against this?" He responded to this question by saying, "Actually, there are plenty of things that I could do; for example, go to a meeting, watch a game, or call my therapist." Next, he asked himself, "Are there other ways of looking at this? Do I really mean there is nothing to do?" His response was, "No, it is not true that there is nothing to do, but the pain of boredom makes it difficult for me to see other things that I might be able to do." He then asked, "If true, what are the realistic consequences?" He responded, "Well, if it is true that there is nothing to do, then the consequences will be that I will feel bored, and, although the boredom is painful, it's not the end of the world. The consequences are that I will feel bored and even that will go away." Jim's next question was, "If true, what are the drawbacks to my continuing to dwell on these thoughts?" He responded, "The disadvan-

DAILY THOUGHT RECORD

Directions: When you notice your mood getting worse, ask yourself, "What's going through my mind right now" and as soon as possible jot down the thought or mental image in the Automatic Thought Column.

DATE/TIME	SITUATION Describe: 1. Actual event leading to unpleasant emotion, or 2. Stream of thoughts, daydreams or recollection, leading to unpleasant emotion, or 3. Distressing physical sensations	AUTOMATIC THOUGHT(S) 1. Write automatic thought(s) that preceded emotion(s). 2. Rate belief in automatic thought(s) 0–100%.	EMOTION(S) 1. Specify sad, anxious/angry, etc. 2. Rate degree of emotion 0–100%.	RATIONAL RESPONSE 1. Write rational response to automatic thought(s). 2. Rate belief in rational response 0–100%.	OUTCOME 1. Re-rate belief in automatic thought(s) 0–100% 2. Specify and rate subsequent emotions 0–100%.
	Sitting at home, my hand broken, and I can't go to work. There is money in my pocket. Thinking about some old drug buddies and the last time I used cocaine. Start craving for cocaine.	"There is nothing to do" "I can't stand this boredom."	Bored Anxious (95%)	"Actually, there are plenty of things I could do; for example, go to a meeting, watch a game, or call my therapist." "It is not true that there is nothing to do but the pain of boredom makes it difficult for me to see other things that I might be able to do." "If it is true that there is nothing to do, then the consequences will be that I feel bored, and although the boredom is painful, it's not the end of the world. The consequences are that I will feel bored and even that will go away." "The disadvantage of continuing to dwell on these thoughts is that I feel helpless, which in turn, leads to the desire for cocaine." "I can go get a newspaper and read the sports page until it's time for a meeting." (90%)	10% Bored (30%) Anxious (20%)

Questions to help formulate the rational response: (1) What is the evidence that the automatic thought is true? Not true? (2) Is there an alternative explanation? (3) What's the worst that could happen? Could I live through it? What's the best that could happen? What's the most realistic outcome? (4) What should I do about it? (5) What's the effect of my believing the automatic thought? What could be the effect of changing my thinking? (6) If (friend's name) was in this situation and had this thought, what would I tell him/her?

FIGURE 10.1. Jim's Daily Thought Record.

tage is that I feel helpless, which, in turn, leads to the desire for cocaine." The patient's last question, "What constructive action can I take?" led to the response, "I can go get a newspaper and read the sports page until it's time for a meeting." Jim's belief in his rational response was 90%. In the last column, we see that Jim has re-rated his belief in the automatic thoughts at 10%. This indicates that the rational response has had a significant impact on modifying Jim's belief in that automatic thought. We also see that his level of boredom and anxiety has diminished, going from 95% for each to 30% for boredom and 20% for anxiety. This level of diminishment indicates a reduction in the degree of intensity for these emotions, which, in turn, may help to reduce the likelihood of Jim's using cocaine to cope with the boredom and anxiety.

In addition, by using a 0–100 rating scale on the standard DTR form (regarding the level of confidence about the thoughts), the patient understands that the automatic thoughts are not necessarily objective realities. Patients can learn to use the rating scale to gauge changes in their perceptions as they apply cognitive and behavioral techniques. The 0–100 rating scale serves therefore as a useful cognitive barometer.

Craving is an idiosyncratic experience made up of cognitive, affective, behavioral, and physiological components. Therefore, by identifying its various components patients can be more objective about the craving experience, and thus diminish the subjective intensity.

Later, through the use of subsequent DTRs, the therapist was able to help Jim to be more objective about craving. The trigger (e.g., a sense of extreme boredom or anxiety) activated the beliefs, "I can't cope without cocaine" and "The craving makes me do it," represented by the automatic thought, "I can't stand this." His physiological responses, tension, excess sweating, and urge to seek relief represented the sequence of events that Jim originally labeled "craving." The therapist then helped Jim see that interventions could be made, for example, becoming aware of the automatic thought and being able to respond rationally to it, thus diminishing the urge to use cocaine.

In addition, it is important to help patients to cope with the craving by teaching them to test their idiosyncratic *predictions* about the duration and intensity, as well as the patients' mastery, of the craving phenomenon. This result can be achieved by teaching them to monitor the intensity, frequency, and duration of craving in order to attack their dichotomous or catastrophic view of the craving phenomenon (Horvath, 1988, in press; Tiffany, 1990).

Examples of such catastrophic predictions are the following:

- "If I don't use something right now, I won't be able to face going to work; I'll lose my job."
- "Without the drug, I'll be a nervous wreck all day. Everyone will think I'm having a breakdown."
- "I'll never have a normal life again. I'm a slave to the drug. I simply have to have it to get through the day."
- "If I resist taking the drug now, I'll just need twice as much later to feel normal later. I might even overdose if that happens."

Activity Scheduling

Patients who have a long history of drug abuse often engage only in activities that center around the use or the procurement of drugs. Oftentimes, their entire social network is drug related. When patients are trying to control their substance use they often find that initially it is beneficial to stay away from the people, places, and things associated with their former lifestyle (O'Brien et al., 1992). As a result, recovering patients may be faced with a great deal of idle time on their hands. The boredom that accompanies this state can spell trouble for patients' abstinence unless new activities are substituted.

Activity schedules are helpful in this regard. First, the activity schedule is used to gather baseline data on how patients actually spend their time. Activity schedules can also be used proactively to structure the patients' day in a constructive way. Many drug-abusing patients have forgotten some of the activities they once enjoyed prior to their drug-using days. The scheduling of activities can revive some of these old, enjoyable, prosocial activities, the likes of which may assist the patient in rebuilding a drug-free life (Hall, Havassy, & Wasserman, 1991).

Such activities serve two purposes. Some of them help patients in the short term to deal with the immediate crisis of coping with urges. Other activities on this list are long-term alternatives to patients' previous drug-related behaviors. In general, the purpose of these substitute activities is to give patients something to do other than the short-lived and deceptively positive experience of using drugs. This is not to say that these activities would be equal to the immediate, intense pleasure received from using such drugs as cocaine; however, these activities do have many long-term advantages.

While it is vital to teach drug-abusing patients to find alternative, *nondrug* sources of reinforcement, therapists must bear in mind that this may require a great deal of training and practice. The difficulty lies in the fact that taking drugs requires no particular skills, but the alternative nondrug activities may require considerable skills (Stitzer et al., 1984). Therefore, therapists must not take for granted that patients have the know-how to schedule positive activities and must be prepared to deal with patients' low self-confidence, high frustration, marked hopelessness, and passive avoidance surrounding this technique.

Relaxation Training

Another technique that we have also found to be useful is relaxation training (Bernstein & Borkovec, 1973). Relaxation training gives patients a tool that they can use to help cope with such feelings as anxiety and anger, which, for some patients, can be triggers for cravings (see Chapter 15, this volume).

When introducing relaxation techniques to patients, it is important to offer them a rationale for the use of this intervention. For example, relaxation training is a method for reducing tension that, left unchecked, might trigger cravings. Relaxation training also helps one to develop an improved general sense of well-being, and to lower one's sense of stress in day-to-day life. In addition, a relaxed individual is less likely to act impulsively and out of a sense of desperation.

It is important that patients understand that relaxation is a skill that can be learned like any other skill. The more they practice their relaxation training, the better they will become at evoking a deep state of relaxation. We recommend that the first relaxation exercise take place in the therapy session, under the therapist's supervision, in order to ensure that the patients are doing it properly.

SUMMARY

The three main goals of this chapter were: (1) to focus on the importance of dealing with urges and cravings, (2) to understand better the patient's subjective experience, and (3) to describe techniques that can help patients to cope better with urges and cravings.

Uncontrolled urges and cravings are a major factor contributing to treatment failure. Therefore, it is imperative to teach patients early in treatment how to monitor and deal with urges and cravings.

CHAPTER 11

Focus on Beliefs

Beliefs are relatively rigid, enduring cognitive structures that are not easily modified by experience. In cognitive therapy it is generally maintained that beliefs have a profound impact on feelings and behaviors. For example, depressed patients have global, negative views about themselves, the world, and the future that contribute to their feelings of despair, guilt, and sadness (Beck et al., 1979). Negative beliefs also contribute to such depressive behaviors as isolation and withdrawal. In cases of anxiety disorders, patients have negative, apprehensive beliefs about some future threat that contribute to avoidance, anxiety, and perhaps panic (Beck et al., 1985).

There are at least three types of beliefs pertinent to the patients' addiction to drugs: anticipatory, relief-oriented, and facilitative or permissive. As described in Chapters 2 and 3 (this volume), anticipatory beliefs involve some expectation of reward, such as "The party tonight will be great. I can't wait to go get high!" Relief-oriented beliefs are those that assume that using drugs will remove an uncomfortable state, for example, "I can't stand withdrawal. I need a hit." And finally, facilitative or permissive beliefs are those that consider drug use acceptable, in spite of the potential consequences, for example, "Only weak people have problems with drugs. It won't happen to me." Permissive beliefs also have much in common with what are more commonly known as "rationalizations." Patients have thoughts that seem to "justify" their drug-using, such as "I *have* to use cocaine or I won't be able to concentrate on my work." Such thinking is tantamount to self-deception.

The following examples illustrate the addictive beliefs of two individuals who are cocaine-dependent. (These case examples will be used throughout this chapter to illustrate important points.)

"Louise" is a 21-year-old unemployed, single parent who has been using cocaine for two years. Most people who encounter Louise can see that she has had a "rough life." When Louise cannot afford to purchase cocaine, she turns to prostitution to acquire money. She holds the following addictive beliefs about cocaine and herself:

"I need drugs to numb the pain."

"I might as well do drugs since my life won't ever improve anyway."

"Getting high is the only thing I look forward to."

"I'm tough; I can handle drugs."

In contrast to Louise, "Bill" is a 39-year-old successful sales executive who has been using cocaine for the past 3 years. He "loves to party" with his friends and coworkers. Bill holds the following addictive beliefs:

"I work like hell all week. I deserve to get high on the weekends."

"I can't keep up the pace without an occasional 'pick-me-up' [cocaine]."

"I've never failed at anything, so drugs won't hurt me."

"I'm basically a pretty decent guy."

At first glance, Bill and Louise appear to be quite different from each other. However, as we examine them more closely we see that they each fall prey to anticipatory, relief-oriented, and permissive beliefs that perpetuate their addictions.

In contrast to *addictive* beliefs, individuals may have *control* beliefs. Control beliefs are defined as beliefs that decrease the likelihood of drug use and abuse. The following are examples of control beliefs:

"Drugs are dangerous to my well-being."

"I am capable of withstanding the urges."

"If I tolerate this craving for awhile, it will go away."

"If I resist the urges, I will feel stronger."

"It is in my best interest to stay drug-free."

An addicted person may maintain contradictory beliefs. For example, a drug-dependent person may hold the addictive belief "I love the feeling of being high." Simultaneously, the same person may hold the control belief "This is killing me." As a result of these contradictory beliefs, drug-dependent persons often feel a great deal of ambivalence about their habit. They may find themselves, for example, awakening in the morning and "swearing off" drugs. By noon they may be seeking treatment for their addiction, although by evening they may be using again. (Contradictory beliefs are also common, of course, among people who have tried to diet or quit smoking.)

When addictive beliefs are more salient than control beliefs, a drug-dependent person is more likely to use drugs. Of course, the opposite is true: when a person's control beliefs predominate over addictive beliefs, that person is more likely to abstain from drugs. An ideal goal for the cognitive therapist is to identify and eliminate the patient's addictive beliefs, replacing them with more adaptive control beliefs. More realistically, the goal of cognitive therapy is to facilitate a process whereby the patient's control beliefs become more salient than his or her addictive beliefs. The result, of course, will be that the patient abstains from, or at least diminishes, drug use. The following is a list of specific methods to address the drug-abusing patients' problematic belief systems:

1. *Assess* beliefs.
2. *Orient* the patient to the cognitive therapy model.
3. *Examine and test* addictive beliefs.
4. *Develop* control beliefs.
5. *Practice* activation of control beliefs.
6. *Assign homework* that addresses beliefs.

In the remainder of this chapter, these methods are described in detail.

ASSESS BELIEFS

In order to modify addictive beliefs, the cognitive therapist must first have an accurate understanding of the role of these beliefs in the patient's life. Thus, a careful assessment must take place for each patient. This assessment may be accomplished in two ways: through therapist–patient interaction during psychotherapy sessions and standardized questionnaires.

The following open-ended questions are examples of those useful for eliciting information about patients' beliefs:

"What are your thoughts about _____ ?"

"What was going on in your head when _____ happened?"

"How do you explain _____ ?"

"How do you interpret _____ ?"

"What does _____ mean to you?"

"What's your 'rule of thumb' here?"

"How did you size up the situation?"

As the patient responds to these questions, the therapist verbally reflects what the patient has said, with particular emphasis on the beliefs expressed by the patient. At various points in the interview, the therapist provides "capsule summaries" of what has been discussed, with strong emphasis placed on the patient's thoughts. To illustrate this process we present the following dialogue between a patient and her therapist, taken from their first session. Louise was referred for therapy by a primary care physician who treated her at a county health clinic for gonorrhea.

TH: Hello, Louise. What would you like to talk about today?

PT: I don't really even know. I was sent here by that doctor at the clinic. I figured I had to be here.

TH: You must have some concerns . . . some things that are bothering you.

PT: Yeh, I guess. But I don't know what good it will do to talk to you.

TH: You doubt that this will be helpful.

PT: Yeh, that's right.

TH: What other thoughts do you have about being here?

PT: Well I've been in treatment before, but as you can probably guess, I'm on the shit again.

TH: What do you mean by "on the shit"?

PT: Oh come on, man! You know what that means! I'm doing drugs!

TH: Does "on the shit" mean that you are doing drugs daily? weekly? monthly?

PT: To me it means doing any drugs at all!

TH: So any slip and you consider yourself "on the shit"?

PT: Yeh! I was clean for a month and then last week I had a really bad time with my old man. I went right out on a two-day binge.

TH: And what have you done since then?

PT: If you mean drugs, I have been clean since then, but I don't suppose it will last.

TH: So when you slip, even once, you see yourself as having a relapse.

PT: Right.

TH: And when you say "I don't suppose it will last" I get the impression that you don't feel fully capable of staying off drugs.

PT: No, not really. Sometimes it seems pretty easy to stay clean and sometimes it's really impossible.

TH: So from what you have said so far, you are skeptical about being here. You doubt that I can be helpful. You see yourself as having fully relapsed, based on a two-day binge. And generally you see yourself as being somewhat helpless to control your drug use.

PT: Yeh, that's it in a nutshell!

In just the first few minutes of the initial interview the patient revealed some of her addictive beliefs. She did not appear to possess salient control beliefs. The therapist continued to construct a database of her addictive and control beliefs, which later played an extremely important role in therapy.

In addition to the interview process, several questionnaires are available to collect data about an individual's beliefs. Some are designed to evaluate general beliefs (e.g., Dysfunctional Attitude Scale; Weissman & Beck, 1978); some are designed to assess mood (e.g., Beck Depression Inventory; Beck et al., 1961); while others (recently developed at the Center for Cognitive Therapy in Philadelphia) are designed specifically to assess drug-related beliefs (e.g., Craving Beliefs Questionnaire, Beliefs about Substance Use, and Automatic Thoughts about Substance Abuse).

These questionnaires are given to the patient at the beginning of therapy to provide baseline information. They are also completed on subsequent visits to assess changes that may have occurred over the course of treatment. During the therapy process, these questionnaires help the therapist to understand the patient's "belief status" as it relates to problems and progress. For example, during her third visit, Louise stated that she wanted to start using cocaine again. On examining her Craving Beliefs Questionnaire, the therapist saw an increase in Louise's addictive beliefs about craving. She indicated on the questionnaire that she *strongly* believed the following:

"The craving is totally out of my control."

"Craving can drive you crazy."

"I'll always have cravings for cocaine."

"The craving makes me so nervous I can't stand it."

"Since I'll have the craving the rest of my life I might as well go ahead and use cocaine."

"If the craving gets too intense, cocaine is the only way to cope with the feeling."

"I can't stand the panicky feeling when craving cocaine."

"The craving frightens me."

In addition to providing these data to her therapist, Louise also completed a Beck Depression Inventory (BDI) prior to this session and her therapist noted that she had a BDI score of 20, suggesting moderate depression. Louise endorsed the following items:

"I feel sad."

"I feel I have nothing to look forward to."

"I am dissatisfied or bored with everything."

"I am disgusted with myself."

"I blame myself all the time for my faults."

"I feel irritated all the time now."

"I have lost all of my interest in other people."

"I have to push myself very hard to do anything."

"I have lost interest in sex completely."

Together, these questionnaires alerted the therapist to Louise's present state of dysphoria and its potential effect on her drug treatment program. It became more apparent during the interview that Louise was struggling with a vicious cycle (see Figure 11.1): she was having strong urges to use cocaine; she believed that she could not control these urges; she believed that they would never go away; she further believed that there was nowhere to turn for support, since "all" her "friends" used cocaine; she believed that her lack of friends meant that she would never be happy again; she felt depressed; she believed that only cocaine could make her happy again, which led to further urges; and so forth. From this assessment of Louise's beliefs, her therapist was able to help her address and begin to modify these beliefs.

ORIENT THE PATIENT TO THE COGNITIVE THERAPY MODEL

Many addicted individuals have an externalized view of their addiction. They may believe the following: "I have no control, whatsoever," "I just need to submit myself to the doctors. Maybe they will beat it this time," or "This treatment probably won't work since nothing else has." Thus, it is important that patients be oriented to the cognitive therapy model in the initial stages of therapy. Ori-

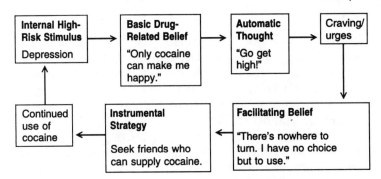

FIGURE 11.1. Cognitive model applied to Louise.

enting patients involves modifying their beliefs about their addiction from an externalized orientation (e.g., "Control is beyond me") to an internalized orientation (e.g., "I am responsible for my drug use and for my recovery from addiction").

As part of the process of orienting the patient, key terms are defined, including "addictive beliefs," "control beliefs," "automatic thoughts," "stimulus situations," "craving," "lapse," and "relapse." Next, the interrelationships between these phenomena are explained, with special emphasis on the role of beliefs in the addictive process.

In the following dialogue, Bill's therapist introduced him to the cognitive therapy model.

TH: Bill, let's talk about the development of your addiction. How do you think you became addicted to cocaine?

PT: When I began to use cocaine with my friends it was an innocent thing.

TH: What do you mean by "innocent"?

PT: Well, when I began using cocaine I could control it. It would enhance a good time with my friends. Now it seems to control me.

TH: What do you mean when you say "it controls me"?

PT: Sometimes it just feels like I have no choice about whether or not I am going to use drugs.

TH: Are you saying that you have no control over the urges and craving; that they seem involuntary and irresistible?

PT: Yes, most of the time.

TH: So perhaps you believe that the chemical properties are like a magnet, drawing you involuntarily towards continued use of drugs.

PT: Right.

TH: OK, let's consider another perspective. What I am about to show you is the model I use to understand addiction. Let's start with a diagram. (*therapist draws the diagram* [presented in Chapter 3, this volume]) First, let's define the terms on this diagram. A stimulus is an internal or external circumstance that may stir up feelings and beliefs. A belief is an established idea you have about the stimulus or about how you might respond to the stimulus. Your belief, in turn, triggers some automatic thoughts, which themselves trigger urges and craving. Do you have any questions so far?

PT: I'm not sure I know what you mean.

TH: OK. The importance of this model is that it focuses on your thoughts and beliefs as playing a major role in your urges and craving. Previously, you believed that your urges were purely a result of a biological process over which you had no control. Alternatively, it is useful to think of urges as being influenced by your thoughts, which are ultimately under your control.

PT: Then if I am in control of my thoughts, and if my thoughts control my drug use, and if my drug use is so bad for me, then why do I continue using?

TH: That's a good question, Bill. When you do use cocaine it's partly because you believe that the immediate advantages of using outweigh the long-term disadvantages.

PT: I just realized that another reason why I keep using is that I don't believe that bad things will ever happen to me.

TH: Right. So, Bill, in cognitive therapy you can expect me to focus heavily on your thoughts and beliefs. Specifically, I will help you to modify your beliefs so that you are less vulnerable to drug use. What do you think of that?

PT: It sounds pretty good to me.

TH: What "sounds pretty good" about this model?

PT: Well, it gives me more hope about controlling my urges and behaviors, rather than having them control me.

EXAMINE AND TEST ADDICTIVE BELIEFS

Addictive beliefs develop over an extended period of time. As a result they become overlearned and extremely resistant to change. The drug abuser collects data supporting such beliefs as "drugs are fun and very exciting," "cocaine greatly enhances sex and many other activities," and "nothing is quite like using cocaine." Many drug abusers have tried to quit using drugs at one time or another; however, their difficulty in doing so provides them with validation for the belief "It's useless to try to control my addiction."

Given the resistant nature of addictive beliefs, the process of modifying them is quite a challenge. After the therapist has assessed the patient's beliefs and oriented the patient to the cognitive therapy model, an examination and testing of addictive beliefs should begin. Examination of addictive beliefs involves asking patients probing questions that test the validity of these beliefs. This process is known as the "Socratic method," or "guided discovery." The following are examples of questions appropriate for this process:

"What is your evidence for that belief?"

"How do you know that your belief is true?"

"Where is that written?"

"Where did you learn that?"

"How confident are you in that belief?"

As the patient considers these questions, his or her addictive beliefs should begin to "loosen" slightly. That is, he or she should begin to consider the possibility that the addictive beliefs are not necessarily true. The following dialogue between Bill and his therapist illustrates this process.

TH: Bill, let's talk about your beliefs about using cocaine.

PT: You want to know the truth? It has been three weeks since my last hit and . . . I have to be honest here . . . I really miss it.

TH: What do you miss about using?

PT: I miss it all: my friends, the parties, the rush of it all.

TH: So you associate cocaine with socializing and having fun.

PT: Of course. There is nothing as much fun as sitting around with a bunch of friends getting high.

TH: So you don't believe that *anything* is as much fun as getting high?

PT: (*thinking*) Hmm . . . (*shaking his head vigorously, smiling*) . . . No!

TH: Nothing?

PT: (*still smiling*) Nothing *I've* ever done!

TH: Let's look at that belief carefully. First of all, how confident are you that there is *nothing* as much fun as getting high?

PT: Maybe there is *something* more fun, but I don't know what it is.

TH: Bill, prior to using cocaine, what would you do for fun?

PT: Hmm . . . *(long pause)* . . . maybe that was partly why I began using cocaine. I remember being bored quite a bit. Actually, I was really in a rut . . . bored with my job and my life generally.

TH: So you initially turned to cocaine to escape the boredom and the monotony of your life.

PT: Yeh.

TH: It sounds like you were in a fairly unsatisfying and even unhappy period in your life.

PT: Definitely.

TH: And you were looking for a simple, instant solution.

PT: Maybe.

TH: Maybe?

PT: Well, I do think I have a tendency to seek quick and easy solutions.

TH: Let's go back to your original belief: "Nothing is as much fun as getting high." When you began to use cocaine back then, what other avenues had you explored for dealing with your boredom and stagnation?

PT: Well, maybe I really didn't give much else a chance.

TH: So, what evidence do you have that using cocaine is really the only fun you can have with your friends?

PT: Actually when you put it that way, and when we look at my life, I guess I got into it at a time when any escape would have looked good.

At the beginning of this dialogue Bill was confident that nothing was as rewarding as cocaine use. However, his therapist's questions led him to reconsider this belief. As the patient's confidence in his addictive beliefs began to wane, he could begin to replace these beliefs with more adaptive control beliefs.

DEVELOP CONTROL BELIEFS

Generally, the Socratic method provides an excellent strategy for having patients examine their dysfunctional beliefs and replace them with more constructive, alternative beliefs. In the case of cocaine addiction, the Socratic method stimulates patients to examine their addictive beliefs and to replace them with control beliefs. Some specific questions that introduce control beliefs are the following:

"What would you do if the drug weren't available?"

"What are the disadvantages of using the drug?"

"How else can you look at this situation?"

"What else could you do to achieve the same end? What else?"

The previous discussion with Bill illustrated how guided questioning can loosen previously held beliefs about the benefits of taking cocaine. In this section, we continue Bill's dialogue to illustrate how the therapist helped him to develop control beliefs.

TH: Bill, you now seem less dead set in believing that nothing is as much fun as getting high.

PT: I'm not sure what to believe now.

TH: What do you mean?

PT: Well, I still think that getting high with my friends was lots of fun, but maybe it wasn't the perfect high I made it out to be.

TH: Bill, what else could you have done with your friends that would have been fun?

PT: Well, I don't know about these guys, but with other friends in the past I could have gone to a baseball game, or played racketball, or done something like sports or something.

TH: What else?

PT: I guess there are lots of things . . . but none seems as exciting as doing cocaine.

TH: Let's try to think of some more things. What gave you the biggest thrill before you began using cocaine?

PT: Well, I was an adventurous guy. When I was much younger I would go camping and hiking and rock climbing, but I'm in no shape for that now.

TH: What do you mean when you say "I am in no shape for that"?

PT: I guess I'm just skeptical that I would enjoy that kind of thing anymore. It's just been so long since I last did it.

TH: What would it take for you to try doing those things again?

PT: I guess I'd just have to do them.

TH: What were some of the feelings you had in the past when you would go camping or hiking or climbing?

PT: I felt great . . . really alive!

TH: How did that feeling compare to the cocaine high?

PT: (*pause*) . . . I guess, in some ways it was better.

TH: What do you mean?

PT: Well, I really *earned* the high I got from those activities. There were no shortcuts then. It was a super feeling.

TH: So perhaps you now have a control belief to replace the old addictive belief: "I can experience a super high without using cocaine."

PT: Yes, I just need to remember that thought.

Another strategy for examining and testing addictive beliefs is the Daily Thought Record (DTR; Chapter 9, this volume). The DTR is a standardized form for listing and modifying maladaptive thoughts. In the case of cocaine addiction, it is useful for modifying addictive beliefs that lead to urges and craving. Specifically, the DTR has five columns: situation, emotions, automatic thoughts, rational response, and outcome. When the patient experiences an urge or craving, he lists the addictive belief that precipitates or fuels this craving. Then, in the rational response column he lists alternative control beliefs. For example, if the addictive belief is "I can't stand the stress without cocaine," the patient might list the alternative control response "Yes I can! In fact there are many days when I feel better because I *didn't* do drugs."

Another strategy for developing control beliefs is the advantages–disadvantages (A–D) analysis. People use drugs because they view the advantages of doing so as outweighing the disadvantages. Thus, the purpose of the A–D analysis is to redirect the patient's attention to the disadvantages of using drugs and the advantages of abstaining. The patient is helped to construct a four-cell matrix where the advantages and disadvantages of two alternative decisions are compared. Regarding cocaine dependence, the two alternative decisions are using cocaine and abstaining from cocaine. Louise's therapist utilized this strategy as follows:

TH: I would like to help you evaluate the advantages and disadvantages of using versus abstaining from cocaine. As you can see, I am drawing a four-part box. (*draws the matrix*) Along the left side we write "advantages" and "disadvantages." Along the top we write "using" and "abstaining." Let's give this a try. What are the advantages of using cocaine?

PT: It's a break from the bullshit . . . and it's a good time.

TH: (*writing*) So it's a break and it's a good time. What else?

PT: It's a chance for me to be with my friends.

TH: (*writing*) Time with friends. What else?

PT: It makes sex a whole lot of fun.

TH: (*writing*) Sex is more fun. Any other advantages?

PT: I'm sure there are . . . I'll think of them.

TH: OK, if you think of any more, let me know. Let's move on to the disadvantages of abstaining. What comes to your mind?

PT: Oh that's easy; I'll have to give up the things I just listed: the break, the fun, time with friends, great sex.

TH: (*writing*) So you'll have to give up the "quick fix."

PT: Yeh, that's another way to look at it.

TH: What about the disadvantages of using cocaine?

PT: I could get busted, I guess.

TH: (*writing*) You could get busted. What else?

PT: It's pretty dangerous out there. I've seen people get pretty badly hurt messing around with that shit.

TH: (*writing*) Danger of getting hurt.

PT: Yeh. There's also the crash. Sometimes I feel like dying would feel better . . . (*long pause*) . . . And when I really think about it, I get to feeling really out of control on the stuff. I guess another disadvantage is that I don't like being dependent on anyone or anything.

TH: (*writing*) Let me get that all: crashing after a high, feeling out of control, being dependent on people and on the drug . . .

PT: It's hard admitting to these things, but they're all true.

TH: Any other disadvantages to using?

PT: Yeh, I know you won't believe this, but I really love my little girl. Each time I get high, I risk losing her.

TH: (*writing*) So another disadvantage of using is that you might lose your daughter. Anything else?

PT: Isn't that enough?

TH: These all seem like pretty major risks. What about the advantages of abstaining or quitting?

PT: They go along with the disadvantages of using: I will avoid having the problems of getting busted, or hurt, or losing my little girl, and on and on.

	USING	ABSTAINING
ADVANTAGES	Break from "bullshit" It's a good time Time with friends Sex is more fun	Gains: self-respect respect of others Avoids: 1. Getting busted 2. Getting hurt 3. Crashing 4. Loss of control 5. Being independent

DISADVANTAGES	Danger of getting
	    busted
	Danger of getting hurt
	Crashing is awful
	Feeling out of control
	Dependency on others
	Danger of losing
	    daughter
		No more quick fix

FIGURE 11.2. Advantages–disadvantages analysis for Louise.

TH: And what will you *gain*?

PT: Self-respect . . . and the respect of others.

TH: OK, that completes our analysis. Let's review what I have written. (*shows the matrix* [Figure 11.2] *to Louise*) What do you see here?

PT: I see a lot of things I don't like.

TH: What do you mean?

PT: This makes me uncomfortable. I didn't realize it, but I really don't like thinking about the problems with using cocaine.

TH: And yet it is those thoughts, called "control" thoughts, that will help you to remain abstinent.

PT: I understand that. It's just easier to ignore control thoughts when I am using cocaine.

PRACTICE ACTIVATION
OF CONTROL BELIEFS

On completing the exercises (guided discovery, rational responding via the DTR, and the A–D analysis), the patient was much more attentive to the disadvantages of using cocaine. She successfully developed control beliefs to strengthen resolve against future cocaine abuse. However, it is quite possible that she will not access these control beliefs when faced with "temptation," especially since she has overlearned her addictive beliefs. (This becomes especially evident in the Louise's last comment: "It's just easier to ignore control thoughts when I am using cocaine.") Hence, special attention must be paid to the activation of control beliefs as part of therapy. There are several methods that serve this purpose. Two methods presented in this section are flashcards and programmed practice in sessions. In the final section of this chapter we introduce "homework" as the ideal opportunity to practice activating control beliefs.

After the patient has developed control beliefs, flashcards can be used to reinforce and activate these newly developed beliefs. For example, on completing the A–D analysis the patient writes the disadvantages of using cocaine (i.e., control beliefs) on one or several 3" × 5" index cards. Louise's flashcards might list the following control beliefs:

"Getting high is fun but it has many disadvantages."

"Getting high could get me busted or killed."

"When I use cocaine, I give up control of my life."

"When I use cocaine, I become dependent on the drug and on others."

"When I use cocaine, I run the risk of losing my daughter."

In using the flashcards, Louise was encouraged to review her control beliefs on a daily basis and access them whenever she has an urge to use cocaine.

Programmed practice (or "covert rehearsal") in sessions, via imagery, is another tool for helping patients activate control beliefs. The patient is encouraged to imagine a tempting drug-related situation. As this situation evokes craving in patients, they activate control beliefs in the session in order to dampen the craving. The following dialogue between Louise and her therapist early in a session illustrates this technique:

TH: Louise, at the end of our last session you said that it was easy to ignore control beliefs when you are using cocaine. Today I would like to help you practice activating control beliefs so that they come more naturally when you find yourself in high-risk situations.

PT: That's a good idea, since those are the last thoughts on my mind just before I take a hit.

TH: I'd like you to imagine and then describe a typical tempting situation where you would be likely to use cocaine. Be as detailed and as vivid as possible in your imagination and description. When this is done correctly it is common for people to start craving cocaine. Don't be afraid or surprised if this happens. Actually, it is desirable; I want you to crave cocaine for the purposes of this exercise. When that happens we will practice activating your control beliefs, which should reduce the craving.

PT: Wow, that's weird. If you insist . . . (*long pause while Louise concentrates on images*) . . . OK, I've got it. A common scene is that I am at my mother's house with my daughter and my mother is ragging on me for not having a job. She is calling me all kinds of names: "lazy," "worthless," you know the list. Anyway, I feel this urge to run, but I know there's nowhere to go. I want to hit her but of course I don't. I want to cry, but I wouldn't give her the satisfaction of seeing that she has hurt me. And finally I start thinking about going to Michelle's house. She always knows were to find some shit. I think: "That's the one thing that will get me feeling better." I know that I can leave my daughter with my mother while I go out to get high. I also think about what I'll do if I don't find Michelle. If she's not around, I'll just go downtown and turn a quick trick. And then I get more intense feelings of wanting to get high . . . (*attention returns to therapist*) . . . Well, you've succeeded in making me crave the shit. Now what are you going to do?

TH: You are craving cocaine now?

PT: Damn straight!

TH: OK, now start reviewing your control beliefs out loud; you know what they are.

PT: The disadvantages?

TH: Yes, but say it with feeling! Take out your flashcards if you like.

PT: No, I don't need the flashcards. (*she begins tentatively at first, but then builds her enthusiasm*) I am *not* going to get high; my baby *needs* me. The stuff is *killing* me. It really doesn't make *anything* better. I'm better off without it. I can stay clean if I want to. I *can* make a life for myself and my baby if I *stay clean*! (*she smiles*)

TH: What are you thinking right now as you smile?

PT: That I can do it!

TH: Great!

In this dialogue, Louise succeeded in creating a strong urge to use cocaine, but she successfully countered that urge with control beliefs. This process was repeated several times over the next few sessions with Louise. For homework, she was encouraged to practice this exercise *in vivo*, as drug temptations naturally arise.

ASSIGN HOMEWORK THAT ADDRESSES BELIEFS

As in all other applications of cognitive therapy, homework involves applying the skills learned in therapy sessions. Thus, homework is a vital extension of therapy (Burns & Auerbach, 1992; Persons et al., 1988). As a long-term goal of homework in cognitive therapy, patients should learn to use self-guided Socratic questioning spontaneously in their lives; for example, "What evidence do I have for that belief?" "How else can I look at this situation?" "What are the consequences of my beliefs?"

Homework is an opportunity to practice applying control beliefs in the "real world." It may involve having patients practice activating control beliefs in the face of tempting high-risk stimuli, since they will never succeed in avoiding all tempting stimuli. Louise, for example, is unlikely to change her mother's behavior, although she can learn to cope more effectively with her. A specific homework assignment given to Louise, therefore, might be to practice control beliefs in response to her addictive beliefs and automatic thoughts when in the presence of her mother.

Homework may also involve testing addictive beliefs to evaluate their validity. For example, Bill might be challenged to try various methods for having fun, in order to test his belief that "there is nothing more fun than using cocaine."

As explained in Chapter 6 (this volume), homework is assigned at the end of each session and it is reviewed at the beginning of each follow-up session. Initially, homework is quite structured. For example, patients are instructed to complete DTRs on a daily basis. Later, however, homework can be less formal, as the patient develops new, more adaptive, patterns of thinking.

SUMMARY

The basic beliefs and automatic thoughts about drugs may account for much of their use. There are at least three types of drug-related beliefs that contribute to urges, craving, and ultimate use of drugs: anticipatory beliefs, relief-oriented beliefs, and permissive beliefs. The role of the cognitive therapist is to assess, examine, and test these beliefs with the patient, in order to ultimately replace them with control beliefs. There are many cognitive strategies that facilitate this process, many of which were presented in this chapter.

CHAPTER 12

Managing General Life Problems

Patients rarely enter treatment for drug addiction or dependence on their own accord in the absence of general life problems (Carey, 1991). When patients are in an early phase of their drug use, they are typically quite pleased with the effects of the drugs. This is so either because the drugs produce a state of unmatched excitement and euphoria or because they offer the abuser an artificial respite from the demands, pressures, ennui, and emotional pain that they may be suffering. At such times, patients operate under the assumption that the use of mood-altering chemicals offers a workable, viable option to functioning in a drug-free state of mind.

However, as the drug user becomes more regularly active in seeking, achieving, and repeating the "high" experience, a number of problems surface. Such problems include, but are not limited to, (1) the realization that drug use does not help the actual demands, responsibilities, and troubles of everyday life magically to go away; (2) the development of a physiological tolerance to the drugs, and therefore the need to expend more time, energy, and money in the search for the ever-elusive "high"; (3) the exacerbation of neglected life concerns, thus increasing stress and the desire to escape through the use of psychoactive substances; and (4) fallout from worsening habits, in terms of damaged relationships, vocational and/or academic failure, and serious medical and legal complications. It is in this advanced state of psychosocial difficulties and life crisis that the individual may be regarded as a drug abuser and will most likely appear for psychological treatment.

The therapist is faced with the daunting task of helping such patients not only to arrest and ameliorate their drug addictions, but also to deal with many serious real-life difficulties. While many of these problems are similar to those of any other diagnostic category of patient, there are many that are particularly salient to the drug-abusing population.

It is imperative that therapists be aware of the typical life problems that the drug-abusing patient presents at the start (and during the course) of treatment. It is equally important that these problems be given adequate attention in therapy, in spite of the temptation to focus solely on the substance abuse disorder. With this in mind, the current chapter presents an overview of the most common life issues that the cognitive therapist will need to address in the treatment of this challenging population.

"CHICKEN AND EGG" CONUNDRUM: WHICH COMES FIRST, SUBSTANCE ABUSE OR ASSOCIATED LIFE PROBLEMS?

An important assessment question concerns whether the patient's major life problems precede or postdate the onset of the substance abuse disorder. (Similarly, it is crucial to note whether the patient's antisocial behaviors are primary or secondary to the drug addiction. See Chapter 16, this volume, for more details.) Information regarding the chronology of life problems and drug abuse patterns can shed light on the "function" of the patient's use of psychoactive substances, as well as elucidating the factors that serve as triggers for the abuse of drugs.

For example, "Marla" presented with a crack addiction that had originally begun two years previously, in the aftermath of the violent death of her younger sister. After being arrested for possession, Marla spent the next three months in various inpatient rehabilitation facilities. When she was discharged, Marla was convinced that she would never "pick up" (resume using drugs) again, and that she was on the right track. However, shortly thereafter she was struck another blow when one of her best friends died. Almost immediately, she resumed her use of crack and once again found herself back in court. After a brief stay in jail she was released on parole, on the condition that she receive ongoing treatment. It was at this time that Marla entered cognitive therapy.

In Marla's case, grief and loss were powerful triggers for drug abuse. Since she had no history of drug abuse prior to the death of her sister, her prognosis was quite hopeful. It was clear that she had had many years of experience as a well-functioning, responsible person. Furthermore, her life was fairly well ordered, and her stressors were not out of the ordinary realm of everyday life. However, in order for therapy to be complete, it would be necessary to help Marla come to terms with the deaths of her sister and friend and her concomitant belief "I'm all alone."

Additionally, the therapist would need to teach the patient to use cognitive therapy skills in a preparatory fashion in anticipation of episodes associated with loss. For example, the illness of a significant other might be sufficient to induce Marla to have catastrophic expectations of that person dying. Such an extreme worry would put Marla at risk for relapse, as her anxiety at the thought of losing someone (and feeling alone) might induce her to self-medicate with crack cocaine. Similarly, the calendar became a source of negative cues that had to be anticipated, and that served as a therapeutic call to action. Major holidays, birthdays, and anniversaries of the deaths of loved ones had become capable of arousing upsetting automatic thoughts and emotions, the likes of which could trigger a resumption of drug abuse.

As it turned out, Marla learned the skills of rational responding, scheduling activities, and problem-solving quite well, and she survived the "anniversary phenomenon" without incident. However, when she was "blind-sided" by her boyfriend's decision to leave her, she suffered a temporary drug lapse (a single binge episode). Another interpersonal loss had triggered a need to blot out her emotional pain through the use of crack cocaine.

Marla's case seems straightforward—life problems preceded the onset of substance abuse. On the other hand, we see cases where the onset of serious life difficulties seems to occur as a result of the substance abuse. Until the time that "Roland" began using drugs in high school he seemed to have a fairly unremarkable life. He was an average student, came from an intact family free of substance abuse, and he had a circle of regular friends. After being introduced to marijuana, Roland began to skip classes and to disengage himself from his family, many of his friends, and most of his normal recreational activities.

As his drug use came to involve "harder" substances such as quaaludes and cocaine, he incurred more and more serious concomitant life problems. For example, although he somehow managed to graduate from high school, Roland did not pursue further education or vocational training, nor did he seek employment. His sole source of income was through petty drug trafficking. His parents, recognizing that something was dreadfully wrong, pressured Roland to "clean up his act" and to get a job. This frequently led to screaming and shoving matches between son and father. Finally, after Roland's parents were frightened by two incidents when drug associates came to the door in the middle of the night, Roland was told to leave the house. Shortly thereafter, Roland was arrested for driving while intoxicated, as well as for possession of a controlled substance.

Roland's steadily increasing problems with substance abuse led to academic and vocational stagnation, family conflicts, loss of his primary domicile, and legal troubles. His main interests and activities were reduced to procuring, using, and selling illicit substances. His chief associates were drug users and dealers, and he had no friends who led a drug-free lifestyle. Roland's drug use had led to numerous negative consequences in his life, yet his sense of helplessness in dealing with these mounting difficulties, coupled with his desire to "forget all his troubles" through the use of drugs such as cocaine, perpetuated his drug-related lifestyle. These were problems that had to be addressed when Roland ultimately entered therapy, in addition to his problematic abuse of drugs per se.

Although the cases of Marla and Roland seem quite distinct in that the former suffered identifiable life troubles as a precipitating factor to the onset of her drug abuse, while the latter produced the majority of his own life problems as the result of his apparently "unprovoked" recreational use of drugs, the two cases have at least one very important similarity.

Both patients eventually became trapped in a *vicious cycle*, where the dual problems of drug abuse and general life problems began to exacerbate each other. For example, Marla's use of crack cocaine, originally the result of her grief, became the cause of her arrest and incarceration. Aside from the obvious negative impact that this had on her life in its own right, Marla further suffered from an inability to find employment as a result of her criminal record. In her anger and frustration, she once again resorted to the use of crack cocaine. Renewed legal troubles soon ensued, and the vicious cycle was complete.

Roland's vicious cycle of substance abuse and life crises was even more entrenched and self-perpetuating than Marla's. His "druggie lifestyle" led to numerous personal, financial, and legal complications. He had no stable relationships, no sense of trust for others, no sense of self-esteem when he came off his high, no legal source of income, no healthy sources of stimulation and pleasure, no treatment for numerous medical problems, and a constant nagging fear of criminal apprehension. All these concerns were quickly "fixed" by using drugs such as cocaine, thus keeping him firmly ensconced in his drug lifestyle. Drugs were a major source of his chaos and crises, yet he continued to view them as his only "solution" to deal with these problems. Later, when Roland began treatment, he would not only have to overcome his addictions, he literally would have to "get a life" as well. (Roland's personality disorders also played an important role with regard to his drug use and general life problems. For more on this, see Chapter 16, this volume, on the interaction between substance abuse and personality disorders.)

In either of these prototypical cases, the life problems represent broad "stimulus situations" that both trigger and are worsened by the patient's continuing abuse of substances. Figure 12.1 illustrates the beliefs and automatic thoughts that feed into this process.

As depicted by Figure 12.1, the patient's chronic unemployment serves as a stimulus situation that sets off a chain of beliefs, automatic thoughts, and actions that lead to drug use. The patient's drug use then contributes to his or her becoming less employable (less motivated, less reliable, etc.), and the cycle continues.

This chapter focuses on the major areas of *chronic* life stress that plague so many substance abuse patients. (See Chapter 13, this volume, for examples of common *acute* crises and emergencies, many of which are related to the issues described later.) Some of these are more likely to be precursors to a drug problem, while some are more clearly the sequelae to drug abuse. In either case, it is important to bear in mind the way that these trouble spots become part of a vicious

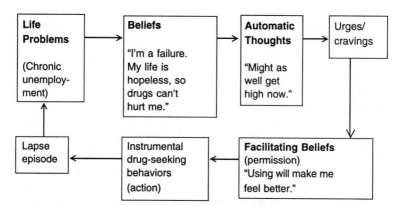

FIGURE 12.1. The vicious cycle of life problems and drug abuse.

cycle that has spiraled out of control. The following life problems are described in detail here: marital and family problems, socioeconomic problems, daily stressors, legal problems, and medical problems.

MARITAL AND FAMILY PROBLEMS

As noted earlier, it is vital for patients to be aware of the "people, places, and things" that they associate with the using of illicit substances. In the early stages of treatment, it is wise for the substance abuser who is trying to remain drug-free to avoid needlessly coming into contact with stimuli that might provoke strong cravings or facilitate the obtaining of drugs. (Later in treatment, however, it is important to teach patients to apply and practice self-help techniques in the face of those kinds of drug-related stimuli that may be unavoidable in their everyday lives.) When the "people" and "places" are impersonal acquaintances and out-of-the-way locations, it is reasonably straightforward (under the proper motivational and coping conditions) for the patient to steer clear of these stimuli. The picture is decidedly more difficult when the people and places are the patient's own family members, in the patient's own residence. Substance abuse amongst one's relatives poses a serious problem for the patient. In terms of etiology, a person whose parents or siblings abuse drugs is at risk for modeling these behaviors (Gomberg & Nirenberg, 1991; Lang, 1992). The patient may have easy access to drug paraphernalia, and may have knowledge of family members' secret stashes.

In terms of maintenance and relapse, the patient may have a particularly difficult time turning away from the continual lure of drugs when family members are high, when these family members encourage the patient to get high as well, and when drugs and money are so blatantly available at all hours of the day. Furthermore, there may be strong social pressures to conform to the "drug subculture" in the household. One of our patients, Dee, was taunted unmercifully by her two substance-abusing brothers for her attempts to stay away from drugs and to attend therapy and support group meetings. They attempted to "bring her down" by ripping into her for her "holier-than-thou" attitude, hoping that she would succumb to their barbs by joining them in their smoking binges. Luckily for Dee, these brothers lived a block away, so she did not have to deal with them on a constant basis. As it was, however, a great deal of time and energy in therapy was spent in learning how to assert herself effectively to her brothers, and to respond rationally to her own initial automatic thoughts. These thoughts included "If you can't beat 'em, join 'em,"

"I have to get them off my back," and "I have to prove that I ain't stuck up."

Rational responses that were generated in response to these automatic thoughts included the following:

1. "If they [the brothers] want to be losers, that's their business. I'm doing the right thing by staying straight."
2. "I'd rather that my brothers hate me than go back to using and have my kids hate me." My kids are much more important."
3. "I'm not stuck up. I'm trying to be humble and know my limitations. My brothers are the ones who are being stuck up, only they're so stoned they don't see it."
4. "I can't change my brothers, so why should I let them change me?" and,
5. "I've dealt with worse hassles before. I'll just remind myself that everything they say is just bullshit, and I'll get back to my own business."

Dee was able to defend herself from her brothers' attempts at heavy-handed peer pressure, but the fact that her two "favorite" siblings had drug problems was a considerable source of stress for her. Dee believed that her brothers' drug problems signified that she came from a family of "losers," each member of which (including herself) inevitably would have a life filled with troubles. Furthermore, she believed that she would need to stay away from her brothers as much as possible, thus depriving her of what had once been enjoyable and companionable sibling relationships. This exacerbated her sense of loneliness.

It is generally unrealistic for patients to expect that they can solve the substance abuse problems of family members. It is generally wisest to focus on cognitive coping skills that enable patients to gain some distance from the problem, and to stay focused on their own recovery. Toward this end, support group meetings can be recommended as an adjunct to cognitive therapy, especially when patients feel overly guilty for family members' drug problems. The negative experiences that these patients have had during their upbringing in alcohol and drug-using households can be discussed as part of treatment as well. This builds rapport between patient and therapist and helps to elucidate implicit dysfunctional rules about substance abuse and family relationships that the patients may have learned.

To have a mate who is self-absorbed in drug abuse entails tremendous stress for a patient. Problems include the partner's (1) having erratic mood swings, (2) being financially and sexually reckless and irresponsible, (3) risking major medical and legal consequences, (4) endangering the patient with regard to AIDS and other sexually transmitted diseases, and (5) seducing the patient into relapsing into substance abuse once again. When a drug-addicted mate refuses to acknowledge a problem or to get help, it is often necessary for the patient either to leave the household or to induce the mate to leave. Such a strategy may be the best way to maintain a home environment that is conducive to recovery. In order to maximize the chances that patients will be willing be go along with such a strategy, therapists can emphasize that it may not be necessary to leave the relationship permanently, but that such a move may be needed at present.

The drawbacks to the above strategy, in the mind of the patient, may be compelling. The patient may be loath to confront a potentially violent partner, and may not have the resources to make a clean start in another domicile. Furthermore, the patient is forced to face the loss of a significant love relationship—a daunting realization, especially if the patient has dependent personality characteristics (see Chapter 16, this volume). When this is the case, the therapist may notice that the patient seems excessively emotionally attached to the substance-abusing partner, no matter what the personal cost. In short, the patient may love the partner deeply, in spite of this person's drug abuse. The patient may go to great lengths to excuse or cover up the partner's transgressions, because the prospect of losing the partner (or even of hearing negative feedback about the partner) is too much to bear. Even worse, the patient may collude with the partner to use drugs together in secret and to provide cover for each other. Such phenomena have been written about extensively in recent times under the rubric of "co-dependency" (cf. Lyon & Greenberg, 1991).

In such cases, cognitive interventions must focus heavily on adaptive problem-solving (Platt & Hermalin, 1989), and on the patient's exaggerated guilt and fears of loneliness. For example, the patient may believe erroneously that the significant other would use more drugs if left alone, when in reality the significant other is demonstrating an escalating drug problem whether the patient is there or not. Similarly, the patient may believe that he or she could not bear the loneliness of being without the drug-using partner, when in actuality the patient already is coping with being functionally alone, as the drug-using partner is emotionally absent. Additionally, it is vital to teach the patient to expand his or her social network of nonusers, so that the substance-abusing mate is no longer the dominant source of interpersonal reinforcement.

At the same time, patient and therapist must be ever vigilant to the patient's own vulnerabilities to using drugs. It is important to pay close attention to the way that the patient's chronic life problems and substance abuse feed into each other, rather than looking at each problem in isolation. For example, in the case of the patient whose significant other is abusing drugs, the belief that "if I stay off drugs I will have to give up the person I love and be all alone" may prime the patient to resume using drugs.

"Walter" had told his therapist many times that the love of his children was one of the only things he cared about in his life. Therefore, the fact that he was now not permitted to see them was a source of tremendous distress. As a result, he escalated his drug bingeing—partly out of a belief that "a greater amount of drugs is needed to blot out a greater amount of suffering," and partly out of a desire to make a suicidal gesture that would attract attention and care—and soon wound up in the hospital due to overdose-induced convulsions. His failure to handle his distress without the use of chemical substances led to an accentuation of his sense of loss (his children), which in turn brought about a life-threatening exacerbation of his drug abuse.

Following his release from the hospital, and his resumption of outpatient cognitive therapy, a great deal of time in session was spent in reviewing the pros and cons of various strategies for coping with interpersonal loss. Among the most favored therapeutic suggestions were seeking the support of others, such as family, friends, and therapist, and focusing on work-related activities, especially those that required a great deal of strenuous physical labor. Additionally, Walter was instructed to respond to his urges to buy and use drugs by conjuring up images of his children, the people he most wanted to be proud of him. These images were to serve as strong deterrents to his initiating the search for drugs (however, they were less effective in stopping him from using once he had the drugs and paraphernalia in his hands).

Ongoing marital discord (or discord in any love relationship) can serve as a powerful stimulus for drug cravings and drug abuse. We have seen patients use drugs in such cases for a variety of purposes. Such "functions" of the drug use include (1) reviving a chemically based, false and temporary boost in self-esteem; (2) exerting control in the relationship by defying the spouse, and by inducing a self-protective state of apathy or invulnerability; (3) "soothing" the anger that is felt toward the spouse, especially if the patient has the belief that not using something will lead to an escalating physical confrontation; and (4) finding an emotional escape from marital unhappiness, especially if the drug-abusing spouse believes that there is no way to solve the marital problem or to leave the marriage. In general, unhappiness and anger in a relationship feed into patients' feelings of helplessness and loneliness, which in turn may lead to a wish for immediate relief. The result may be a craving for drugs, followed by their use.

It is not surprising to note that the use of drugs within the context of a marriage will likely affect the relationship adversely. If the marriage is already disturbed, the substance abuse will exacerbate matters, thus contributing to yet another vicious cycle. The situation is perhaps most dire when the abuse of substances leads to physical, psychological, and/or sexual assault. In contrast to the oft-held belief (alluded to above) that the use of drugs can "soothe" the angry spouse, drug use actually more often than not serves to disinhibit and to activate the potential for violence (Amaro, Fried, Cabral, & Zuckerman, 1990). Therefore, the therapist must be ever vigilant to possible signs of domestic violence in the life of the substance-abusing patient. Along with this vigilance, it is wise for the therapist to have ready access to information about crisis hotlines and shelters for victims of physical and sexual abuse.

If the patient is primarily a perpetrator of such violence, the therapist must do all that is possible to contract with the patient to deal with this problem as a number one priority in treatment. As discussed previously in Chapter 4 (this volume), the limits of confidentiality that exist when the patient is a threat to the well-being of others need to be spelled out. At the same time, great therapeutic skill must be employed to keep the patient positively engaged in the process of therapy and to keep the patient's trust.

An examination of the patient's personal and family history may demonstrate that physical, psychological, and sexual abuse during the patient's childhood and adolescence played a significant role in the development of the patient's drug problem. (Note: In order to highlight patterns and relational configurations in the patient's family, it is sometimes useful to map out a family tree on paper. Such a tree can indicate separations, divorces, deaths, abusive relationships, persons who abused alcohol and drugs, and the like.) This may be true for any number of reasons, such as (1) the aversive conditions at home force patients to spend more and more time on the streets, thus exposing them more to the drug culture; (2) the perpetrators of violence in the family may be drug abusers themselves, thus modeling the behavior for the victims to emulate; (3) the use of drugs may be viewed as the only means of escape from an intolerable situation at home; and (4) the loss of self-esteem that is incurred over years of being abused creates an increased addictive vulnerability in victims, as they search for quick ways to produce good feelings and to obtain a crowd of associates who will validate them and do the same.

These background factors produce such beliefs as "Using drugs is a natural way of life," "Violence—particularly when under the influence—is acceptable," "Using is the only way of blotting out unpleasant feelings," and "I am weak and inferior and can feel good (and accepted) only by using."

In treating such patients, self-esteem issues become a central component to the therapy. Therapists can help their patients begin to develop a stronger internal deterrent to drug abuse if they find (and work to build) evidence that dispels the patients' notions that they are worthless, deserving of a troubled life, and incapable of meeting their own needs through more socially acceptable and healthier means.

SOCIOECONOMIC PROBLEMS

Substance abuse disorders frequently occur against the backdrop of socioeconomic problems. For example, in the last decade we have witnessed a significant increase in the prevalence of cocaine abuse among the impoverished of our inner cities (Closser, 1992; O'Brien et al., 1992). Crack cocaine in particular has become more and more frequently abused within this milieu (Gawin & Ellinwood, 1988; Smart, 1991). As the people of this segment of society grow more and more disillusioned with their chances of improving their lots in life through standard long-term means (e.g., finding quality education, staying in school, and working one's way up a ladder of vocational success), they may be more inclined to turn to nonstandard, short-term fixes (e.g., using drugs for a boost in mood and selling drugs for an increase in income).

It has been argued that it is quite difficult to steer children, adolescents, and adults alike away from drugs when so few alternatives for finding enjoyment exist in the immediate environment. Additionally, it is equally difficult to stay focused on the distant rewards of schooling, or the modest remuneration of low-level employment, when the distribution of drugs can produce staggering material rewards in a relatively short space of time. Furthermore, the risks of arrest and incarceration, overdose and poisoning, and violence are less of a deterrent against using drugs when there is a prevailing sense that the future holds no promise anyway. This is especially so for vulnerable individuals who have developed core beliefs of hopelessness and helplessness.

For these reasons and others, therapy with lower socioeconomic status substance abusers poses considerable challenges to the therapist. Walter typified this type of patient. When the therapist made an attempt to appeal to Walter's sense of pride and self-worth (in order to counteract his belief that he was a helpless victim) by asking if he could be "strong enough to be a man and walk away from his dealing friends," Walter replied, "I don't feel strong when I walk away from drugs. I feel like nothing, like I always do. I only feel like I'm worth something when I use a little something [usually cocaine or heroin]. That's the only time I feel like a big shot." In order to combat this drug-abuse-fostering attitude, the therapist focused Walter's attention on how he felt after he came down off his high, which was lower, weaker, more helpless, and less adequate than ever. This fact was reviewed time and time again, so as to deromanticize the false sense of pride that the use of drugs seemed to induce temporarily.

Another critical component of treatment in this instance was to help Walter to recognize things in his life in which he could take pride while in a drug-free and alcohol-free state of mind. These included his skill as a longshoreman, his physical strength, and the love and pride of his children. Still, Walter had difficulty focusing on these factors, especially when he felt frustrated in reaching his goals. At times of despair and anger, he would lapse into all-or-none thinking, believing that he had nothing worth living for. Walter liked to make a point of this by quoting Bob Dylan's immortal line, "When you ain't got nothing, you ain't got nothing to lose." This saying activated the belief that "I have nothing and I am nothing," and fostered his tendency to turn to drugs when he would suffer a disappointment. It therefore became critical to (1) discuss the precious things he did indeed have, such as the love and respect of his children, and (2) how he would lose them if he were to indulge in drug abuse. It should be noted that one of the most important opportunities for producing changes in basic beliefs occurs when those beliefs have been activated, as by a disappointment or frustration.

On the other end of the socioeconomic spectrum we see affluent patients who have become substance abusers. Some common rationales proffered by more financially successfully substance abusers resemble those of lower socioeconomic status patients, revolving around core beliefs of being ineffective or socially undesirable. One patient stated that he began his cocaine use at a time (ten years earlier) when it was still considered "cool" to get high, and when cocaine was viewed as a drug of particularly high status amongst those on the fast track. He noted that the drug accentuated his feelings of power, attractiveness, and invulnerability—feelings that were not only pleasing to him but also congruent with his view of what a corporate vice-president should be. Although he started as a social user, his continued usage led to physiological and psychological tolerance, which necessitated that he increase the quantity and frequency of his usage. As a result of his financial affluence he was able to continue his habit unabated. In this sense, his wealth served as a contributory causal factor in the development of his full-blown cocaine dependence.

Ultimately, his performance at work deteriorated and he was unceremoniously fired. Following this event, he was unable to attain another position at the same level. The patient hypothesized that he had been blackballed within the local corporate community. At this point, he found himself in financial crisis, as he had not diminished his lavish life-style or cocaine usage, although he had ceased to have an income. As a result, he fell into a state of considerable crisis, with a serious cocaine dependence, and faced the threat of bankruptcy. It was only at this advanced stage of life difficulties and cocaine abuse that he sought therapy. At this time, he has succeeded in remaining free of cocaine for a number of months, although he is still moderately depressed about his significant loss of status, money, and friends. Therapy continues to focus on (1) problem-solving with regard to earning a livelihood, (2) dealing with continuing cravings for cocaine (although they have diminished somewhat over time), and (3) rebuilding his self-esteem, which deflated when he lost his high-profile lifestyle and had to look at himself without the masked feelings provided by cocaine.

Another high socioeconomic status patient reasoned that he began using cocaine in order to increase his energy and confidence. He came to believe that he would be unable to perform his job without the "boost" that he received from using the drug. He also enjoyed the temporary sense of a release of pressure, and therefore was convinced that cocaine was a stress reducer. Predictably, as his habit grew, his perceptions of the quality of his work became distorted and inflated way beyond reality. He became less productive, and more and more interpersonally aversive due to his advanced symptoms of paranoia and impulsive anger outbursts. In similar fashion to the patient mentioned previously, he lost his job and incurred financial debts. Additionally, he was shunned by his friends and lover after he repeatedly rejected their suggestions that he receive help for his problems.

A factor that both high and low socioeconomic status drug-abusing patients have in common is a vulnerability to peer pressure. Lower socioeconomic status patients are frequently confronted by friends and associates who urge them to use, share, and sell drugs. Such patients may come to believe that they will be deprived of meaningful social contact if they avoid every substance abuser they know. As we witnessed in the case of Dee, the razzing that her brothers gave her for not joining them in their smoking binges provided a strong temptation for her to use again. In this case, it was vital to help her to seek and develop contacts and friendships with people who were abstinent from drugs and alcohol.

Other lower socioeconomic status patients may feel pressured by their associates to prove that they are "one of the gang," or that they have the "guts" to use drugs heavily. Walter told his therapist that he was challenged to shoot up a powerful combination of cocaine and heroin by a couple of guys he knew at a junkyard where he often hung out. When the therapist suggested some typical "middle-class liberal" (patient's description) assertive comments that he could make in response to their challenge, Walter replied, "You can't talk that kind of intellectual crap in my neighborhood. Maybe it works in your neighborhood, but not in mine." With this, the therapist adjusted the intervention by putting the responsibility for generating "proud, drug-free comebacks" onto Walter's shoulders. This episode highlights the role that socioeconomic characteristics play in conceptualizing problems and designing interventions.

The peer pressure may take on a different form among the upper socioeconomic status patients, but it exists nonetheless. For example, a patient at an exclusive party may become convinced that he must join in with the "recreational" cocaine users in order to be considered one of the "beautiful people." Fortunately, this distorted, over-romanticized view of the wealthy cocaine user has more recently fallen into disfavor, as the extent and ramifications of the nation's cocaine problems have come to light since the latter half of the 1980s.

In another vein, the more affluent cocaine user may be motivated by a need to gain even more money, more power, and more success as a way to gain acceptance by the perceived upper echelon in his or her profession or community. In this drive to succeed, the patient may resort to a chemical stimulant such as cocaine in order to give him or her a sense of increased productivity and sociability.

When peer pressure (in any form) is a factor that contributes to substance abuse, it becomes necessary to address the patient's excessive need for social acceptance. In this regard, self-esteem issues come to the fore. Furthermore, therapist and patient must work together to help the patient learn more adaptive social problem-solving skills, so that drugs are no longer considered part of the "solution."

DAILY STRESSORS

Mundane problems or stressors can serve as triggers for patients' drug use. The daily hassles that people face, such as working at a job that entails pressure and deadlines, or one in which they feel trapped for financial reasons, or dealing with two or three unruly toddlers on a continual basis without a respite, can create feelings that exceed a person's tolerance for discomfort. An accumulation of such stressful events and feelings, experienced day after day, can serve as factors that encourage a person to resort to drugs in order to "get through the day."

"Dee" was a patient for whom the management of everyday concerns was central to her maintaining abstinence. An important therapeutic priority for Dee entailed helping her cope with taking care of her infant son. As a single parent, Dee was confronted with a great deal of change in her daily life when her son was born. She had been happy working long hours as an assistant in a nursing home; now she had to curtail her hours considerably. She had also been used to coming and going as she pleased, as her older children were adolescents who could be trusted to take care of themselves in their mother's absence. Now, Dee's freedom of movement was restricted, and she had to plan her activities with her baby's care in mind. In addition, Dee was very troubled and annoyed by her son's nocturnal crying spells. In sum, the everyday demands of being responsible for the well-being of an infant reinforced in Dee a sense of inadequacy (as a mother), helplessness (in taking care of all her responsibilities), and hopelessness (in ever enjoying life again). These core beliefs were sources of marked anger, frustration, and sadness, the likes of which touched off thoughts and cravings to smoke crack as her "only" source of pleasure and "freedom."

It was clear that keeping Dee away from the lure of drugs would necessitate lessons in coping with her new life as the primary caregiver for a helpless child. Among other therapeutic strategies, problem-solving and the planning of daily activities (working a few hours, arranging baby-sitting for her child, attending a support group meeting, spending time with her baby, reading, etc.) were reviewed and employed. In addition, much time was spent in using Daily Thought Records to counteract Dee's thoughts that suggested to her that her life would now be intolerably restricted. Indeed, she was encouraged to consider rational responses that focused on various potential benefits that she would now receive as a result of her newborn's arrival. For example, she would have the opportunity to disprove all the critics who told her that she would not be able to raise this child due to her drug habit. Naturally, this rational response was a powerful positive motivator to engage in the process of cognitive therapy; however, it also gave rise to another automatic thought. Specifically, Dee worried that a lapse into drug use would lead to everyone's giving up on her, judging her negatively, telling her "I told you so," and taking her baby away from her.

In order to safeguard against this possible eventuality, Dee and her therapist worked on strengthening her reactions to her areas of greatest vulnerability. Specifically, Dee was taught how to better deal with her baby's crying fits (which perturbed her very much). In session, Dee was instructed to close her eyes and to imagine being at home at a given time when her baby was crying without letting up. When Dee indicated that she could indeed "hear" her baby crying, she was encouraged to express her automatic thoughts. Given Dee's aptitude for vivid imaging, her automatic thoughts truly represented her "hot" (i.e., affectively charged) cognitions. These included "I can't stand it anymore. I have to get out of here," and "I'm going to go out and pick up again [use drugs again], and then my aunt will have to come and take care of my son. Then I'll be free again." After reciting these thoughts, Dee was then instructed to imagine what her life would be like in the aftermath of these events. With this, she would become remorseful, and would begin to express rational responses to override the hot cognitions elicited above.

As the exercise continued, Dee spontaneously generated more automatic thoughts that further explained her negative emotionality in response to her baby's crying. She thought, "My baby doesn't love me. My baby doesn't want to be with me. He'd rather be with the sitter. He'd rather be with my aunt." These thoughts fed into Dee's sense of rejection. In response, Dee was encouraged to consider alternative meanings to her son's crying, such as "He's trying to tell me he's uncomfortable—that he's hungry, or cold, or needing to be changed," and "He's just being a baby. He's not telling me he doesn't love me. He doesn't even understand stuff like that yet. He's just being a baby."

Still keeping her eyes closed, Dee was then told to imagine the self-satisfaction she would feel if she resisted the temptation to use drugs, and instead proved to herself and others that she was capable of taking care of this child. In addition, Dee was assisted in imagining the distant future, when her then grown-up son would love her and think highly of her, because she was always there for him and because he saw her as a positive role model. These techniques, repeated in different variations over the course of a number of sessions, were highly efficacious in helping Dee to see herself as being a person worthy of love, and effective in dealing with the stressors of life. As her core beliefs of helplessness and unlovability diminished, Dee became more consistent in remaining abstinent from drugs and alcohol. In turn, her mothering skills improved.

Stressors of daily living can include any events that trigger a sense of frustration, anxiety, anger, fatigue, and loneliness. When such events occur frequently, or involve chronic conditions such as living in a noxious home environment or in an undesirable neighborhood, then the therapist needs to help drug-abusing patients to anticipate and adaptively respond to their maladaptive reactions to these situations. In this way, patients may learn to become adept at coping with (and solving) the commonplace triggers that put them at daily risk for substance abuse.

LEGAL PROBLEMS

Where there is illicit substance abuse, there is the threat of criminal apprehension. This is so not only because of the patient's drug use itself, but because drug use often leads to additional illegal activities as well. For example, Dee was first arrested when she was caught trying to cash forged checks. Walter's criminal conviction resulted from his hijacking and fencing stolen goods from the docks where he worked. "Charleen" was apprehended when she sold crack to an undercover officer.

When a patient enters treatment as a condition of parole or probation, the therapist needs to be aware not only of the difficulties that the patient will have in trying to stay away from drugs, but also of the difficulties that the patient will have in coping with the constraints and stigma associated with being in legal limbo. Charleen often expressed her consternation at having to be monitored by both the therapist and the parole office. For her, almost every therapy session and urinalysis served as a reminder that her life was not entirely her own. As she dwelled on all the drawbacks of this situation (e.g., loss of freedom), her anger grew, and with it her defiant desires to renew her drug use as well. Figure 12.2 represents one of the Daily Thought Records that Charleen worked on in order to quell the anger and cravings associated with such negative thoughts about her parolee status. Until she used the Daily Thought Record, Charleen had never considered the advantages that her legal and psychological monitoring provided for her—namely, added support and incentive to remain drug free.

Walter also experienced a significant degree of dysphoria in reaction to automatic thoughts about his legal status. In particular, he was frustrated and angered by the limitations set on his traveling by the terms of his parole. He believed that most of his problems had to do with his family members and his neighborhood acquaintances who abused drugs. He rationalized (not to be confused with rationally responding!) that he would stand a better chance of staying away from drugs if he could move upstate to a more rural area. In fact, he applied

Directions: When you notice your mood getting worse, ask yourself, "What's going through my mind right now?" and as soon as possible jot down the thought or mental image in the Automatic Thought Column.

DATE/ TIME	SITUATION Describe: 1. Actual event leading to unpleasant emotion, or 2. Stream of thoughts, day-dreams or recollection, leading to unpleasant emotion, or 3. Distressing physical sensations	AUTOMATIC THOUGHT(S) 1. Write automatic thought(s) that preceded emotion(s). 2. Rate belief in automatic thought(s) 0–100%.	EMOTION(S) 1. Specify sad, anxious/ angry, etc. 2. Rate degree of emotion 0–100%.	RATIONAL RESPONSE 1. Write rational response to automatic thought(s). 2. Rate belief in rational response 0–100%.	OUTCOME 1. Re-rate belief in automatic thought(s) 0–100% 2. Specify and rate subsequent emotions 0–100%.
	I'm on the bus going to my therapy session. I have to go. I don't have a choice or I'll mess up my parole and I'll have to go back to jail.	1. I hate this, I hate this, I hate this! 2. Why do I have to be watched like this? 3. I hate being monitored. I hate ruining my day to go see my parole officer and my therapist. It makes me mad. 4. I should be allowed to live my own life. 5. I'm being treated like a criminal and a baby. 6. I want my freedom back now!! (100% for all thoughts)	1. Hate (100%) 2. Anger (100%) 3. Frustration (100%)	I have to be watched like this so I won't go back on drugs again and mess up my life again. (80%) I may hate it, but it's better than being a crackhead and going to jail. (100%) Being monitored makes me more careful to stay off drugs, so I guess it's helping me. (60%) My parole officer and my therapist want me to be OK. I guess they care about me, even if they annoy me sometimes. (100%) I guess these meetings could have a good reason. (50%) I'll get my freedom soon enough! (100%)	1. Hate (50%) 2. Anger (50%) 3. Frustration (80%) 4. Calmed down (50%)

Questions to help formulate the rational response: (1) What is the evidence that the automatic thought is true? Not true? (2) Is there an alternative explanation? (3) What's the *worst* that could happen? Could I live through it? What's the *best* that could happen? What's the *most realistic* outcome? (4) What should I do about it? (5) What's the effect of my believing the automatic thought? What could be the effect of changing my thinking? (6) If _____ was in this situation and had this thought, what would I tell him/her?
(friend's name)

FIGURE 12.2. Charleen's Daily Thought Record.

to the parole office for a change of venue, but was told that he would have to wait a considerable length of time before this could be approved. Walter reacted with a sense of hopelessness, along with cynicism and anger. Now, every time he came into contact with the "problem people" he alluded to above, Walter would think that he was now justified in using drugs. His rationalization was, "Hey, I tried to get away from these people, but the cops wouldn't let me. If I fuck up, it's on their heads." Naturally, the therapist in this case spent considerable time in getting Walter to modify his views on this matter, and to find alternative methods for steering clear of these "people and places."

Another legal concern that drug-abusing patients sometimes face is loss of custody of their children, either to an ex-spouse, a relative, or to child protection services. Dee was one such patient. Her aunt in Baltimore had taken care of Dee's baby son for two months while Dee went through an inpatient drug abuse rehabilitation program. Dee knew that her aunt was waiting in the wings to assume custody of the child if Dee were to relapse. In fact, Dee's aunt had stated that she would seek to become the child's legal guardian if Dee were to demonstrate that she were an unfit mother. Rather than viewing her aunt as a safety net, she saw her as a threat, and often got herself agitated over the possibility that she would lose her baby. Such a perception produced added pressure on Dee, which exacerbated her urges to resume her use of crack cocaine.

In this case, Dee was confronted with the very real possibility of losing custody of her child. The therapist aimed to help Dee to view this as a motivator to stay straight, rather than as a sword of Damocles hanging over her head. Furthermore, rather than suspiciously treating her aunt as an evil adversary, Dee was taught to cooperate and work with the aunt. It was noted that they both shared a common concern—namely, the welfare of the baby.

It should also be noted that therapists who treat drug-abusing populations are confronted with more legal and ethical questions than are those who treat most other groups. For example, the association between drug use and domestic violence means that therapists have to be especially vigilant to situations that would require a duty to warn an intended victim, or a duty to contact agencies that monitor child or spouse abuse cases. Managing such situations, while also maintaining a constructive therapeutic relationship with the patient, requires considerable skill indeed.

Another legal–ethical situation that we have encountered occurs when a patient attends a therapy session in an intoxicated state. Whether or not the therapist chooses to continue with the session is subject to personal choice and/or case-by-case decision-making. However, if the therapist chooses to interact with the patient, it is imperative that the therapist assess whether the patient has driven a vehicle to the therapist's office. If the patient has in fact driven to session, the therapist should make every effort to keep the patient off the highway until such time as he or she is sober. In one case, we required a patient to remain in the waiting room for two hours before permitting him to leave the Center. Other alternatives include calling a cab, using public transportation, or contacting a relative who could give the patient a lift.

MEDICAL PROBLEMS

Drug abuse is associated with a myriad of chronic medical conditions (O'Connor, Chang, & Shi, 1992). Even when the patient has given up drugs altogether, the medical consequences of the abuse may linger indefinitely, causing pain, worry, hopelessness, and renewed urges to "self-medicate" via the use of illicit drugs. This phenomenon is well illustrated by a scene in the film *Bird*, the story of the legendary jazz saxophonist Charlie Parker. Parker, whose hard-drinking, hard-drugging, and hard-driving lifestyle led to the development of excruciating gastric ulcers, used heroin to deaden the pain. This habit only served to hasten his death at the age of 34. In one scene, he tearfully tells his drug-free friend, Dizzy Gillespie, "Ain't it a bitch . . . I go to the doctor and pay him $75, and it don't help me . . . but I go to some 'cat' and pay him $10 for a bag of shit [heroin], and my ulcers don't hurt, my liver don't hurt, my heart troubles is gone . . . and you tryin' to tell me that *this* is the man I'm supposed to stay *away* from? Mr. Gillespie, my comrade in arms, that is what I call a paradox."

Therapists need to be aware of the medical issues involved in substance abuse, so as to be able to educate the patient about such matters, as well as to be able to detect physical signs that indicate that the patient may have relapsed.

A patient who is actively abusing hard drugs such as cocaine, heroin, or amphetamines, may be a malnourished and sleep-disturbed patient as well. Charleen had the misconception that the use of crack cocaine produced a beneficial weight loss. She lamented her weight gain during her recovery and treatment period, and talked about "the good old days" when she was using and was thin. The therapist taught her that her weight loss reflected a dysfunctional dependence on a drug that in no way substituted for nutrition. He emphasized that weight loss needed to be achieved through exercise and sensible eating habits, not through drug-induced loss of appetite.

It is common for patients who go on drug binges to be awake all night (while they are using), and to sleep most of the day. Another variation of sleep disturbance involves the patient's remaining awake for days at a time, and then crashing for a number of days. In either case, the body's natural sleep cycle has been badly disrupted, and normal vocational and social functioning ceases to be possible.

It is noteworthy when a patient misses an afternoon therapy session due to "oversleeping," or sounds groggy on the phone in the middle of the day. These are some of the telltale signs of substance abuse (Gawin & Kleber, 1988). In fact, a number of high-profile athletes who were discovered to be cocaine abusers were first suspected as a result of oversleeping for important team practices, meetings, or travel obligations.

Whenever practically feasible, we like to schedule our most difficult patients for the earliest appointments. A 9:00 A.M. appointment minimizes the likelihood that a patient will be able to mask the fact he or she used drugs the day before. At times when an early therapy session cannot be arranged, early-morning phone checks can be utilized. For example, a patient may be instructed (as part of his homework assignment) to call the therapist each day at a specified midmorning time, just for a minute. When a patient complains that a session or a telephone call is too early to comply with, we respond by saying, "If you can't attend a therapy meeting at 9:00 A.M., will you be able to keep a job that requires you to be there at 9:00 A.M.?"

In the same way that drug-abusing patients are often less than maximally compliant with therapy, they too are frequently noncompliant with medical advice. When the patient has a steady physician, it is important to obtain the necessary releases so as to have ongoing contact with the doctor. When the patient is on public assistance, and therefore may not see the same doctor with each medical visit, the situation is a bit more convoluted. Nevertheless, it is important to make every effort to keep apprised of the patient's medical conditions and treatments.

One of our most stubborn cases of medical noncompliance was "Ray," who suffered from a serious case of diabetes and was insulin-dependent. His maladaptive approach to his condition was a continual cause for concern in treatment. During one period in the course of therapy, he refused to inject himself with his required daily dosage of insulin, saying that he could control his blood-glucose level simply by watching his diet carefully. When this was questioned, Ray added that the use of a needle (to inject insulin) would be a powerful inducement for him to shoot up "something a little harder than insulin." Needless to say, this posed quite a dilemma.

To make matters worse, Ray refused to consult with his physician on this matter. The therapist attempted to appeal to the patient's sense of reason, and expressed a great deal of personal concern for Ray's life, all to no avail. It was only after Ray began to experience significant physical malaise that he finally relented and contacted his doctor.

Once there was open communication between patient, therapist, and physician, the next phase of treatment could begin. This entailed having Ray bring his insulin and needles to session, so that intensive rational responding could be practiced in the presence of the stimuli that elicited his most severe hot cognitions and cravings. Although this intervention involved a degree of risk for relapse, it was deemed by all parties to be less risky than the possibility of diabetic coma. Before long, Ray was successfully administering his own insulin shots, albeit sporadically. Ray's insulin compliance would need to be checked throughout the course of cognitive therapy.

One of the most serious medical problems associated with the abuse of cocaine is the increase in prevalence of expectant mothers who are regular users. We have witnessed a rise in the number of cases where babies are born prematurely, with life-threatening complications, and with physiological addictions to cocaine, as a result of their mother's habits during pregnancy (Closser, 1992; Grossman & Schottenfeld, 1992; Smart, 1991; Stimmel, 1991). (Additionally, there is recent preliminary evidence that traces of cocaine bind to sperm, thus also implicating fathers in transmitting the harmful effects of cocaine to their unborn children.)

Again, education plays an important role in treatment. The therapist can explain to pregnant patients the risks of drug use (and alcohol use, as well as cigarette smoking) to their unborn children. Such patients also need to be encouraged to receive regular prenatal medical attention. Imagery work can help these patients focus on mental pictures of healthy babies versus those who are seriously ill, so as to help sway the patients away from using drugs when cravings arise. One of our pregnant patients learned to recite a standard rational response to herself when she had an urge to go out and purchase crack cocaine. She would imagine a healthy, happy baby, and she would say to herself, "I'm going to start being a good mother right now. I'm going to start taking care of my baby right now. I'm going to choose health for both of us. I'm not going to go out and use."

Another medical problem related to substance abuse concerns communicable diseases, either by sexual contact or via the sharing of needles. Substance abusers are notoriously reckless in their sexual behavior (e.g., Goldsmith, 1988; Watkins, Metzger, Woody, & McLellan, 1991). For example, they are prone to ignore simple measures of protection, such as the use of condoms. Remember (as stated in Chapter 4, this volume) that Walt stated flippantly that it was against his religion to wear a condom. In extreme cases, people who are addicted to hard-core drugs will trade sex for drugs. This translates to many people having indiscriminate sexual relations with many other people over time. The risks of contracting a wide range of venereal diseases, hepatitis, and the AIDS virus are substantially increased within this population (Chiasson et al., 1989; Fullilove, Fullilove, Bowser, & Gross, 1990; Stimmel, 1991). Given the fact that many of these people are intravenous drug users who use and share unsterile needles (Metzger et al., 1991), the risk of acquiring AIDS escalates even more.

Once again, education is a crucial component of therapy. Three steps toward the goal of safety from transmittable diseases include (1) abstinence from intravenous drug use, (2) practicing safe sex, and (3) remaining monogamous with a trusted partner. We have found that patients are fairly compliant with point (1), considerably less compliant with point (2), and very rarely compliant with point (3), especially if they continue to abuse drugs. It is extremely difficult to help a patient who is actively abusing substances to monitor his or her sexual behaviors. It is far more realistic to get patients to be sexually safer once they become abstinent from drug use. Nevertheless, every effort must be made to address this medical issue, whether or not the patient is using (see Appendix, page 329, for more information on managing patients who are HIV positive, as adapted from Fishman, 1992).

Finally, a most basic and obvious area of medical complication associated with drug use involves the deleterious effects of the drugs themselves (Frances & Miller, 1991). Dangers include damage to the central nervous system, cardiac and respiratory abnormalities, liver atrophy, and death by overdose. Yet another hazard is encountered when the drug is adulterated by foreign substances. In one notorious case in the Philadelphia area, three men were killed when they smoked the poison-laced crack that was smuggled into their prison cells.

SUMMARY

In this chapter we presented an overview of the life problems that typically plague substance-abusing populations. We noted the vicious cycles that occur when such life problems trigger the abuse of substances, which in turn exacerbates the patients' negative life situations.

Common problem areas include family and relationship dysfunction and discord, socioeconomic hardships, chronic, cumulative daily stressors at home and at work, difficulties associated with legal apprehension, and medical conditions and complications. We discussed the roles that these problems play in the course of cognitive therapy, and provided case illustrations that highlight methods of addressing such life crises in the context of a comprehensive outpatient treatment for substance abuse.

We would like to add that we have been struck by the way that some patients are able to make broad-sweeping changes in their lives as a result of their steadfast commitment to the treatment regimen. When positive life changes follow the patient's success in achieving and maintaining a drug-free existence, it behooves the therapist to make certain that the patient understands the nature of this positive feedback loop. In the same way that the therapist teaches the patient to recognize the dangers of the vicious cycles that drug abuse fosters, the therapist reminds the patient to take stock of the beneficial changes that take place as a result of abstinence. When patients fully come to realize how much they can improve their overall life situations, they gain even more motivation to make the most out of therapy and to work at preventing relapse.

CHAPTER 13

Crisis Intervention

A crisis is an unplanned, sudden, and often undesired change in a person's life that typically is associated with emotional distress. The Chinese symbol for "crisis" consists of the combined characters for "danger" and "opportunity." Similarly, in the cognitive therapy of substance abuse, a crisis is viewed as a stressor that simultaneously presents a danger of relapse and an opportunity for learning. To the extent that patients successfully cope with a crisis without using drugs, they increase self-confidence and future coping skills. The individual who does not cope effectively with crises decreases self-confidence, resulting in weakened coping skills and increased potential for future relapse.

Being available to patients in times of crisis is one of the therapist's most important responsibilities. For example, when a patient is acutely suicidal or otherwise in a potentially harmful situation, it is vital that the therapist be accessible for emergency consultation. Furthermore, it is advisable that the therapist be highly skilled in managing such crises. Patients who abuse drugs are especially prone to get into serious trouble, and a typical course of therapy with such patients often involves having to handle a number of critical incidents (Newman & Wright, in press).

For example, it is not uncommon to see a patient who seems to be making therapeutic progress, only to have that patient suddenly stop showing up for therapy sessions, and fail to return the therapist's telephone calls. Sometime later, the patient calls the therapist in a highly agitated state, and it becomes clear that the patient has begun to abuse drugs once again.

Typical crises involve (but are not limited to) renewed drug use, breakups and/or violence in significant relationships, loss of employment, depletion of finances, recurring legal difficulties, criminal involvement, medical emergencies, and overdose and suicidality.

This chapter serves as a blueprint for the therapist in the handling of the acute crises of drug-abusing patients. We review and discuss the most common types of critical incidents, and we explicate some of the therapist's options in dealing with these difficult clinical situations. First, we examine some of the warning signs that should alert the therapist to the possibility of imminent or current crisis in the patient's life.

WARNING SIGNS

Even when patients are not voluntarily forthcoming about serious difficulties that they are encountering, there are a number of common telltale signs that indicate that they may be in crisis. Such "crises" may or may not entail drug use. However, more often than not, *a crisis that starts out as a non-drug-related event, left unmanaged, turns into an episode of drug use, thus compounding the crisis* (Kosten et al., 1986).

One common sign is that the patient is habitually late for therapy sessions, or does not show up at all. When a patient misses a session, especially when he or she has not called to cancel officially, it often spells trouble. We have witnessed many instances when patients not only missed sessions, but literally seemed to disappear for long stretches at a time. When the patient is incommunicado in this manner, the chances are high that he or she is actively using drugs, or is embroiled in other serious difficulties.

After a patient has failed to show up for a session, the therapist should attempt to contact that patient as soon as possible. If the patient is easily reached by telephone, the therapist can ask the patient directly what is happening (e.g., "Do you know why I'm calling? Did you know that we were scheduled to meet a half hour ago? Can you tell me what's going on right now?").

A more problematic scenario occurs when the patient cannot be reached following a missed session. This scenario is typified by the patient's (1) telephone ringing at all hours of the day and night without being picked up, (2) not returning the therapist's telephone messages, and (3) relatives or housemates sounding hostile, giving cryptic answers in response to queries about the patient's whereabouts, or giving lip service to their willingness to pass on messages to a patient who ultimately does not return the call.

In a high percentage of cases in which the patient drops out of sight for more than a few days at a time, drug use has been involved. As such, missed sessions provide the therapist with a conspicuous red flag.

Another warning sign that the patient may be in crisis is the patient's demonstrating a marked change in mood or behavior. Examples include (1) a patient who ordinarily speaks clearly and articulates his thoughts well sounds oddly incoherent or otherwise cognitively disorganized during a telephone contact; (2) a patient who almost routinely scores zero (i.e., no self-reported pathology) on such questionnaires as the Beck Depression Inventory suddenly endorses the most extreme symptom items (e.g., "I would like to kill myself"); (3) a patient who has generally been cooperative and amicable evidences hostility toward the therapist; (4) a patient evidences labile affect in session, such as shifts between agitation, crying, and "silliness"; and (5) a relative of the patient telephones to say that the patient is acting "out of control" and pleads for the therapist to intervene immediately. Although these examples are the most typical, they by no means represent an exhaustive list.

Whenever possible, pronounced changes in patients' functioning should be addressed as soon as possible. A skilled mixture of accurate empathy and frank confrontation is called for in such instances. In this manner, the therapist may strengthen the therapeutic relationship while also making strides to stabilize the patient and begin to deal with the sources of the crisis in a constructive manner.

Yet another red flag for the therapist to notice and address is the patient's sounding or looking abnormally groggy, on the telephone or in person, especially during the middle of the day. One of our patients used the excuse that she had worked "the late shift" the day before a session in which she appeared extremely fatigued and subdued. The excuse seemed plausible at first but began to lose credibility when she began to miss sessions and then answered the therapist's telephone calls in similar states of retardation, regardless of the time of day that she was called. Furthermore, when asked to schedule her sessions in such a manner that she would not have to arrive after working "the late shift," this patient was unable to produce a work schedule of any sort. At this point, the therapist told her point blank that he believed that her drowsiness was drug or alcohol related, and that this was a very serious problem indeed.

Patients rarely are eager and enthusiastic to report on renewed drug episodes or their concomitant crises, but they may be more willing to discuss "close calls." When a patient spontaneously reports that he "almost used drugs this past week", it is a sure-fire bet that he will have at least another close call this week. More than likely, he has actually already used drugs during the past week, and will probably use even more drugs in the coming week. When this topic comes to light in session, the therapist must be alert to make it the number-one priority item for the session. The rest of the session must involve a concentrated effort to plan an emergency strategy to ward off drug use once the patient leaves the office.

When the patient does not mention near-miss drug episodes on his or her own, the therapist may choose occasionally to ask, "Have there been any times this past week when you were tempted to use drugs? What's the closest that you came to using?" Such questioning may lead to the discussion of problems and potential crises that the patient may not have volunteered to discuss.

When therapists are aware of the warning signs of renewed drug use and other crises, they stand a much better chance of keeping their drug-abusing patients in treatment. In doing so, they may also succeed in nipping major problems in the bud, and dealing with full-blown emergencies before they lead to harm or incarceration (Newman & Wright, in press).

CRISIS SITUATIONS

In the sections that follow, we discuss some common crises that are often directly related to the use of alcohol and illicit drugs. These crises include overdose and suicidality, loss of domicile, disappearance, loss of employment, loss of close personal relationships, medical emergencies, criminal involvement, and violent confrontation with the therapist.

Overdose and Suicidality

Whether by accident or in a deliberate attempt to harm one's self, an overdose of illicit drugs (perhaps in combination with alcohol or legal controlled substances) represents a potentially life-threatening situation.

In many instances, the therapist of a patient who overdoses will not know about the episode until after the damage is done. For example, Dee called her therapist from her hospital bed, saying that she would not be able to keep her therapy appointment due to her hospitalization for a severe asthma attack. Later, when the therapist consulted with the physician on her case, it was learned that her attack was induced by cocaine intoxication, and that Dee had nearly asphyxiated.

On rarer occasions, a patient will call the therapist to inform him or her of a drug overdose. When the overdose is an accident, the patient will likely be in a state of panic and confusion. An attempt should be made to confirm the patient's location, and to explain that the therapist will be calling "911" in order to have an ambulance sent. If a friend or relative is on hand, that person may be asked to do the same. In cases in which the patient is alone and is too incoherent to provide an address, the therapist will need to have handy such basic information about the patient. A simple solution is for the therapist to keep copies of all patient telephone numbers and addresses both at work and at home.

When the overdose is a suicidal gesture or attempt, the same need for an ambulance exists. (Needless to say, under such conditions the therapist does not have an obligation to protect the patient's anonymity; therefore it is appropriate to break confidentiality in order to save the patient's life.) However, if possible, it is important to keep the patient on the line. This is particularly necessary when the patient is unwilling to reveal his or her whereabouts. When Ray called his therapist at home (and reversed the charges) on Thanksgiving Day, he claimed that he had taken enough heroin and cocaine "to kill an elephant." He refused to say where he was, save to note that he was at a telephone booth. Luckily, the therapist had two telephone lines at home and was able to write a message to his wife, signaling her to call an operator from the other line in order to trace Ray's call. Although the therapist kept the patient on the line for 50 minutes, the trace was unsuccessful. The therapist proceeded to call the police directly, giving a description of the patient and recommending places that he could most likely be located. Fortunately, Ray's claim was exaggerated, and the "suicide attempt" merely made him sleep for most of the next 24 hours.

When the suicide call comes directly to the therapist's office, it may be possible to contact a colleague in the same manner that the therapist in the above example contacted his spouse.

In sum, the therapist should (1) determine the patient's location, (2) keep the patient on the telephone, or in the office as the case may be, (3) assess the degree of severity of the suicidal behaviors, and (4) contact the police, an ambulance, or another person in the vicinity who can do this for the therapist while the therapist gives the patient undivided attention.

In the case of a suicidal emergency where drugs have not already been ingested, but rather the patient is making threats that have not yet been carried through, the therapist can afford to respond a bit more cautiously and methodically. If a patient is feeling hopeless as a result of renewed drug use, or has suffered a loss as a result of the abuse of substances, the suicidal wishes may be reduced by attacking the hopelessness directly. If successful, the therapist may not have to contact the police or an ambulance. Instead, a face-to-face therapy appointment should be arranged as soon as possible (e.g., same day or first thing the next morning).

The situation becomes a bit more cloudy when the patient is suicidal while under the influence of drugs or alcohol. Even when the patient has not taken an overdose the intoxication still may result in an irrational exacerbation of the patient's intentions to self-harm by other means (Marzuk et al., 1992). Under these conditions, the patient may not be capable of following the therapist's instructions, or of understanding the therapist's attempts to help. If the therapist senses that this is the case, it is necessary to take the safest course of action. This may entail contacting and instructing a relative of the patient to admit the patient to hospital or the therapist's calling for an emergency vehicle directly.

Loss of Domicile

Another drug-related crisis entails the patient's being expelled from his or her household, usually by a spouse, parent, housemate, or landlord who has gone beyond the limits of toleration for the substance abuser's extremely maladaptive behaviors. In some instances the patient has an alternative place to go, such as to another relative or a friend. Unfortunately, unless the patient changes his or her behavior, the same sequence of events may recur. Ultimately, such patients may find themselves with no place to go but out on the streets, in shelters for the homeless, in drug houses, or (if they are lucky) an inpatient facility.

When a therapist becomes aware that a patient has been forced out of his or her domicile, it is advisable that the therapist elicit permission from the patient to consult with the patient's parole officer or with a social worker. This allows the therapist to improve the patient's chances of gaining admission to an inpatient drug abuse rehabilitation program. Although the inpatient setting may provide only a short-term solution to a long-term problem (Cummings, 1993), it is far better for patients to be receiving medical supervision than to be languishing on the streets. Furthermore, the patient's participation in an inpatient program may help him or her to regain favor with family members, as well as to reestablish a program of outpatient cognitive therapy after discharge.

Disappearance

At times, crises emerge not when patients are forced to leave their homes, but instead when they suddenly disappear from their residences. As noted earlier, this usually indicates that the patient is on a drug binge, and may be taking shelter with others who are also "on a run." This type of crisis is one of a variety about which patients do not contact their therapist. Although patients who "disappear" to places such as crack houses (for days at a time) may be losing money, jobs, family ties, physical health, and other important facets of life, they typically do not realize their own states of crisis until after the run is over. At this point, the patients are forced to face the devastation that they have wrought. They have to face their lack of money; their now accentuated drug urges; their poor physical hygiene and condition; their irate relatives, employers, and landlords; and possible legal consequences, especially if their parole officers track them down.

When patients leave their homes to go out on a drug run they may be almost impossible to locate. Still, it is important for therapists to continue to try to reach them by telephone or by mail, and to be prepared to resume treatment with them once they return (or once they are apprehended).

Therapists of patients who reappear following their binges may feel particularly frustrated, disappointed, and angry at the patients over their self-defeating and antitherapeutic behaviors. A common automatic thought we have shared in response to this very type of situation might translate to the following: "After all the work I've done with this patient, he has some nerve leaving therapy to go out on a binge! How dare he ruin all the painstaking work we've done together, just for a temporary high. Now he expects me to pick up all the pieces for him again!" Such automatic thinking needs to be counterbalanced by rational responses that highlight the patient's genuine state of desperation, the therapist's opportunity to continue to offer earnest professional help even under conditions of adversity (thus, hopefully strengthening the therapeutic relationship), and the realization that the therapist does not have to "pick up all the pieces." It is significant just that the therapist demonstrates a willingness to continue to work with the patient. However, much work will need to be done to minimize the risk of a repetition of such an episode. This includes emphasizing the importance of the patient's contacting the therapist on a regular schedule, and whenever cravings for drugs are elevated.

Loss of Employment

Persons who are actively abusing drugs rarely make good employees. Often, drug use leads to the patient's arriving late for work, missing days of work, doing inefficient work, and at times losing the job altogether. A patient who loses a job may react with anger, anxiety, frustration, hopelessness, accentuated reductions in self-esteem, and a wide range of other negative emotions. These feelings, along with their concomitant automatic thoughts and beliefs, represent significant threats to the patient's abstinence. For example, a patient who derived most of his self-worth from his job will probably react quite adversely to being laid off. He may then believe that he has nothing to lose (including his pride, which has already been damaged) by going out and getting "stoned." In this scenario, the patient might think "I worked so hard to stay off drugs, and look what it got me—nothing but trouble! If that's the way it's going to be, I might as well just go out and get messed up!"

When a therapist learns that a drug-abusing patient has lost a job, swift and concerted effort is called for to help the patient solve this life-disrupting problem. Obtaining new legal sources of income becomes a high priority agenda item. Such sources include unemployment insurance, public assistance, or another job. Newly fired patients must not be given tacit permission to give up, to abdicate all financial responsibilities to their families, to anesthetize themselves with more drugs and alcohol, and to seek money through illegal means. Naturally, the substance abuse problem per se will continue to be addressed; otherwise the patient's resultant poor work habits will result in further losses of jobs.

If the patient states that he or she no longer can afford to attend therapy, the therapist would do well to show sympathy for this position. However, the therapist should impress upon the patient the importance of attending at least one session in order to address this crisis in a productive way. The therapist may then wish to consider making special arrangements for the patient to continue with treatment, such as a reduced fee (when possible) and/or reduced frequency of sessions. In the case of parole-office-referred patients, or research cases, unemployment should have no bearing on the patient's continuing with therapy, as the expense typically is covered by a third party. The two focal points of the session should involve (1) assessing and modifying the negative feelings, thoughts, and drug urges that may have arisen as a result of the loss of the job, and (2) planning and problem-solving with regard to making ends meet financially, while also beginning the process of looking for new employment.

In addition, the therapist needs to engage the patient in an exploration of the possible results of attaining employment. This would involve discussions about such issues as (1) how the patient will "unwind" after work without resorting to drugs or alcohol, (2) how the patient will spend and save money, (3) what kinds of thoughts and beliefs are likely to be triggered as a result of adjusting to a new job, and (4) how to respond rationally to drug urges that may crop up or escalate in reaction to the changes associated with the job.

Loss of Close Interpersonal Relationships

A rift with a significant other represents another crisis that often develops in patients' lives as a result of their substance abuse. We have seen patients become extremely dysphoric, angry, and hopeless when parents have "disowned" them, mates have broken up with them, contact with their children has been denied them (e.g., by an ex-spouse or the courts), and members of their family or circle of friends die. Needless to say, the therapeutic relationship takes on tremendous significance at these points, as patients may infer that they will lose the support of the therapist as well.

Newly broken romantic and marital relationships in particular often put patients at risk for renewed drug use. Patients may seek solace in their drugs of choice, hoping to anesthetize themselves from the pain of interpersonal loss. Even if such patients do not attempt to use drugs as a form of self-medication, they may deliberately engage in self-destructive behavior out of anger, hopelessness, or a desire to manipulate the other party. In one case, a patient started an alcohol and cocaine binge in order to make his ex-girlfriend feel guilty and responsible for his "fall." He admitted later that he believed that she would take him back if he could convince her that the breakup "drove [him] to drink and drug again." In another case, a patient explained that when her boyfriend threw her out of the house she thought to herself that, "Nothing don't matter no more anyway, so I might as well get wasted." Consequently, she spent the night at a crack house and resumed her heavy use of the drug.

A particularly disturbing form of interpersonal crisis related to substance abuse is domestic violence. When the patient is the perpetrator of physical or sexual abuse of a minor, the therapist will be legally obligated to inform child protection authorities. In order to keep the patient in treatment, and thereby help to control this serious problem, we strongly advise therapists to encourage their patients to report themselves to the appropriate agencies while in the therapist's presence. The therapist who is willing and able to remain collaborative under these most trying of circumstances stands the best chance of helping abusive patients work toward change.

When the patient is the victim of violence in the home, the therapist will need to have ready access to telephone numbers of protective shelters and support groups. Therapists should pay particular attention to their female patients who are involved with substance-abusing males, as this type of relationship is significantly correlated with domestic violence, and with the victim's retreat into heavier drug and alcohol abuse as a "coping" mechanism (Amaro et al., 1990).

When patients experience crises in their most important relationships, it is helpful for therapists to provide support and to encourage their patients to discuss their sense of loss, anger, or guilt. Two critical points need to be emphasized to the patient: (1) that the therapist will not abandon the patient, even as others may have cut off emotional ties, and (2) that the patient has some measure of control over these interpersonal losses, to wit, the patient is capable of doing things to precipitate loss, and the patient is also capable of changing behaviors in order to facilitate reconciliation or new relationships. In cases in which reconciliation is impossible, such as when a loved one dies, the therapist must react with great sensitivity to the patient's grief, yet still be willing to call attention to the patient's increased risk for drug use. As with any crisis, the patient's risk for suicide should be assessed.

Medical Emergencies

Patients who abuse drugs and alcohol incur substantially greater risk for acute medical crises than does the general population. Examples include the alcohol abuser who experiences bleeding gastrointestinal ulcers, the pregnant crack abuser who goes into premature labor, the diabetic who neglects his insulin in favor of shooting heroin and then lapses into a coma, the asthmatic woman who begins to asphyxiate after smoking free-base cocaine, and others.

An increasingly prevalent example is provided by "Roland," who discovered that he was seropositive for HIV. He called the therapist in an extreme state of agitation when he received the results of the test, saying over and over again that "I'm going to die, I'm going to die!" The therapist's first response was to offer a great deal of sympathy and to let the patient vent. Next, the therapist assessed whether there was any immediate risk for drug use or suicidal behavior. Finally, after spending 30 minutes on the telephone, the patient was sufficiently calmed down to the point where he could be engaged in looking for signs of hope. Specifically, it was noted that although the patient was seropositive, he was asymptomatic and might remain that way for many years to come. Therapist and patient agreed that in order to maximize this incubation period, Roland would have to live as healthy a lifestyle as possible, including abstention from drugs. In this manner, Roland would increase his chances of surviving long enough to see the day when effective treatments or a cure could be developed.

Later, when Roland arrived for a face-to-face therapy session, he was in a positive enough state of mind to address issues of sexual responsibility to his partners. In the meantime, the therapist continued to show empathy for Roland's medical condition, and disproved the patient's hypothesis that even the therapist would now treat him as if he were a social pariah.

In many instances, therapists will be unaware of their patients' medical emergencies until after an acute crisis has passed, with treatment already received. Here, the therapist's job is not so much to help solve the crisis as it is to reengage the patient in the work of therapy, with special emphasis on the ways that the patient's drug use and unhealthy lifestyle practices may have contributed to the emergency. The new goal is to take whatever steps are necessary in order to minimize the risk of further medical complications.

On those occasions when the patient informs the therapist that a serious medical problem is going untreated, it is imperative for the therapist to encourage the patient to consult a physician, or to go to the emergency room of the nearest (or most appropriate) hospital as soon as possible. When the patient indicates that he or she is incapacitated by the illness, injury, or disorder, the therapist may be required to take the kinds of life-saving steps described earlier in the section on overdose and suicidal crises.

At times, patients will strongly resist the therapist's pleas to seek medical help, either because the patients *want* to worsen the crisis (e.g., due to hopelessness and passive suicidality), because they resent the implied "weakness" or loss of control over their bodies, or because they fear that hospital tests will reveal their active drug abuse. In such cases, when the therapist's attempt at support and reason fall on deaf ears, the therapist may need to call for medical help without the patient's consent, and hope to repair the therapeutic alliance after the medical crisis remits. The therapist should emphasize that this does not spell the end of the therapeutic relationship, but rather a necessary break while the patient receives medical treatment.

Criminal Involvement

When patients slip back into regular drug use they run the risk of getting involved in a wide range of criminal activities, the likes of which will certainly compound a state of crisis. For example, months after Walter precipitously and prematurely dropped out of therapy, it was learned from his parole officer that he had gone into hiding to escape apprehension and beatings at the hands of organized crime figures. It seems that as he resumed his use of cocaine, he began to borrow large sums of money from loan sharks. This was a stark example of his poor judgment and planning skills (especially when under the frequent influence of cocaine), as there was no way that he would ever be able to repay his exorbitant debts. In the end, Walter resorted to committing burglaries in order to attain enough money and goods to pacify the loan sharks. Eventually, he was caught by the police and reincarcerated for a number of months. When he was released, he resumed therapy.

When therapists learn that a patient is actively breaking the law, they must first determine whether other parties are at risk of being harmed. If so, there is an obligation to alert the police, as well as the intended victim. Ideally, this can be avoided if the patient is either willing to work with the therapist to cease and desist from the criminal activity in question or willing to voluntarily come clean to his parole officer or voluntarily commit himself to hospital for inpatient or day hospital psychiatric and drug abuse treatment.

If no others are at risk, the therapist and patient must work to find and implement problem-solving behaviors in place of the illegal behaviors. Cognitive techniques can help the patient to generate viable options, and to combat beliefs that "There's nothing I can do about this problem," or "There ain't no way out of this situation except [to engage in the illegal activities]."

Violent Confrontation with the Therapist

Another related crisis—that we have been fortunate enough rarely to have encountered at the Center for Cognitive Therapy—is one in which the patient threatens the therapist with bodily harm. If the threat is purely verbal, and the patient has no weapon and does not make physically menacing gestures toward the therapist, the therapist may be able to defuse the situation simply by showing a sympathetic interest in understanding the reasons for the patient's anger. When the patient has calmed down a bit, the therapist can explain that there is no need for the patient to make threats toward the therapist. For example, the therapist can say, "Mr. Smith, it's okay that you're angry with me. I want to know why, and I want to work things out between us so that we can continue to work together. However, it is extremely unhelpful if you say you're going to hurt me, because then I have to turn my attention away from your needs and onto my own need for safety and self-defense. If we are going to continue to work together, I must insist that you never make any threats or take any harmful actions toward me again. Does this make sense to you?"

When the threat is more serious, such as when a patient assaults the therapist or produces a weapon, the therapist has to choose quickly whether to flee from the situation (if possible) or to muster all his or her empathic skills in order to mollify the patient until the acute threat has passed. Under such conditions it is appropriate to enlist the assistance of colleagues and/or the police, and it is also within the therapist's ethical prerogatives to choose to discontinue seeing this patient (principle of self-preservation). If the therapist is out of danger and the patient is still present, the therapist may also choose to go on with the therapeutic contract after explaining the ground rules as noted previously. Fortunately, we have found the incidence rate of such crises to be especially low in an outpatient setting.

SUMMARY: GENERAL PRINCIPLES IN MANAGING CRISES

When patients respond to crises by using drugs, it is highly advisable that they contact a helper in order to prevent the episode from progressing to a full-blown relapse. Therapists should stress to their patients that a lapse into drug use may serve as grist for the therapeutic mill, and therefore may be used advantageously in treatment. They can explain to their patients that the renewed use of drugs does not mean that the patients are "failures" in treatment, and that the therapist still will be willing to help. Therapists can tell the patients that it is not necessary—indeed, it is often harmful—to isolate themselves from helpful others after using drugs.

Once the therapist has succeeded in establishing contact with a patient during or following a crisis, there are at least four important principles that the therapist must follow. First, the therapist has to be aware that in such instances the patient will probably want to resort to the abuse of drugs as a "coping" technique. Therefore, along with offering support and accurate empathy, the therapist must assess the patient's intentions to use drugs in this manner. A great deal of therapeutic work will be required in order to help the patient to remain drug-free under these conditions.

Second, it is imperative that the therapist be alert to the patient's hopelessness and fatalism (e.g., "I'm always going to be jinxed. Why should I even try to get my life back together again? It won't do any good anyway."). Unless vigorously combatted, such an outlook will put the patient at risk for drug use, flight from treatment, and other self-defeating behaviors.

Third, the therapist can help the patient to use the current crisis as an opportunity to practice coping skills without using drugs as an escape or crutch. Here, the therapist assists the patient in viewing his or her predicament as a "test" that, if passed, may signal true progress toward recovery. There is also the added benefit of the patient's gaining a sense of self-efficacy with each such crisis that is handled successfully without the use of psychoactive substances.

Fourth, in order to prevent treatment from being reduced to focusing on one crisis after another, therapists can look for the common dysfunctional beliefs and common problematic behaviors that underlie a seemingly disparate set of crises. For example, a patient's repeated interpersonal rifts (with spouse, family of origin, employer) may all be linked by a common theme, such as the patient's resistance to being told what to do and what not to do. In such a case, the therapist can help the patient to spell out the dysfunctional beliefs; for example, "If I listen to someone's advice, it means that I'm being controlled," and "If I'm being controlled, I'm not a real man." By focusing on these beliefs and their concomitant problematic behaviors, the therapist can maintain better structure and continuity in therapy.

As therapists are human, they are not immune to being stymied by crises that patients present to them. At such times, we strongly recommend that therapists consult with other professionals, including case workers, parole officers, and fellow clinicians. For example, when legal problems have arisen, we have held therapy sessions that included the patient's parole officer. On occasion, this has provided an interesting "good cop–bad cop" scenario, with the parole officer reading the patient the riot act while the therapist intervened to reengage the patient in some serious and concerted therapeutic work in order to stay out of further trouble.

Finally, we would like to reiterate a rather sobering as well as hopeful point. Substance abuse patients, as a group, will almost certainly experience and present with more crises than do most other types of patients. This means that the therapist will rarely be able to rest easily with such cases, no matter how well things may seem to be going in treatment. On the other hand, therapists who are prepared to handle such crises, and who persevere in teaching patients to deal with them, have the opportunity to make significant positive impacts on their patients' lives. There is a great sense of intrinsic reward in seeing patients through their toughest times, and in witnessing them turn their lives around for the better.

CHAPTER **14**

Therapy of Depression in Addicted Individuals

Mood disorders are a frequent concomitant of substance use disorders. The comorbidity ranges from 13.4% in alcoholism to 26% among general drug disorders (other than alcoholism) (Regier et al., 1990) to 30.5% specifically for cocaine abusers (Rounsaville et al., 1991). It is important to be aware of the presence of depression: first, because it may be a profound source of suffering for a given patient; second, because it reduces the prognosis for recovery from substance abuse; and third, because it is a clear-cut indication for interaction by a trained professional rather than a counselor (Woody et al., 1983).

It should be noted that it may not be possible in some cases to make an absolute diagnosis of depression for several months after a drug-addicted individual has completed a detoxification program since the use of drugs may in itself produce a clinical picture similar to a mood disorder or some other syndromal disorder. However, a careful history and clinical evaluation based on an instrument such as the Structured Clinical Interview for DSM-III-R Disorders (SCID: Spitzer, Williams, & Gibbon, 1987) and the Beck Depression Inventory (BDI: Beck et al., 1961) may help to tease out a true depression. In any event, the negative thinking and beliefs typical of depression ("depressotypic") should be addressed as part of the therapeutic regimen.

APPLICATION OF THE COGNITIVE MODEL OF DEPRESSION

The approach to depressed drug abusers can be formulated in ways similar to depression in general (Beck et al., 1979;

Carroll, 1992). It is helpful to inquire about the negative cognitive triad (Beck, 1967): patients' view of themselves, their immediate life situation, and their future. Much of this negative triad has a particular coloring relevant to drug use but, in most respects, it is the same for the drug-dependent depressive as for the nonabuser depressive. The depressogenic automatic thoughts and beliefs of each are phrased in similar or identical words and the thinking disorder and pervasive negativity are the same.

Individuals who see themselves as trapped in a situation over which they have no control, believe that they are helpless or socially undesirable, and can see only a wall of difficulties and disappointments ahead are likely to (1) feel sad, (2) express pessimism about the future, (3) consider suicide as the only solution, (4) experience a subjective loss of energy, (5) lose motivation to attempt any constructive activity ("because it is useless and I will only fail"), and (6) lose satisfaction from sex, eating, or other formerly pleasurable activities. In addition, such individuals are likely to become dependent and indecisive. Each of these symptoms can become a target for therapeutic intervention (see Beck et al., 1979). Because of the high risk of suicide in depressed drug abusers and alcoholics (Mirin & Weiss, 1991), special attention must be directed toward suicidal wishes.

BELIEFS ASSOCIATED WITH DEPRESSION

Certain negative beliefs are typical of depression but also are observed in some addicted individuals who are not depressed. As described in Chapters 2 and 3 (this volume), these dysfunctional beliefs have a powerful effect on the addicted individual's thinking, feeling, motivation, and behavior. The kinds of beliefs that are typical of depressed individuals who abuse drugs or alcohol are listed below.

NEGATIVE SELF-CONCEPT
"I am helpless (because I can't control using)."
"I am weak (because I can't resist craving)."
"I am unlovable."
"I am defective."
"I am worthless/disgusting (because I have a 'dirty' habit)."
"Everything I do is wrong."
"I am a failure."
"I am trapped."
"I don't have the will power to stop using."

NEGATIVE VIEW OF PAST

"I have never done anything right."

"Nothing has worked out for me."

"I have always been unhappy."

"I have messed up my whole life."

"My whole life is a big failure."

NEGATIVE VIEW OF LIFE SITUATION

"People despise me for my addiction."

"My family has given up on me."

"There are so many demands on me, I can't handle them."

"My family is watching me all the time."

"My neighborhood is impossible."

"My job is dull and depressing."

NEGATIVE VIEW OF THE FUTURE

"If I try something, it won't work out."

"I will never get what I want."

"My future is hopeless."

"Things can only get worse."

"I will never be able to stop using."

"I don't have anything to look forward to."

"I don't deserve anything better in life."

These beliefs can be subjected to exploration by the therapist in a series of maneuvers such as (1) looking for evidence to counteract the dysfunctional belief, (2) examining the logical relation of these beliefs to actual experiences, and (3) testing the beliefs in planned experiments. The preceding checklists should be used to help focus on the specific negative beliefs and also to monitor the patient's progress. Therapists should note that it is particularly important to assess and modify patients' beliefs about their "complete inability" to overcome their drug abuse, especially in light of research that suggests that self-efficacy beliefs profoundly affect treatment outcome and maintenance (Burling, Reilly, Moltzen, & Ziff, 1989).

THERAPEUTIC APPROACH

Timing of Intervention

By preparing a comprehensive formulation of the patient's depression (see next section), the therapist can make tentative decisions as to the type and timing of interventions. In deciding which strategies to use initially, the therapist should consider the following questions:

1. Is the depression so painful that the emphasis should be on symptom relief rather than on an immediate confrontation of the using or drinking problem?
2. Is it likely that relieving some of the symptoms will reduce the pressure to use?
3. Will providing the structure (inherent in cognitive therapy) for controlling the craving and using itself reduce the depression?
4. Can the therapist use the drug control and antidepression programs concurrently?
5. Are the suicidal tendencies and hopelessness sufficiently strong to warrant robust antisuicidal intervention and precautions?

Certainly, if the patient is acutely depressed and suicidal, the therapist's attention should be focused on this serious clinical problem. By focusing on improving the patient's mood, the therapist not only reduces the patient's risk of suicide, but also may help the patient to feel better equipped to manage the drug problem (Hall et al., 1991).

Case Formulation

The case formulation is as important in treating depression as it is in treating drug abuse in general. The following symptomatology should be covered: (1) cognitive, (2) affective, (3) physiological (e.g., sleep disturbance), (4) motivational (giving up, avoidance, lack of drive, ambivalence, suicidal wishes), and (5) behavioral ("retardation," inertia, agitation).

The cognitive symptoms in particular should be identified—specifically, the automatic thoughts and the types of distortions. The therapist should also try to link up the automatic thoughts with the consequent affective or motivational symptoms. For example, the thought "It's useless to do anything, I'll only feel worse" can be linked to the patient's loss of motivation and consequent avoidance or inactivity. The thought "Everything is hopeless. I can never get what I want" can be linked to patient's suicidal wishes. The thought "I am all alone; nobody cares" can be tied to sadness. The thought "I have messed up my life" can be tied into the patient's self-criticisms.

As the patient's life history unfolds, the therapist can construct a diagram such as that shown in Figure 14.1. In this case, the patient attempted to break the rigid pattern of blind obedience to the group's demands, but by becoming isolated he experienced his childhood-based belief in his unlovability and became depressed.

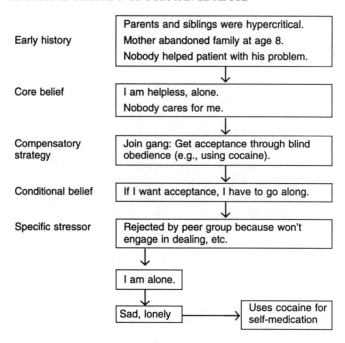

FIGURE 14.1. Relationship of developmental factors to basic beliefs and using.

The therapist should prepare a conceptual diagram such as that shown in Figure 14.1. At an appropriate time, the therapist should show it to the patient and explain the sequence of external events and external reactions.

SELECTING TARGET SYMPTOMS

It is difficult to specify in advance which problems should be selected for intervention during an interview and at what level these problems can be approached most effectively. In general, for the moderately to severely depressed user, the focus of the therapeutic intervention is at the level of symptoms ("target symptom level"). The target symptom is defined as a component of the depressive disorder that involves suffering or functional disability. The specific target symptoms may be divided into five categories (see Beck, 1967, for a more complete description):

1. *Affective symptoms.* Sadness, loss of gratification, apathy, loss of feelings and affection toward others, loss of mirth response, anxiety.

2. *Motivational.* Wish to escape from life (usually via suicide), wish to avoid "problems" or even usual everyday activities.

3. *Cognitive.* Cognitive errors such as dichotomous thinking, overgeneralization, selective abstraction, personalization; errors are frequently linked to harsh self-criticisms (e.g., "I am a worthless person" or "I am no good and don't deserve to get any satisfactions").

4. *Behavioral.* Passivity, (e.g., lying in bed or sitting in a chair for hours on end); withdrawal from other people, retardation, and agitation; total reliance on drugs or alcohol to escape or moderate dysphoria.

5. *Physiological or vegetative.* Sleep disturbance (either increased or diminished sleeping); appetite disturbance (either increased or decreased eating).

The therapist (in collaboration with the patient) makes a determination as to which of the target symptoms should be addressed on the basis of many factors:

1. Which symptoms are the most distressing to the patient?
2. Which symptoms are most accessible to therapeutic intervention?

In general, the techniques may be classified as predominantly behavioral—engaging the patient in specific activities or projects, which, in themselves, help to ameliorate some of the suffering; and predominantly cognitive—in which the major focus is on the patient's thinking.

When the patient's depression is less severe, the therapeutic focus is often on the kinds of problems that are related to the precipitation or aggravation of the depression. These problems include difficulties at home, school, or work. Many users become depressed after a loss, such as a disruption of a close personal relationship, particularly the death of a close person. Personal losses also occur through legal, financial, and medical problems associated with use. In severe depression, in which the patient feels totally out of control over drug using, the therapist might want to focus on ways to help the patient to control his craving and to structure his day in such a way as to distance him from his craving.

Some depressed users engage in nondrug activities but derive little pleasure from them. This failure to derive gratification may result from (1) an attempt to engage in activities that were not satisfying even prior to the depressive episode, (2) the dominance of negative cognitions that obscure any potential sense of pleasure, (3) selective inattention to actual experiences of pleasure, or (4) a belief that none of these activities can ever replace the high that once was achieved by drug use. Other depressed drug users may not engage in very many non–drug-related activities, due to lack of skills, inattention to the existence of such activities, a sense of apathy, or the sheer time-consuming nature of finding, using, and responding to drugs. Therefore, simple attention to the cessation of drug use is an incomplete therapeutic strategy. It is *imperative* that such patients develop sources of *nondrug* positive reinforcement, such as work, hobbies, and prosocial recreation (Stitzer et al., 1984).

Eliciting Automatic Thoughts and Beliefs

Some depressed patients find it difficult—or may be unwilling—to bring up topics for discussion in session; which may be the consequence of the depression itself. Among the depressive factors that may account for patients' lack of productivity are the following: difficulty remembering specific problems since the last session, a general passivity and slowing down that interferes with their discussing their problems, avoidance of painful subjects, and inhibition due to concern of the therapist's possible disapproval.

One way to elicit relevant material is to review specific responses to items on the Beck Depression Inventory or the Beck Hopelessness Scale. For example, the therapist's questioning of the patient regarding the reasons for endorsing a particular alternative may start up a flow of information:

PT: I have nothing to talk about today. Nothing important has happened since last week.

TH: (*examining the Beck Hopelessness Scale*) I see that you have checked the item "My future seems dark to me." When did you have that thought during the past week?

PT: Well, last week my girlfriend said she'd break up with me unless I stopped using.

TH: Yes . . . ?

PT: Well, I don't think I can stop.

TH: What did you feel when she said that?

PT: I felt bad . . . hopeless.

TH: What thought went through your mind when she said that?

PT: If we break up, I have nothing.

TH: And if you have nothing, what then?

PT: There's no sense in going on.

At this point, the therapist demonstrates the relationship between the sad feeling and the thought "I have nothing." The therapist then explores the basis for his beliefs "I don't think I can stop" and "If we break up, I have nothing." (Both beliefs, of course, contribute to the patient's hopelessness and suicidal tendencies.)

The therapist could infer from these ideas that the patient has a set of core beliefs centering around "I am helpless (weak, defective)" and "I am unlovable." Without necessarily explicitly addressing the core beliefs at this time, the therapist could then utilize specific interventions to undercut the dysfunctional beliefs and, thus, to some degree defuse the depressive feelings and suicidal tendencies. The therapist, for example, might initiate a line of inquiry as follows:

TH: You have shown a lot of control in the past—and, in fact, you haven't been using for several weeks now. What makes you think that you will not be able to continue [to abstain]?

PT: I just feel I don't have any will power any more.

TH: I respect your feeling. But remember you felt that way several weeks ago but you were able to apply the techniques and show control.

Addressing the sense of loneliness and dependency on the girlfriend might start with a question:

TH: At the moment, your girlfriend seems to be devoted to you. But, if for some reason she did leave you, why does it follow that you are nothing?

PT: But I feel like nothing.

Depending on the interchange, the therapist might then proceed with a series of questions such as:

TH: Did you feel like nothing before you met your girlfriend?

PT: I felt OK then.

TH: Did you have a girlfriend then?

PT: No.

TH: So it seems that you don't need to have a girlfriend in order to feel like something.

PT: I suppose. . . . But I still feel like nothing.

TH: Just because you may feel like nothing, does it follow that you *are* nothing?"

The therapist may then continue with the type of Socratic questioning described in Chapter 6 (this volume). The therapist should keep in mind that the ultimate goal of questioning patients' interpretations of a particular event is not simply to disqualify an interpretation but also to undermine the basic negative beliefs leading to that interpretation or conclusion.

As noted in the above excerpts, many depressed patients are influenced largely by their unpleasant feelings. They "read" these feelings to mean that they are all alone, that they are nothing, and that things are hopeless. The feelings are taken as a source of information to which the patients attach considerable credibility. The therapist needs to reduce the patients' tendency to accept their feelings as a factual representation and to help them turn to objective, verifiable evidence to form their conclusions and interpretations.

One of the distressing aspects of the ideation in depressed drug abusers is its saturation with themes of self-deprecation relevant to the meanings attached to the addiction. For example, a patient may apply the following labels to him- or herself: weak character, bad, worthless, immoral, sick. These notions are woven into the patient's belief that he or she is the helpless victim of the addiction, that he or she is defective for having the craving and not exercising will power. The patients consequently may be severely self-critical for their presumed faults ("I'm worthless," "I'm disgusting," etc.). Such thinking is apt to perpetuate both depressive symptoms and drug use. It is therefore not surprising that there is an association between depression and rates of drug relapse (e.g., Hatsukami & Pickens, 1982).

The therapist addresses depressotypic beliefs through explanations and reframing. The therapist, however, needs to use judgment to decide whether an explanation is indicated in a given case and how it should be presented to the patient. Table 14.1 illustrates this procedure.

Dealing with Suicidal Ideation

The therapist needs to be alert to covert suicidal tendencies and to deal with them frankly. A number of interventions are available (see Beck et al., 1979, Chapter 10). As in the preceding illustration, the therapist needs to address the underlying hopelessness and negative self image.

Another approach is to list the reasons for living as opposed to

TABLE 14.1 Examples of Beliefs and Explanations and Reframing

Belief	Explanation/reframing
I am a bad person.	Drug abuse is a pattern of behavior that becomes self-defeating. The effects, thus, are bad but the addicted person is not necessarily bad or immoral.
I am defective because I can't control the habit.	Your problem is a technical one. You need to understand more about the working of your addiction and then learn special techniques to bring it under control.
Life is painful, empty, without using.	The painful empty feelings are due in part at least to your personal problems and in part to your dependence on drugs for relief. We can work together to help solve the problems and develop other ways to get satisfaction.

the reasons for dying. This strategy requires considerable skill because it presupposes that the reasons for living will outweigh the reasons for dying. Another strategy is to get the patient intrigued by the therapeutic process and the interesting questions that are raised—so that the patient will be motivated to return to the upcoming sessions in order to get some of the answers. Also, the patient can be instructed to call the therapist when the wish to escape via suicide is the strongest. The therapist might say, for example, "You may feel better when you are here but you may feel worse later. That is the time when you can get the most out of therapy. If you call me then—or at least write down your thoughts—we can help you the most." The therapist should also bear in mind the need to notify the patient's family and consider hospitalization if the suicidal drive is not controllable. Above all, the therapist must appear confident, reasonably upbeat, and in control of the situation.

Negative Reactions to Therapy

A disruption of the therapeutic collaboration may occur in therapy if the patient lacks objectivity toward his or her negative thoughts. For example, patients often experience new disappointments or frustrations due to traumatic environmental events.

When this occurs, they may be flooded with a stream of negative cognitions that they automatically regard as valid without subjecting them to further considerations. Consequently, they are likely to experience increasing depression and hopelessness. This symptomatic exacerbation may lead them to decide that cognitive therapy is ineffective and that their addiction is incurable. This is often a critical point for a relapse. Patients may also feel disillusioned with their therapist.

Any of these reactions may lead the patient to stop cooperating, resist carrying out assignments, miss appointments, or drop out of therapy. Their reactions may be compounded if the therapist unquestioningly accepts the patient's negative construction of his or her progress. If the patient begins to miss appointments, the therapist is advised to contact the patient and clarify the dysfunctional thinking that is disrupting the therapeutic collaboration. Also, the missed appointment may be due to a relapse, which needs to be investigated.

Ironically, there is some evidence that patients diagnosed with antisocial personality disorder (ASPD) actually may be *more* likely to seek out and cooperate with therapists when they are most depressed (Alterman & Cacciola, 1991; Woody, McLellan, & O'Brien, 1990). In such cases, the patients' desire to feel better outweighs their characteristic autonomous need to defy authority figures. By helping these ASPD/depressed drug abusers to improve their mood, therapists may be able to form an interpersonal alliance with patients who otherwise would not form a bond with a helper.

Symptomatic recurrences of depression are common during treatment (Rawson, Obert, McCann, Smith, & Ling, 1990; Ziedonis, 1992). The therapist should prepare the patient early in treatment to expect to have negative fluctuations. Such exacerbations provide a valuable opportunity to apply cognitive techniques and skills. Further, they provide "practice" to deal with the problems that inevitably occur after termination of treatment.

The therapeutic focus for the depressed addicted person also is directed to external problems that are related to the precipitation or aggravation of the depression (cf. Kosten et al., 1986). These problems may include stresses or difficulties at home, work, or school. They frequently involve friction in close relationships, difficulties in reference to work, or financial or legal problems. Thus, for example, the therapist and patient may work on helping the patient to make important decisions regarding a problem contributing to or maintaining his or her depression, discuss specific techniques to help to cope better with a difficult life situation, and consider ways of relieving stresses or external demands.

This type of approach (concentration on external problems) is also used after the patient's acute or severe symptoms have been relieved. The therapist should bear in mind that situational problems, drug use, and depression may aggravate each other. This multiple reciprocal interaction may be modified to improve both the external stresses and the depressive symptomatology.

APPLICATION OF BEHAVIORAL TECHNIQUES

Cognitive Change through Behavioral Change

The cognitive *therapy* of the depressed abuser is based on the cognitive *theory* of depression (as well as the cognitive theory of addiction). Working within the framework of the cognitive model, the therapist can vary his or her therapeutic approach according to the specific needs of a given patient at a particular time as long as the treatment is based on a cognitive formulation of the case (cf. Persons, 1989). The therapist is conducting cognitive therapy even though he or she is utilizing behavioral techniques.

In the early stages of cognitive therapy with depressed users, it is often necessary for the therapist to concentrate on restoring the patient's functioning to the predepressed level. Specifically, the therapist attempts to induce the patient to counteract his or her withdrawal and to become involved in more constructive activities. Often the important people in their life have given up on the patient. These significant others may attribute the patient's low mood and impaired performance to drugs and conclude that the patient is no longer capable of carrying out his or her expected functions as provider, homemaker, spouse, parent, or student. Furthermore, the patients can see no hope of gaining satisfaction from those activities (other than using) that had previously brought them pleasure.

The depressed users are caught in a vicious cycle in which their reduced level of activity leads to labeling themselves as ineffectual or worthless. These negative self-evaluations often reflect the opinions of those around them—as well as society at large. These self-inflicted put-downs lead to further demoralization and ultimately to a drift into a state of immobility. In severe cases, it is difficult to carry out intellectual functions (such as reasoning and planning) as well as performing complicated acts requiring specialized skill and training. Since these forms of behavior are generally instruments for achieving satisfaction and maintaining one's self-esteem and the esteem of others, the disruption of these functions as a result of diminished concentration, fatigability, and low mood produces dissatisfaction and a reduction of self-esteem.

The role of the therapist is clear. There is no easy way to "talk patients out" of their beliefs that they are weak, inept, or undesirable. Patients can observe that they simply are not doing those things that once were relatively easy and important to them. By helping patients change certain depressive behaviors (avoidance, passivity), the therapist may *demonstrate* to them that their negative self-evaluations are biased views and can help to restore their morale. Once a patient begins to get involved in constructive activities, the therapist may show the patient that he or she has not, in fact, irretrievably lost the ability to function at his or her previous level. The therapist points out that the patient's discouragement, pessimism, and giving up make it difficult to mobilize resources to make the necessary effort. The goal is to get the patient to recognize that one of the prime sources of the problem is a cognitive error: The patient *thinks* (absolutely) that he or she is weak, helpless, and worthless, and those beliefs seriously impair his or her motivation and behavior.

The term "behavioral techniques" may suggest that the immediate therapeutic focus is exclusively on the patient's overt behavior; that is, the therapist simply prescribes some kind of goal-directed activity. In actual practice, the reporting of the patient's thoughts, feelings, and wishes remains a central factor for the successful application of the behavioral techniques. The ultimate aim of these techniques is to produce positive change in the dysfunctional negative attitudes so that the patient's performance will continue to improve.

In a sense, the behavioral methods can be regarded as a series of small experiments designed to test the validity of the patients' negative hypotheses or ideas about themselves. As the negative ideas are contradicted by these "experiments," the patient gradually becomes less certain of their validity and is motivated to attempt more difficult assignments.

Scheduling Activities

Many depressed users report an overwhelming number of self-debasing and pessimistic thoughts when they are withdrawn and inactive. They criticize themselves for being "vegetables," for being addicted, and for having withdrawn from other people. At the same time, they may justify their withdrawal on the basis that activity and social interaction are meaningless or that they are a burden to others. Thus, they sink into increasing passivity and social isolation.

Depressed patients tend to interpret their inactivity and withdrawal as evidence of their inadequacy and helplessness and they are caught up in a vicious cycle. Individuals with a drug problem tend to relapse readily if their life is not structured.

The prescription of special projects is based on the clinical observation that depressed patients find it difficult to undertake or complete jobs that they accomplished with relative ease prior to the depressive episode. When depressed, they are prone to avoid complex tasks, or, if they do attempt such tasks, they are likely to have considerable difficulty achieving their objective. Typically, the depressed patient avoids the project or stops trying soon after he encounters some difficulty.

Negative beliefs and attitudes appear to underlie the tendency to give up. Patients often report, "It's useless to try," for they are convinced they will fail. When they engage in goal-directed activities, they tend to magnify the difficulties and minimize their ability to overcome them and carry out the task.

The use of activity schedules (see Chapter 9, this volume) serves to counteract the patient's loss of motivation, inactivity, and preoccupation with depressive ideas. Scheduling the patient's time on an hour-by-hour basis is likely to maintain a certain momentum and prevent slipping back into immobility. By focusing on specific goal-oriented tasks the patient and therapist obtain concrete data on which to base realistic evaluations of the patient's functional capacity.

As with other cognitive techniques, the therapist should present the patient with a rationale for scheduling activities. Often patients are aware that inactivity is associated with an increase in their painful feelings. At the very least, the therapist can induce patients to engage in an "experiment" to determine whether activity diminishes their preoccupations and possibly improves their mood. The therapist and patient determine specific activities and the patient agrees to monitor his or her thoughts and feelings while engaged in each task. If the patient is reluctant, the therapist may seriously question the patient, "What have you got to lose by trying?"

The therapist may choose to provide the patient with a schedule to plan his or her activities in advance and/or to record the actual activities during the day. A "graded task" hierarchy should be incorporated into the daily plan.

Planning specific activities in collaboration with patients may be an important step in demonstrating to them that they are capable of utilizing their time constructively. Severely depressed patients may report a sense of "going through the motions" with the notion that there is little purpose in their activities. By planning the day with the therapist, they are often able to set meaningful goals. Later, the patient's record of the actual activities (compared to what was planned for the day) can provide the therapist and patient with objective feedback about the patient's achievements. The record also provides a reference to self-ratings of mastery and satisfaction for successful attainment.

It may challenge the therapist's ingenuity to get the depressed user sufficiently involved in the idea of carrying out a program of activities or even filling his or her activity schedule retrospectively. Thus, the therapist (1) explains the rationale (e.g., that people generally function better when they have a schedule), (2) elicits the patient's objections or reservations, and (3) then proposes making a schedule as an interesting experiment. The therapist should emphasize to the patient that the immediate objective is to attempt to follow the schedule rather than to seek symptomatic relief: Improved functioning frequently comes before subjective relief.

When patients engage in various activities, it is useful to have them record the degree of mastery and pleasure associated with a prescribed activity. The term "mastery" refers to a sense of accomplishment when performing a specific task. "Pleasure" refers to pleasant feelings associated with the activity. Mastery and pleasure can be rated on a 10-point scale with 0 representing no mastery/pleasure and 10 representing maximum mastery/pleasure. By using a rating scale, the patient can recognize practical successes and small degrees of pleasure. This technique tends to counteract the patient's all-or-nothing thinking.

SUMMARY

The approach to the depressed user or alcoholic is similar to the approach to depression in general with the added feature that the typical depressive negative bias against the self often revolves around the patient's reaction to being on drugs or alcohol. Thus, patients may be filled with contempt for themselves, may consider themselves lacking in character, and may perceive themselves as helpless, defective, and rejected by other people and by society in general. Given the negative bias against the self and the profound hopelessness that often accompanies it, individuals with the combination of depression and addiction constitute one of the highest-risk groups for suicide (Marzuk et al., 1992; Mirin & Weiss, 1991; Ziedonis, 1992). Consequently, the possibility of suicidal wishes must be addressed early in therapy. Aside from the attention to the suicidal wishes, the therapist can follow the usual guidelines:

1. Conceptualize the case.
2. Apply behavioral strategies if the patient is motorically regressed.
3. Utilize cognitive strategies to undercut the hopelessness and negative self image and suicidal tendencies.
4. Help the patient to acquire greater control over the cravings (see Chapter 10, this volume)—a strategy that in itself may help to stem the tide of the depression.

The specific techniques include structured activity scheduling, greater task assignment, and improved time management as a way of counteracting patients' regressive tendencies. In addition, Socratic questioning and the use of daily thought records may help patients gain more distance from their dysfunctional thinking. As with the standard treatment of the addict, it is ultimately necessary to come to grips with patients' beliefs that are driving both their drug abuse and their depressive tendencies.

CHAPTER **15**

Anger and Anxiety

Unnecessary or exaggerated anger presents a major problem in human relations, whether intimate or casual. The fact is that people tend to overreact to disappointments, hurt, fancied slights, and imperfect behavior of others. This phenomenon is particularly apparent in substance abusers (Ellis et al., 1988; Walfish et al., 1990). Hostility takes its toll not only in its undesirable effects on other persons but also in terms of its effect on the person who is angered. Substance abusers are prone to act out hostile impulses when they are under the influence of drugs or alcohol. Although they are particularly prone to use or drink to dampen unpleasant feelings of anger, the substance paradoxically may increase the likelihood of the expression of anger via disinhibition.

The angry reaction is greater if the "noxious action" by another person is perceived as avoidable, unnecessary, intentional, and attributable to a failing in the other person; the reaction is less (or not all) if the same event is viewed as unavoidable, necessary, unintentional, and not blameworthy. If individuals perceive that they (or somebody they are attached to) have been wronged, they may become angered to a degree that greatly exceeds the degree of damage or discomfort. Much of the anger is the result of the symbolic meaning that is attached to the event, the cognitive mechanism involved in magnifying its impact, and the degree of responsibility attributed to the other person.

LOW FRUSTRATION TOLERANCE

One of the most common conditions prompting an addiction-prone individual to seek relief through substance use is a feeling of frustration. Patients with low frustration tolerance (LFT) are hypersensitive to any thwarting, nonfulfillment, or interference with their goals, wishes, or actions. The typical patient with LFT goes through life judging situations in terms of the following: "Am I getting what I want?" or "Are people getting in my way?" Because of the "internal" pressure to attain the objectives of fulfillment of wishes or completion of a particular task, patients overreact to situations that interfere with satisfying their wishes or reaching a goal. Thus, they tend to be chronically impatient, intolerant, and uneasy.

Wish-oriented patients operate under the "now dimension": They experience continuing craving for immediate "reinforcement" (encouragement, praise, recognition) or help. Stuck in the receptive mode, they consider it imperative that their cravings and desires be satisfied without delay. Behind this pressure lurks a fear clothed in dichotomous thinking: "It's now or never." Patients react as follows: "If I can't get what I want right now, I *never* will." Consequently, any delay in satisfaction is particularly distressing. The fear that they will be prevented from getting what they want arouses anxiety. Any interference with or interruption of an enjoyable activity is perceived as a major deprivation and causes pain. Either pain or anxiety (or both) can lead to anger if the individual holds another person responsible for the deprivation or interference.

"Lil," a young woman, told by her landlady to lower the volume of her stereo, felt a sharp pang of disappointment over being deprived of one of her pleasures (high-volume music). She generalized this disappointment to "Nobody ever lets me do what I want." Consequently, Lil became angry, stomped around the apartment, and started to drink. As Lil's actions demonstrate, rapid, fleeting experiences of disappointment or anxiety trigger and are overshadowed in the patient's awareness by anger toward the thwarting or disappointing individual.

It should be noted that a rather subtle mechanism operates between the initial feeling of disappointment (or anxiety) and the experience of anger. This mechanism involves attributing responsibility for the disappointment to the other person in a fashion akin to blame. Attribution of responsibility may be a focus for discussion in therapy. Patient and therapist can explore whether the attribution of responsibility is reasonable.

Since these patients have not learned to modulate their wishes and urges, they tend to experience them as "needs" that demand prompt fulfillment. These demands on themselves and others are experienced as dire needs ("I must") or imperatives ("people should"). Since the needs have a "do or die" quality, their nonfulfillment is experienced as a threat or painful deprivation. The intolerance for frustration is paralleled by intolerance for the dysphoria produced by disappointment. The distress is compounded by thoughts such as "This should not have happened. They have no right to treat me this way."

The claims, expectations, and demands on these patients and others are not only imperative but also rigid and unrealistic. Karen Horney (1950) refers to these phenomena as the "tyranny of the shoulds"; Albert Ellis (1962) applies the term "musturbation." These individuals impose the shoulds on themselves as well as on other people. Individuals driven to achieve success may experience a sense of being dominated by an internal "slave driver." Such individuals often experience stress symptoms (Beck, 1993) and may turn to drugs and/ or alcohol to relieve these symptoms.

Action-oriented individuals with LFT operate according to the same rules as the wish- or receptive-oriented individual. They act on the assumption that they must attain a goal promptly. Any delay is perceived as interminable; any interference as unconscionable. The principle underlying sensitivity appears to be concerned with "the conservation of energy." Impediments to the forward progress of such individuals are experienced as an unacceptable drainage of power or energy, which leads to impatience and restlessness.

Wish-oriented and action-oriented people are disposed to ascribe negative motives to other people. They operate on the following premise: "Anyone who does not help me or facilitate my goals is selfish; others' noncompliance with my wishes is the equivalent of opposition." The LFT individual interprets lack of support or help as signs of indifference, negligence, or irresponsibility. Ironically, these individuals are not cognizant of the fact that their behavior is controlled by their inner dictates (cravings, demands, imperatives) but perceive themselves as controlled and victimized by other people who are indifferent to their "legitimate needs."

Since the patient's pattern of frustration is crude, inflexible, and indiscriminate, the thinking mechanisms are equally crude. Such patients tend to catastrophize and overgeneralize when their wishes are not met: "I will never be able to get the job done." "Others never cooperate with me." "People always get in my way."

In order to ward off the threats and prevent pain, patients with LFT attempt all the more strongly to control their environment and to impose regulations and expectations on other persons. However, the harder they try to compensate for their sense of inner vulnerability, the more likely they are to be frustrated. As their demands and claims on others escalate, they are prone to feel let down, disappointed, or blocked. Thus, the strategy of hypercontrol of others is ultimately self-defeating. The social environment simply will not conform to these continual demands and expectations. Sooner or later, other people will fail to respond satisfactorily to their wishes or drives.

At a deeper level, patients with LFT perceive themselves as powerless or helpless. Any obstacle to a goal that the patient encounters primes the sense of powerlessness and produces a transient feeling of weakness. The next step is attributing responsibility to the "frustrating" individual and wanting to punish that person for his or her transgression. This sequence leads, of course, to the most notable characteristic of LFT, namely, explosive rage over relatively trivial incidents. An action-oriented person is enraged by a slow driver in front of him and aggressively and dangerously passes him—with his thumb pressed firmly on the horn. A husband rails over delays in meals or unsatisfactory food; a wife is incensed at being kept waiting while her husband works late at the office. In each instance, the patient attaches an overgeneralized meaning to the "offense": "She doesn't care about me" or "He treats me like a servant." These highly personalized meanings attached to the event—not the event itself—lead to the inflammatory reaction: the sense of being wronged. This tendency to "personalize" situations, to interpret neutral behaviors as a perceived affront, is a hallmark of LFT.

The generation and expression of anger and hostility serve several related purposes. They constitute a robust attempt to establish control over other persons by "punishing" them for their action or inaction. When the expression of hostility is effective, there is no form of behavior that exerts as powerful an influence on other people, particularly if the offended individual is in a position of strength. The patient assumes that punishment, whether in the form of a complaint, a reproach, or a tantrum, will help to shape the other person's future behavior properly. The implicit punishment will supposedly be a "learning experience" for the offender. Further, the punishment contained in the reproach in some vague way undoes or compensates for the damage to the patient's self-esteem: A person is not "a helpless, vulnerable wimp" if he or she can inflict pain on another person.

Most important, the expression of anger gives a subjective sense of *power* (even though fleeting). By acting in a forceful, aggressive way, the patient is able to neutralize the sense of powerlessness activated by the delay in gratification. Since frustration or disappointment accentuates the perception of the self as ineffective, the expression of hostility shifts the self-concept from "I am helpless" to "I do have power."

Of course, punishing other people as a consequence of one's own "neediness" or sense of inadequacy is ultimately self-defeating. Other people are pained and often angered when reproached and are prone to retaliate. Further, the frustrated individual is drawn into a power struggle with others over the issue of who will control whom. The individual gets tangled in a vicious cycle of increasingly futile attempts to control others, leading to increasing disappointment and rage.

LFT individuals are prime candidates for addiction (Ellis et al., 1988). Using drugs and/or drinking can serve several purposes. First, these substances satisfy the desire for instant gratification. Second, they reduce the anxiety and sadness engendered by frustrations. Finally, they can give a transient euphoria and sense of mastery to compensate for the feeling of helplessness and sense of inadequacy.

It is important for the therapist to recognize that patients with LFT often are deficient in perceiving important social cues or recognizing the rules that govern human behavior and allow people to interact with a minimum of friction. They are frequently unaware of and overstep the usual boundaries between people. Lil, for example, had no recognition of the fact that the loud noise from her stereo would bother the other boarders. Some patients addicted to drugs have Attention Deficit Disorder (Gawin & Kleber, 1986; Glantz & Pickens, 1992; Weiss, 1992) and may rely on cocaine, for example, to sharpen their focus and increase their guarded awareness of other people.

CHECKLIST FOR EVALUATING LFT

1. The patients' desires are viewed as imperative needs that require prompt fulfillment.

2. Delays, interference, and blocks have idiosyncratic meanings such as "I may not finish this job" or "I can't get what I want."

3. The frustration is overgeneralized to notions such as "I never get what I want" or "People always get in my way."

4. Patients personalize such frustrations as though the frustrations are deliberately directed against them, and they regard the alleged agent of the frustration as culpable. Patients manifest the usual thinking errors associated with emotional distress: all-or-nothing thinking, selective abstraction, overgeneralization, catastrophizing, and personalizing.

5. Because of dichotomous thinking ("It's now or never"), patients build up arbitrary rules (shoulds and musts) to enforce their wishes, expressed as rights, entitlements, and claims: "People have no right to withhold what I want," "Others are wrong to get in my way," and "I should be able to work without interruption."

6. The absolutistic expectations and demands are driven by catastrophizing: The consequences of a delay, obstacle, or difficulty are expected to be disastrous.

7. The patients' rules and demands also represent attempts to control others and prevent problems. When controls break down (a rule is violated, a demand is unfulfilled), patients experience anxiety or hurt resulting from catastrophizing or exaggerated sense of loss.

8. The expression of anger is legitimized: "I have every right to be angry."

9. Underlying the low threshold for frustration is a core belief such as "I am helpless" or "I am unlovable." Any delay, interference, or problem related to attainment of wishes or goals can evoke the sense of helplessness or unlovability, lead to catastrophizing, then distress, and, finally, to anger.

10. The accumulation of anxiety and anger and the mobilization to punish the offender lead to tension which patients attempt to relieve with drugs. In this context, drug-taking beliefs may take the following forms:

"I can't stand the anxiety, sadness, or anger and must relieve it right away."

"People want to stop me from using or drinking because they consider me weak and want to control me."

"They are wrong and bad for wanting to control me."

"I will regain control by drinking or using when I want to."

11. People may be overly frustrated by their own mistakes, ineptitude, or deficiencies and will manifest extreme self-criticism. This mechanism is especially prominent in the addicted patient with low self-esteem (Tarter, Ott, & Mezzich, 1991).

LFT AND SUBSTANCE ABUSE: A CASE VIGNETTE

"Charlotte," a 35-year-old single woman, was in outpatient cognitive therapy following a 30-day inpatient stay for crack cocaine abuse at a nearby hospital. Charlotte and her cognitive therapist identified many situational and cognitive triggers for her urges to use crack, including family disputes, worries about money, thoughts about deceased relatives, news about old boyfriends, and dissatisfaction with her employment situation. These triggers tapped into a great sense of loss (e.g., "I don't have anything meaningful in my life anymore, so I might as well drown my sorrows in alcohol and cocaine") and helplessness and hopelessness ("Everything I do to try to help myself gets messed up in the end anyway, so there's no point in planning for a future").

Charlotte's dysfunctional beliefs (noted above) underlay her low tolerance for frustration. For example, when she tried to reach her new boyfriend by telephone one evening to talk about some upsetting things that happened on her job interview that day, she found that nobody was home. She tried to call numerous times within the following hour, but he still did not answer the telephone.

Charlotte became quite agitated and she felt an increasingly strong urge to go out and find a crack dealer. In retrospect, her thoughts included:

"I need him *now*. If I can't talk to him now, I'll go out of my mind." [Imperative: equating wish with need]

"I *can't stand* being alone when I'm hurting. My only alternative to feel better is to get high." [Myth of intolerability of pain]

"Why isn't he home when I need him?" [Excessive demands]

"I can't wait any longer!" [Intolerance for frustration]

"Maybe he's out with another woman. Maybe he's cheating on me." [Catastrophizing]

"If that's true, then I don't have any reason to stay straight anymore." [Justification]

Charlotte noted that all of these thoughts transpired within only 90 minutes of trying to reach her boyfriend at home. Rather than attempting to solve the problem—calling him back at a later time, calling the therapist, or trying to utilize her own coping skills—she became very upset that she could not find her boyfriend *right at the time she "needed"* him. This frustration led her to the premature and maladaptive conclusion that she had no choice but to go out and get high. She believed it was *justifiable* to do so; after all, if you are alone (as she believed), helpless, and have no future, why *shouldn't* you find a way to feel better *now* by any means possible, including drugs?

This vignette demonstrates how LFT is based on a thinking style that justifies impulsive and self-defeating behavior, and therefore feeds into urges to use drugs. The LFT patient is constantly in danger of exaggerating temporary inconveniences and upsets as indicative of (or equivalent to) unremitting denial of the most important goals in life—forever. Therefore, the LFT patient is likely to conclude that drug use (a short-term "solution") is necessary, given that long-term solutions are unseen or dismissed.

DEALING WITH SPECIFIC ISSUES

Imperativeness of "Needs"

Patients require *practice* in delaying satisfaction of desires—whether in terms of resisting the desire to use or drink or of demands on others for their help, reassurance, and praise.

1. From a practical standpoint, patients should be coached to *monitor* their wishes: write down the specific desire, note its intensity, and determine how long it takes for the desire to be reduced. This procedure enables patients to distance themselves from the desire and, thus, to control it better.

2. *Distraction*—for example, getting involved in an absorbing activity such as conversing with another person—often helps to reduce the imperativeness of the need.

3. By *delaying* their demand for instant gratification, patients can become aware of the exaggerated importance they attach to a particular desire. Their desires for affection and recognition are similar to the cravings for drugs and alcohol. When an individual is frustrated in his or her yearning for affection (or expects to be frustrated), for example, he or she may channel this yearning into a craving for a drink or a "fix." The kind of pleasure from the chemical agent is perceived as a substitute for the pleasure desired through a loved one's affection.

Meaning of the Event: Hidden Fears

By delaying the expression of anger or impatience (acting out the frustration), the individual has an opportunity to become aware of (1) the immediate cognitive reaction to an event (e.g., a specific fear of disappointment) and (2) the immediate affective response such as anxiety or sadness. For example, the wife who railed at her husband for not coming home when she expected had an initial fear, "perhaps something happened to him," and felt considerable anxiety. When he did appear, she was angry at him for "causing" her distress rather than for being late—although she scolded him for being late. In therapy, she recognized that the initial fear was related to her childlike concern of being abandoned. Thus, the therapy was directed toward her confronting her sense of vulnerability, which was aroused by his tardiness. In this case, her hostility served to punish him for making her feel vulnerable and, at the same time, gave her some sense of power.

When an unpleasant event occurs, patients with LFT practically simultaneously assess the consequences and attach responsibility either to themselves or to others (or occasionally simply to bad luck). The expectation of negative consequences is not a thought-out, reflective, rational procedure but is molded to a large degree by a tendency to exaggerate. This tendency may take the form of foreseeing the possibility of catastrophic consequences or by exaggerating the current loss. The catastrophizing may be heralded by a "What if . . . ?" prelude; for example, "What if I hadn't caught the mistake in time. . . . It could have cost me a large sum of money." The sense of loss places a great premium on the supposed diminution of some resource; for example, "They are costing me valuable time by their inefficiency" or "I am forced to waste my energy answering stupid questions."

Issue of Responsibility

The attribution of responsibility occurs almost at the same time as the estimate of loss or threat. The individual determines that some person is responsible for the loss or threat. The patient's reaction is to fix accountability on the other person as the *cause* of the frustration. This attribution of responsibility is evidenced in expressions (or thoughts) such as "You *should* have known better" or "You never pay attention." Words such as *should, should not, never,* and *always* are often expressions of attribution of responsibility and simultaneously of reprimand.

A more subtle process is also discernible. Noxious events are likely to evoke a sense of helplessness in the LFT-prone patient. If such patients can fix responsibility on another and mobilize reproach, they can regain some of the sense of lost power. By blaming another person, the patient in a sense is saying, "I'm not so weak and helpless. I am strong enough to punish you." Of course, if such patients perceive themselves as the cause of the problem, they criticize themselves and feel even more helpless.

Issue of Control

The problem of control is particularly pertinent to the treatment of drug abusers since the therapy involves, in essence, the therapist's attempting to control patients' behavior. This problem has been exacerbated in many instances in which patients have been subjected to threats, coercion, and criticism by other well-intentioned persons trying to enforce abstinence or, at least, continence. These attempts by others can produce a chronic resentment in the substance abusers. Most significant from the therapeutic standpoint is the impact of such interventions on the individuals' self-esteem. They are likely to respond covertly to the criticism with an increased sense of inadequacy, even helplessness, isolation, and unworthiness, although overtly they may devalue the other party.

Many of these patients will become infuriated at their "tormenters" and will attempt to regain a sense of power by counterattacking and thus alleviating the pain. Others will engage in elaborate deceptions to disguise their using or drinking and to protect their self-esteem from further blows. Thus, the confrontation by the therapist of the patients' deceptions is a delicate procedure since exposure of a pretense may constitute a significant threat to the patients' self-esteem.

Handling Anger Toward the Therapist

Situations in which one person is attempting to influence the behavior of another person embody specific sets of problems. The drug-abusing patient's sensitivity to being controlled is practically a given in the therapeutic situation and is an issue that needs to be addressed by the therapist. As already indicated, the patient's strategy of covering up lapses in order to protect him- or herself from criticism may represent an important defensive maneuver. Consequently, discussions of the patient's drinking and using or of his or her deceptions may arouse the patient's anger and shake the foundations of trust. On the other hand, if the therapist appears to be "taken in" by the patient's deceptions, the therapist may appear to be a "pushover" and will not maintain the patient's confidence.

Patients should be encouraged to discuss their angry feelings toward the therapist. However, while ventilation of the feelings may serve a constructive purpose—up to a point—the therapist must be prepared to set limits to the expression of anger as illustrated below.

"I realize that you are very angry at me and I'm glad that you feel safe to express it here. But before we go any further, it is very important to find out all the factors that are fueling your anger. For example, what were you thinking just before you became angry?"

Often the exploration of the automatic thoughts preceding the appearance of the angry response serves as a distraction, which allows the patient to gain some objectivity. Further, by eliciting the automatic thoughts, the therapist can get a better grasp of the cognitive aspects of the patient's disposition to anger. The anger is often the consequence of a sequence of automatic thoughts relevant to secret fears or hidden doubts. For example: "He's trying to control me" therefore "I won't be able to do anything on my own" (secret fear) therefore "I can't let him get away with this" therefore anger; or "I must be a weakling to allow him to talk to me that way" (self-doubt) therefore "He has no right to treat me that way" therefore anger.

However, this therapeutic strategy is not effective all the time, and many times the therapist has to be prepared to absorb verbal expressions of hostility until the patient's anger subsides.

Abusive Behavior and Control of Anger

Patients with an addictive personality profile are particularly likely to have difficulties in family relationships and may engage in abusive behavior (Amaro et al., 1990). The various steps for anger control are described in *Love Is Never Enough* (Beck, 1988). Briefly, these consist first of being able to recognize the earliest subjective signs of anger, which may simply consist of somatic sensations such as a tightness in the chest or a stiffening of the muscles in the arms. When a patient experiences these premonitory signs, for example, he should then slow down his talking and examine whether he sounds angry. If he is indeed angry, he should stop talking until his anger subsides. If he is still angry, he should leave the room (assuming the hostile interaction is at home). He should then stay away from the targets of his hostility until he has cooled off. At times it may be necessary to leave the house for a while, although it is essential for patients to have a drug-free destination in mind (e.g., the public library).

The therapist should explore with the patient various kinds of *distraction*. While in the heated situation, the patient might try to distract him- or herself by thinking of a pleasant experience. After leaving the room, the patient could get involved in some physical exercise or manual project to "work off" the anger. In order to prepare the patient for using these self-control methods, the therapist should use the therapeutic session to get the patient to practice the techniques. One method is to have the patient recall in vivid detail a recent dysfunctional interaction and then, using imagery, go through the scenario but imagine using techniques of self-control.

Induced imagery is also useful for ascertaining the individual's automatic thoughts (see Chapter 10, this volume). The patient is requested to relive a hostile encounter in imagination and then to pinpoint the automatic thoughts associated with the angry feeling. The material can then be dealt with using the standard way of framing reasonable responses to automatic thoughts.

The therapist may also utilize *role playing* in order to model self-control techniques for the patient. Patient and therapist simulate or recreate a hostile encounter that will provide the patient with an opportunity to recognize his or her anger, detect the automatic thoughts, and rehearse rational responding.

It should be kept in mind that an important facet of patients' anger proneness is their deep sense of helplessness and inadequacy in interpersonal conflict. Compounding this defective self-image is the lack of social problem-solving skills (Platt & Hermalin, 1989) and frequently a lack of assertiveness. In his or her formulation of the patient's difficulty, the therapist needs to diagram the sequence:

"I am helpless/inadequate" therefore "I am vulnerable to being insulted, controlled, etc." therefore "He has taken advantage of me" therefore "I have to protect myself" therefore anger and acting out.

Patients capable of insight often are willing to accept this formulation. The therapist's role then is to help the patient to reinforce a self-image of adequacy without having to prove it by expressing anger or abusing another person. Building up a positive core concept includes not only demonstrating to patients their potential capacity to handle conflicts with other people but also negating their dysfunctional beliefs; for example, "If I don't succeed at something, it shows I'm inadequate" or "If somebody argues me down, it means I'm inferior." Further, the therapist has to communicate to the patient that "feeling helpless" is not an objective representation of reality; people tend to read their feelings as factual. But one can "feel helpless" and still function adequately.

Assertive Training and Problem-Solving

Some patients become unnecessarily provoked because they feel inhibited or lack social skills in presenting their own viewpoint or expressing their own self-interest. Failure to assert themselves effectively makes them feel put upon and helpless and to view other people as controlling and domineering. These patients often have a particular problem with people in authority.

"Steve," who has a history of dependence on alcohol and cocaine, worked as a contract mechanic in a automotive garage. When he and the other mechanics were given jobs by the service manager, he noticed that the other mechanics were assigned the more expensive jobs. Although he realized that they were more assertive than he in asking for the good jobs, he concluded that he was being discriminated against. He was too inhibited, however, to complain to the service manager, whom he perceived as authoritarian and callous.

One day he felt particularly frustrated because a big job on an expensive foreign car was given to one of the other mechanics. He wanted to say something to the manager but was too inhibited. As he left the garage, he became increasingly angry. He thought of going home but he had an image of his children squabbling with each other and that made him feel more frustrated. Although he had previously resolved not to drink or use, he decided to stop at a bar and have a drink to relieve his anger and frustration. After three or four beers he again thought of going home but this time he had visions of his wife scolding him for being late and drinking so when he left the bar he sought out a friend who gave him a joint of crack cocaine. When he got home eventually, he was filled with remorse for his lapse.

The therapist pointed out to him in their session that his lapse was not a full-blown relapse and that they could do something to overcome his repeated frustration and escalating anger. The therapist then engaged Steve in a series of exercises in assertive training (cf. Alberti & Emmons, 1974; Collner & Ross, 1978). He first modeled for the patient how to approach the manager and state his concern in a reasonable, straightforward manner. The therapist then role-played the manager and Steve rehearsed the approach. During the rehearsal, Steve had a number of automatic thoughts such as "He'll think I'm a troublemaker for complaining" or "He'll make me look foolish." (These were his "secret fears" that he became aware of only as a result of the role play.) The therapist discussed these dysfunctional thoughts after the role play was concluded and tried to communicate that the important thing was being able to express a legitimate complaint irrespective of whether it was immediately effective. Also, since the other men seemed to be able to make requests or complaints without being "put down," Steve certainly could try. Finally, Steve agreed that he would be no worse off than he was currently without complaining.

The result was that the manager denied that he was playing favorites and claimed (probably as an excuse) that he thought Steve preferred working on the American cars. Subsequently, the manager began to give him some jobs on foreign cars.

Problem-Solving and Skills Training

Addicted patients have difficulty in solving problems, particularly those dealing with interpersonal conflict (Platt & Hermalin, 1989), for at least two reasons. First, a problematic situation can arouse such a degree of anger that they are driven to punish (scold, criticize) the other person so that the problem, far from being solved, becomes aggravated. Second, because of poor problem-solving skills, the patient is rapidly frustrated in a difficult situation and consequently becomes angry.

It is interesting to note that addicted patients are not always deficient in skills. Many know what to say in situations in which they do not have a strong personal involvement. Also, they may know how to advise others to handle difficult situations. However, when they themselves are involved in a difficult situation, they feel they cannot or do not want to try to resolve the problem other than by berating the other person.

Once the patients label others' behavior as an offense against them, they have slipped into the punishment mode. The remedy is for them to detach themselves from the personalized meanings and address the problem in a way leading to solution. "Bob," for example, became infuriated because a mail clerk denied having a package that Bob knew had been delivered to the mail room of his office. Instead of brainstorming about where the package could be, Bob started to yell at the clerk. The clerk became defensive and retaliated, "You can't speak to me that way." Bob then responded sarcastically and walked away in a huff. He was so upset that he felt inclined to go to the bar next door and have a few drinks. Much later he learned that one of his colleagues had picked up the package and delivered it to Bob's secretary.

In the therapy session, Bob realized that he had "personalized" the problem—as though the circumstances had directed this against him. He also had had a catastrophic thought, "If I don't locate the package, I may lose my job." Once he took the situation personally, it was played out at a level of interpersonal fighting (conflict) instead of mutual problem-solving (cooperation).

Thus, the following steps can be prescribed for situations in which one is angry about a difficulty:

1. Detach self from the personalized meanings (put down, discriminated against, let down).

2. Try to approach the problem cooperatively despite the presence of anger:
   a. Define the problem: the "lost" package and the clerk's difficulty in recalling where it might be.
   b. Experiment with explanations: Ask the clerk where it could have been mislaid. Inquire whether one of the other clerks may have seen it. Could somebody else have picked it up?

Steve had a problem with his children—when they started to squabble, he became furious and wanted to yell at both of them. Applying the rule of "defining the problem," he discovered that the older child was continuously teasing the younger one. Steve then could see the solution clearly: Issue a stern reprimand to the older child to stop teasing.

This may seem to be a minor example, but it was built up into a major problem because of Steve's inner belief, "I am helpless when there is a conflict." This sense of helplessness made him reluctant to go home at the end of work because of his fear of friction in the family. Hence, part of the program of anger management consisted of building up Steve's confidence in his parenting skills.

Dealing with Catastrophizing

The way that the underlying mechanisms of LFT can be increased is indicated in another interview with Steve.

TH: Tell me more about why you decided to use [cocaine] last Thursday.

PT: Well, I came home and I asked my wife whether she had taken the kids to the doctor—like she had promised. She said that they weren't really sick and besides she was too busy today.

TH: What did you feel then?

PT: I felt really mad but I controlled myself and left the room. Then I decided to have a line.

TH: What went through your mind when she said she hadn't taken them to the doctor?

PT: I thought, "Suppose they really are sick? Even getting there a day late could be very serious."

TH: As you look at it now, do you still believe that it was a serious problem?

PT: No, they really weren't sick, but at the time it seemed like they could get much worse.

TH: So that's an example of what we know you are in the habit of doing—catastrophizing—a kind of exaggerated worrying.

PT: Right.

TH: Now, what did you feel in your body when you had that thought?

PT: I felt weak all over.

TH: Where?

PT: Especially in my muscles.

TH: What else?

PT: I felt a heavy feeling in my stomach.

TH: Was this weak feeling like a helpless feeling?

PT: Well, I did feel helpless at the time. Because I told her something to do and she didn't do it.

TH: So now, it seems that you have a tendency to expect a catastrophe when somebody doesn't follow instructions. You start to feel weak and helpless. Then you get mad at the person who you think made you feel that way and you want to punish her.

Steve, of course, was more introspective than many patients and was adept at identifying his catastrophic thoughts and his feelings. But many, if not most, patients can be trained the way that Steve was, to recognize and evaluate these automatic thoughts.

ANXIETY DISORDERS AND SUBSTANCE ABUSE

Background

Anxiety disorders are among the most common of psychiatric disorders. Zung (1986), in a survey of 739 family practice patients, found that 20% had clinically significant anxiety symptoms. In the Epidemiologic Catchment Area study, Regier and his colleagues (Regier et al., 1988; Regier et al., 1990) report that the lifetime prevalence of anxiety disorders in the general public is over 14%. In their study, this rate is exceeded only by substance use disorders, with a lifetime prevalence rate of over 16%.

DSM-III-R distinguishes between seven Axis I anxiety disorders: Panic Disorder, Agoraphobia, Social Phobia, Simple Phobias, Obsessive-Compulsive Disorder, Post-Traumatic Stress Disorder, and Generalized Anxiety Disorder. On Axis II, there are at least two personality disorders characterized by substantial anxiety: Obsessive-Compulsive and Avoidant Personality Disorders. Compared with those who do not have chronic anxiety, people with these disorders may be more vulnerable to abusing certain psychoactive substances (e.g., alcohol, benzodiazepines, and nicotine). They may use drugs in an attempt to cope with anxious feelings (i.e., as "compensatory strategies"). In fact, numerous studies and reviews suggest a significant positive relationship between anxiety disorders and substance abuse (e.g., Beeder & Millman, 1992; Helzer & Pryzbeck, 1988; Hesselbrock, Meyer, & Kenner, 1985; Hudson, 1990; Kranzler & Liebowitz, 1988; Kushner, Sher, & Beitman, 1990; LaBounty et al., 1992; Linnoila, 1989; Mullaney & Trippett, 1979; Quitkin, Rifkin, Kaplan, & Klein, 1972; Regier et al.,

1990; Ross et al., 1988; Schuckit, 1985; Walfish et al., 1990; Wilson, 1988).

According to Kushner et al. (1990), estimates of alcohol problems in anxious patients have ranged from 16% to 25%. In alcohol treatment programs, estimates of patients with coexisting anxiety problems have ranged from 22.6% to 68.7%. From a critical analysis of existing literature, these authors conclude that coexistence of alcohol problems and clinical anxiety is not a simple, unidirectional, causal relationship. Instead, Kushner et al. (1990) state:

> It appears more likely that alcohol has the potential to interact with clinical anxiety in a circular fashion, resulting in an upward spiral of both anxiety and problem drinking. For example, increasing alcohol consumption motivated by the short-term relief of anxiety (or the belief that alcohol can relieve anxiety) may lead to increased anxiety related to autonomic nervous system hyperexcitability and anxiety-inducing environmental disruptions which, in turn, may lead to more alcohol consumption to relieve symptoms. (p. 692)

The Cognitive Therapy of Anxiety

A text on the cognitive therapy of anxiety disorders (Beck et al., 1985) emphasizes the importance of appraisal processes in anxiety. Anxiety is typically precipitated by a situation in which the individual regards himself as vulnerable to some threatening (i.e., unpleasant, dangerous, or harmful) event or situation. Prior to the onset of anxiety symptoms, a person makes a series of appraisals about a potentially threatening event or situation. The first appraisal, called a "primary appraisal," involves the initial assessment of risk. For example, in response to the social encounter, the socially anxious person might make the primary appraisal "I am going to embarrass myself." In response to his rapid heartbeat, a person with a panic disorder might make the primary appraisal "I'm having a heart attack."

After the primary appraisal, an individual makes a "secondary appraisal," followed by a series of "reappraisals." Secondary appraisals involve the assessment of a person's resources for dealing with a potentially dangerous event or situation. The following are examples of positive secondary appraisals that enable an individual to cope effectively: "I have been able to handle situations like this before." "My heart is strong." "These are my friends; I don't need to worry about them." Reappraisals involve "reality testing" and the construction of risk:resources ratios.

The central core of the anxiety process is the individual's chronic sense of *vulnerability* (i.e., uncertainty and insecurity). Anxious individuals tend to have core beliefs about their own helplessness that are activated in potentially threatening situations; that is, they characteristically underestimate their ability to cope with the threat.

As a natural consequence of this appraisal process, the patient with an anxiety disorder will experience an escalation of symptoms of anxiety: increased heart rate, sweating, shortness of breath (i.e., psychological symptoms); increased fear or terror (i.e., emotional symptoms); and increased rumination or obsessive thinking (i.e., cognitive symptoms). The addicted person may respond to these symptoms by using psychoactive substances. For example, a person with a flying phobia may use alcohol as a sedative in order to cope with a necessary flight. A social phobic may use cocaine in order to feel more confident in a social situation. A person with generalized anxiety disorder may smoke cigarettes in order to relax (in spite of the fact that cigarette smoking simultaneously creates autonomic stimulation and sedation).

Treatment of the Anxious Substance Abuser

Case Conceptualization

An essential step in the cognitive therapy of the anxious substance abuser is the case conceptualization. Similar to the treatment of other disorders, the therapist evaluates the patient's typical cognitive, behavioral, and emotional responses to relevant experiences. The therapist traces these responses to earlier life experiences (e.g., familial, social, educational) in order to understand their development. An accurate case conceptualization ultimately facilitates the selection of appropriate techniques.

For example, "Rick" is a 38-year-old unmarried accountant with a history of alcohol dependence and cocaine abuse, who entered treatment as a result of a recent "driving while intoxicated" conviction. He explained that he had been drinking between one and two six-packs of beer per night for several years. He typically drank in the evenings until he would pass out while watching television. Rick admitted to blackouts, absenteeism, hangovers, and severe guilt related to his drinking.

In an effort to develop an accurate and useful case conceptualization, Rick's therapist inquired about his current functioning, his problematic situations, his developmental history, his basic beliefs and typical automatic thoughts, and his behavioral and emotional responses to these thoughts. The therapist related these to the development and maintenance of Rick's alcohol use.

Rick described himself as a "loner." He stated: "I wish I had close friends, but I just get so nervous around people. I would like to get married some day, but I'm terribly uptight around women." Rick specifically described the following thoughts: "I have nothing intelligent to say to people," "I will appear stupid," and "People, and especially women, will reject me." Rick occasionally dated women; however, he reported that he had to get intoxicated to tolerate the anxiety triggered by dating.

Rick admitted to occasional panic attacks prior to social encounters. He viewed these panic attacks as supporting his beliefs about his extreme vulnerability. In fact, Rick dreaded all social encounters and he reported that his heavy drinking began when he was required to conduct financial audits for his company (requiring interpersonal contact with numerous business executives). He explained that his fear of criticism and failure, and his resulting anxiety, seemed to be intolerable until he began drinking.

Although he was self-medicating with alcohol, Rick's symptoms of anxiety heightened as he developed a tolerance for alcohol. He viewed himself as increasingly fragile and vulnerable, until he was avoiding most social situations. As he reflected on his life, he felt increasingly depressed, typified by such global negative beliefs as "I am totally worthless," "I am a loser," and "I am hopeless." Eventually, Rick began using cocaine to cope with his boredom, loneliness, and isolation. His cocaine abuse further supported his global negative beliefs (e.g., "Now I'm *really* worthless!").

Upon inquiring about Rick's developmental history, his therapist learned that Rick's parents were "withdrawn and emotionally unresponsive," only showing appreciation when he received perfect grades in school. Regarding his family history of alcohol use, Rick explained that his parents were "fundamentalists who never drank a drop." Their beliefs about alcohol were global and negative, including "Drinking is evil" and "No booze is good booze." Such messages from his parents taught Rick to have dichotomous beliefs about alcohol. For example, he believed, "If I am going to drink at all, I might as well get totally drunk." As a result of his extreme thoughts about alcohol, Rick had difficulty drinking in moderation.

Rick's anxiety, loneliness, and isolation made him vulnerable to heavy alcohol and cocaine use. He responded to his symptoms with thoughts such as "I need a drink or snort to handle this!" "What the hell!" and "Who cares if I use?" These thoughts resulted in urges and cravings to which Rick responded with permissive thoughts such as

"I deserve this!" and "Besides, it doesn't really matter!" Following this permission, he focused on the instrumental strategies necessary for the acquisition of beer or cocaine. This often led him to drink until he passed out or to use cocaine until he had none left. The sequence for Rick's alcohol use is illustrated in Figure 15.1. A similar sequence occurred in his cocaine use.

Educating the Patient about Anxiety and Substance Abuse

Although most anxious individuals are somewhat aware that their fears are exaggerated, they continue to fear that something unpleasant will actually occur. In cognitive therapy the patient is educated in an alternative, more objective method for understanding his or her problems. Specifically, the therapist teaches the cognitive therapy models of anxiety and substance abuse to the patient as these models relate to the patient.

Rick was taught that his anxiety resulted from his *perception* that he was weak or vulnerable. Further, the therapist taught Rick that his drug-related beliefs, automatic thoughts, and core beliefs fed into his

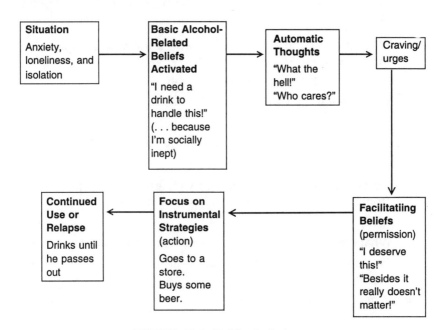

FIGURE 15.1. Rick's alcohol use.

drug use, more than did the environment or his circumstances. The therapist further taught Rick that there were multiple decision points at which he could control his substance abuse, including modifying the anxiety-arousing beliefs, rationally responding to permission-giving beliefs, and finding non-drug-related ways to cope with the anxiety.

Techniques for Managing Anxiety

There are numerous techniques used in the treatment of the anxious substance abuser. The particular technique chosen depends on the patient's presenting problem at each session, as well as the therapist's general conceptualization of the case. The efficacy of selected techniques depends on several factors: the quality of the therapeutic relationship, the accuracy of the case conceptualization, the therapist's appropriate use of the Socratic method, and the patient's socialization to the cognitive model.

In the Socratic method, the therapist asks questions to guide the patient to more realistic conclusions about himself, his personal world, and his future. For example, Rick initially held the belief "I will be rejected if I allow others to see how anxious I am." At the same time, he held the belief "My mistakes are terrible." Using the Socratic method, the therapist asked questions to lead Rick to more adaptive conclusions:

TH: What do you think about when you anticipate an upcoming social encounter?

PT: I know that I'll make a fool of myself.

TH: What do you mean by "a fool"?

PT: I mean that I'll make an idiot of myself.

TH: How do you picture yourself making "an idiot" of yourself?

PT: I see myself having nothing to say.

TH: Do you believe that all people who are quiet in public are "fools," and that they make "idiots" of themselves?

PT: Well, I guess not.

TH: What else are other people likely to think about a quiet person?

PT: They might think that the person is just listening . . . or that the person is just shy.

TH: When you think of yourself as an "idiot" or a "fool," how do you feel?

PT: Upset, nervous, uptight, depressed . . .

TH: And when you view yourself as "just shy," rather than foolish and idiotic, how do you feel?

PT: A little better.

Prior to this dialogue, the patient equated "quietness" or "shyness" with "foolishness" or "idiocy." Through the Socratic method, the therapist helped the patient to objectively examine this maladaptive assumption.

There are five key questions that assist patients in responding rationally to the anxiogenic thoughts that may stimulate cravings and urges for drugs (these questions are applicable to all patients across the diagnostic spectrum): (1) What other perspectives can I take about this situation? (2) What concrete, factual evidence supports or refutes my automatic thoughts? (3) What is the worst that could happen in this situation and how would it ultimately affect my life? (4) What constructive action can I take to manage this situation? and (5) What are the pros and cons of my continuing to have negative automatic thoughts? We summarize the rationale for each question here.

1. *Other perspectives.* Here, patients who might otherwise see things in tunnel vision are asked to broaden their viewpoints in order to ascertain new possibilities. One way to facilitate this process is to ask the following questions: "Could there be a blessing in disguise here?" or "How might this situation not be as bad as it first seems?" This approach helps patients think more divergently and thus opens their minds to more constructive alternatives.

2. *Evidence.* Patients need to learn that their opinions are not necessarily synonymous with facts. Therefore, therapists teach them the importance of looking for information that can be *objectively confirmed or disconfirmed.* Therapists ask patients for evidence *for and against* their automatic thoughts because they want patients to be evenhanded in their evaluation—even if that means finding evidence that supports their negative impressions. One useful way to communicate the nature of "evidence" is to say, "If it wouldn't stand up in court, it's not factual enough to count as evidence."

3. *What's the worst that could happen?* This is not the rhetorical question that people sometimes ask sarcastically when they are minimizing someone's problems. This is a factual question that asks patients to consider a realistic worst-case scenario and then to evaluate the actual implications for their lives. In general, this question serves to decatastrophize many patients' extreme worries, as they come to realize that the worst-case scenario is highly unlikely, and that they can cope with the outcome in any event.

4. *What action can I take?* Even if patients find that their automatic thoughts are borne out, this question reminds them that they can actively engage in problem solving. By asking this question, patients are more likely to apply higher cognitive processes such as planning and decision making, and less likely to lapse into lower-level catastrophizing.

5. *Pros and cons of automatic thoughts.* Some patients seem wedded to their negative, dysfunctional ways of thinking. In such instances, it is useful to ask them what benefits (and drawbacks) they derive from such negativistic thinking. This tactic defuses the patients' resistance in that it respects their reasons for maintaining their points of view, however self-defeating they may be. For example, we have encountered the following "reasons" that patients are unwilling to relinquish their automatic thoughts:

"I don't deserve to think positively."

"Every time I get my hopes up disaster strikes."

"If I think the worst, I won't be disappointed when it actually happens."

"Nobody will take me seriously unless I'm really upset."

Understanding these beliefs helps therapists to conceptualize patients' core assumptions, helps establish rapport, and may provide a window of opportunity to help these patients find some *advantages* to improving the adaptive quality of their thinking.

An example of Rick's completed Daily Thought Record (DTR) can be seen in Figure 15.2. Any and all of the five questions summarized above can be used effectively within the format of the DTR in order to generate rational responses. Not all of the questions need to be used—note that Rick's DTR seems to address the questions "What other perspectives can I take?" and "What constructive action can I take?"

Behavioral Techniques

Behavioral techniques are particularly useful in the treatment of anxiety disorders. Relaxation and assertiveness training (Alberti & Emmons, 1974; Collner & Ross, 1978), for example, provide the individual with behavioral skills for coping with potentially threatening situations. Relaxation skills involve the systematic, progressive relaxation of various muscle groups (Bernstein & Borkovec, 1973) and controlled breathing (Clark, Salkovskis, & Chalkley, 1985), which allows the individual to be more physically comfortable during times of physiologic distress. Assertiveness training involves learn-

Directions: When you notice your mood getting worse, ask yourself, "What's going through my mind right now?" and as soon as possible jot down the thought or mental image in the Automatic Thought Column.

DATE/TIME	SITUATION Describe: 1. Actual event leading to unpleasant emotion, or 2. Stream of thoughts, day-dreams or recollection, leading to unpleasant emotion, or 3. Distressing physical sensations.	AUTOMATIC THOUGHT(S) 1. Write automatic thought(s) that preceded emotion(s). 2. Rate belief in automatic thought(s) 0–100%.	EMOTION(S) 1. Specify sad, anxious/angry, etc. 2. Rate degree of emotion 0–100%.	RATIONAL RESPONSE 1. Write rational response to automatic thought(s). 2. Rate belief in rational response 0–100%.	OUTCOME 1. Re-rate belief in automatic thought(s) 0–100%. 2. Specify and rate subsequent emotions 0–100%.
Friday	Alone at home. Coworkers have invited me to meet them at a restaurant.	"I'll make a fool of myself." (75%)	Nervous (75%)	"I'm generally quiet when I go out, not foolish." (100%)	1. "Fool" (25%) 2. "Relieved" (65%)
		"I don't know how to act around people." (85%)	Anxious (85%)	"I know how to be polite toward others." (90%)	1. "Don't know how to act" (25%) 2. Relieved (65%)
		"Ill be alone for the rest of my life." (50%)	Sad (45%)	"If I take risks, I'll meet someone eventually." (75%)	1. "Alone for life" (35%) 2. Hopeful (50%)

Questions to help formulate the rational response: (1) What is the evidence that the automatic thought is true? Not true? (2) Is there an alternative explanation? (3) What's the *worst* that could happen? Could I live through it? What's the *best* that could happen? What's the *most realistic* outcome? (4) What should I do about it? (5) What's the effect of my believing the automatic thought? What could be the effect of changing my thinking? (6) If _____ was in this situation and had this thought, what would I tell him/her?
(friend's name)

FIGURE 15.2. Rick's Daily Thought Record..

ing direct, adaptive expressive communication. As a result of increased skills, individuals develop a greater sense of competency. The learning of behavioral skills is facilitated by the use of covert rehearsal (imagery) and overt practice (role-play, behavioral experiments).

Rick's therapist, for example, determined that Rick was particularly vulnerable to feelings of inadequacy and rejection in social situations. Specifically, social situations tended to activate Rick's core beliefs about his vulnerability, which in turn activated his autonomic nervous system. His anxiety symptoms (perspiration, racing heart, etc.) then escalated into panic attacks, which he self-medicated with alcohol. To compensate for his feelings of vulnerability, Rick occasionally used cocaine. Ultimately, Rick found that he had great difficulty controlling his cocaine use, which in turn exacerbated his feelings of vulnerability.

In order to treat Rick's anxiety-related substance abuse problems effectively, his therapist began with progressive muscle relaxation and controlled breathing exercises. Such exercises prepared Rick for dealing with the physiological arousal associated with panic attacks. After Rick had mastered relaxation, his therapist asked him to imagine a series of threatening social situations. On becoming physiologically aroused at the thought of such situations, Rick practiced relaxing to decrease his autonomic arousal. Eventually, Rick began to modify his thinking from "I can't handle my anxiety" to "I can at least calm myself to avoid having a panic attack." Rick's therapist also engaged him in assertiveness training in order to provide him with essential communication skills.

SUMMARY

Unnecessary or exaggerated anger takes its toll not only on other persons but also on the person who is angered. Substance abusers are prone to act out their hostile impulses when they are under the influence of drugs or alcohol. Although they are particularly prone to use or drink to dampen the tension associated with anger, their substance use may, paradoxically, increase the likelihood of hostile behavior. Much of the generated anger is the result of the symbolic meaning attached to the provoking event, specifically, the notion "I have been wronged."

Addicted individuals with low frustration tolerance (LFT) are hypersensitive to any blocking of their wishes or actions and are consequently prone to experience excessive and inappropriate anger. They frequently have underlying beliefs such as "If I can't get [or do] what I want right now, I never will" or "Others are wrong to refuse me or get in my way." Stemming from the other two beliefs is the belief "People are wrong and should be punished for blocking me." When activated, this belief leads to anger. Patients with LFT perceive themselves as powerless or helpless. The generation of anger helps restore a sense of control and power by punishing other people. Whether or not they act out their impulses to punish, however, they are more or less stuck with the anger, which can then lead to using or drinking.

Additionally, the physiologic, cognitive, affective, and behavioral correlates of anxiety may place an individual at increased risk for substance abuse. We presented some methods for conceptualizing LFT and anxious substance abusers, as well as some methods for intervening with people who respond to LFT and/or anxiety with substance use.

CHAPTER 16

Concomitant Personality Disorders

The term "dual diagnosis" has been used widely to refer to the coexistence of substance abuse and other psychiatric disorders (Brown et al., 1989; Evans & Sullivan, 1990; O'Connell, 1990). In Chapters 14 and 15 (this volume) we discussed the dual diagnosis of substance abuse and major psychiatric syndromes (e.g., depression and anxiety). In this chapter we discuss the treatment of patients with dual diagnoses involving substance abuse and concomitant personality disorders.

Personality disorders (represented by Axis II of the DSM-III-R classification system) (American Psychiatric Association, 1987), consist of longstanding affective–behavioral–cognitive patterns that are rigid, maladaptive, and resistant to modification.

There have been numerous studies documenting the high prevalence of personality disorders among substance abusers. Regier et al. (1990), in their important comorbidity study, reported on data from over 20,000 subjects in the Epidemiologic Catchment Area study sponsored by the National Institute of Mental Health. These investigators found that of those with alcohol problems (abuse or dependence), 14% met criteria for antisocial personality disorder (ASPD). They found ASPD among those who abused marijuana (15%), cocaine (43%), opiates (37%), barbiturates (30%), amphetamines (25%), and hallucinogens (29%). In accord with these figures, many researchers acknowledge a strong relationship between ASPD and substance abuse (e.g., Grande, Wolf, Schubert, Patterson, & Brocco, 1984; Helzer & Pryzbek, 1988; Hesselbrock, Hesselbrock, & Stabenau, 1985; Hesselbrock, Meyer, & Kenner, 1985; Lewis, Robins, & Rice, 1985; Penick et al., 1984; Ross et al., 1988; Schuckit, 1985; Stabenau, 1984; Wolf et al., 1988). Estimates of the lifetime prevalence of ASPD disorder in substance-dependent individuals vary between 20% and 50%. The high prevalence can be explained, to some extent, by the fact that substance abuse is one of the criteria for the diagnosis of ASPD.

Several studies conclude that a wide range of personality disorders coexists with substance abuse. For example, Khantzian and Treece (1985) studied 133 opiate addicts and found that 65% met criteria for at least one coexisting personality disorder. These investigators reported that "virtually the entire range of personality disorders [was] represented in [our] sample" (p. 1071). Drake and Vaillant (1985) evaluated 369 middle-age inner-city men, followed in a longitudinal study, for the presence of personality disorders and alcohol problems. Of those who had been alcohol dependent, 37% had a concomitant personality disorder.

Borderline personality disorder (BPD) is also commonly associated with substance abuse (Koenigsberg, Kaplan, Gilmore, & Cooper, 1985; Nace, Saxon, & Shore, 1983; Zanarini, Gunderson, & Frankenburg, 1989). These authors report consistently that among drug and alcohol abusers, BPD is second only to ASPD as a concomitant personality disorder diagnosis.

Beck et al. (1990) have applied cognitive therapy to the treatment of personality disorders. The authors describe these patients as "often the most difficult in a clinician's caseload" (p. 5). Personality-disordered patients typically share some of the following common features that make them especially challenging to treat:

1. Their most chronic symptoms are ego syntonic; that is, the patients do not perceive that there is anything substantially "wrong" with their personality. Although they may come into treatment in order to receive help for depression or anxiety problems, they rarely seek help for problems such as self-centeredness, avoidance of responsibilities, lying, lack of empathy for others, lack of conscience, tendency toward violence, interpersonal manipulativeness, defiance of authority, and other chronic aspects of their character that reflect common Axis II disorders.

2. Their behaviors and attitudes typically are noxious to others. Although these patients may feel that they are in emotional pain, it is common to find that they *cause others* a great deal of hardship as well. An example is a patient who bemoans the fact that his wife does not give him respect, but conveniently neglects to mention to the therapist that he steals her money, beats her, and cheats on her.

3. These patients are extremely resistant to change. Although they

may enter therapy hoping to obtain some *relief* from their psychological suffering, they often do not wish to take an objective look at their own shortcomings, nor do they wish to alter their maladaptive behaviors or attitudes. An example is a patient who implicitly expects the therapist to offer him a "magic pill" to make him better, but balks at the idea of dealing directly with his problems at work and at home.

4. Personality-disordered patients have difficulty imagining being any other way. When therapists try to elicit their cooperation in making important changes in life, the patients often respond by saying, "But this is who I am. I can't change," or "I've always been this way. How can I be any different?" or "If you try to change me, I'll cease to exist." For these patients, their problems often are synonymous with their identities. Therefore, they resist change as staunchly as they would fend off personal annihilation.

When a personality disorder contributes to drug use the pattern becomes more rigid and compulsive. Once the drug use has begun, the personality-disordered patient may be more likely to continue the pattern of drug use until it becomes a full-blown addiction. For example, the avoidant personality patient who cannot tolerate emotional discomfort may receive temporary respite from his or her upsetting thoughts about their life situations via the use of crack cocaine. As a result, this patient may choose to continue using (and ultimately abusing) drugs as the preferred method to avoid facing up to problems.

Furthermore, the patient who suffers from a concomitant personality disorder will be at heightened risk for relapse following a period of successful abstinence. As a case in point, we have seen a borderline patient relapse on drugs as a deliberate form of self-destructiveness and interpersonal manipulation in response to arguments with a lover. Another patient, a woman who was diagnosed as having dependent personality disorder, believed that she would not be able to survive unless she had a man in her life. Consequently, she sought out male companionship at all costs, even if the men involved were active substance abusers. Each time she became involved with a new lover, she would subjugate her needs to his and would join him in his drug use. Thus, she knowingly and voluntarily lapsed back into drug use, even after having struggled so hard in therapy to achieve abstinence.

Another ramification of patients' personality disorders is their capacity for cooperating and collaborating with the therapist (Carey, 1991). A substance abuser who does not suffer from a personality disorder may be an amiable and earnest patient with whom to deal in session after he or she has been free from drug use for some time. By contrast, we have seen patients who seem to be staying away from drugs successfully but who have been extremely difficult to manage by virtue of their personality disorders. For example, "Ken" is a parole-office-referred patient who also has been diagnosed as having both paranoid and passive-aggressive personality disorders. In each therapy session, he adamantly insists that he has abstained from drugs in an ongoing fashion, and therefore concludes that his participation in treatment is "an idiotic waste of my time." When the therapist attempts to engage Ken in productive dialogues about the management of general life stressors and maintenance of sobriety, he becomes reticent and projects an air of suspicion. At present, he remains drug-free, but he is not engaged in treatment to an optimal degree. His long-term prognosis, therefore, remains guarded.

We do not mean to imply that the treatment of drug abuse patients with concomitant Axis II disorders is an impossible task, nor do we mean to say that therapy with drug abuse patients without personality disorders is a breeze. The truth, obviously, is less dichotomous and more complex. Nevertheless, it is vital that therapists perform a thorough diagnostic assessment of each substance abuse patient, so that the difficulties associated with the treatment of personality disorders may be anticipated. Treatment plans that address both the patients' drug abuse problems *and* characterological issues are better equipped to keep patients in treatment, and to prepare them for self-maintenance after regular sessions have been terminated (N.S. Miller, 1991).

ASSESSMENT

Personality disorders have been described in a number of ways. One simple formula that clinicians have followed over the years states that patients who have personality disorders cause as much or more grief for *others* in their lives as they suffer themselves (Cummings, 1993). Obvious examples of this are the narcissistic patient, who may be so blindly self-absorbed that he or she completely neglects the physical and emotional well-being of spouse and children, and the ASPD patient, who may be having a "grand old time" while he or she lies, connives, and cheats in order to achieve his or her own ends. Another example is the borderline patient, whose affective lability, self-destructive impulsivity, and excessive interpersonal demands cause much consternation for significant others and for therapists.

If we use this rule alone, however, most substance-abusing patients will look as if they necessarily have personality disorders as well (Carey, 1991). When patients are in the throes of compulsive, addictive drug abuse, the following maladaptive behaviors are not uncommon: (1) stealing from family members, friends, or strangers in order to fulfill a desperate need to purchase and use drugs (symptom of ASPD); (2) inveterate lying, in order to cover one's drug-abusing tracks (symptom of ASPD); (3) almost delusional suspiciousness, a side effect of heavy usage of cocaine and/or amphetamines (symptom of paranoid personality disorder); (4) angry outbursts and violence toward self and others due to overdose or withdrawal symptoms (symptoms of borderline, paranoid, and antisocial personality disorders); (5) withdrawal from social activities into solitary drug use (symptom of schizoid personality disorder); and (6) progressive self-absorption, such that responsibilities toward others become ignored (symptom of narcissistic personality disorder), as well as numerous other behaviors. As we can see, the particular problems that accompany the Axis I substance abuse disorder often look suspiciously like—and need to be distinguished from—full-blown Axis II disorders (cf. Gawin & Kleber, 1988).

In order to clarify the assessment picture, we must look to the criteria of DSM-III-R, and to the diagnostic questionnaires that map onto the DSM-III-R, such as the Structured Clinical Interview for the DSM-III-R (SCID: Spitzer et al., 1987). Here, we are instructed to examine the *enduring* personality traits that exist and persist *apart* from the primary Axis I diagnoses. In this case the question becomes, "What personality traits were present during those times in the patients' lives when they had not yet begun to abuse drugs?" This question is especially useful when the substance abuse problem has an adult onset, and therefore there is an extensive premorbid history.

Another useful source of assessment data comes from previous treatment experiences of patients. It is potentially enlightening to review notes and reports of patients' former therapists, as well as to ask patients themselves about their recollections of therapy contacts (and outcomes) in the past. Such information can shed light on the degree of chronicity of patients' drug problems, "changes" in personality over the course of time as a result of drug use, and clues as to the kinds of interventions that were helpful or unhelpful.

Another useful question is, "What personality traits are present during prolonged periods of abstinence, *between* drug use episodes?" Such an assessment question is salient when abstinence is the norm, punctuated by problematic lapses into drug bingeing.

A simple interpretation of DSM-III-R suggests that a serious concomitant Axis II disorder is less likely to be present when dysfunctional beliefs and behaviors did not predate the onset of the substance abuse disorder, and when they diminish or disappear during times of prolonged abstinence. The non–Axis-II-disordered patient is identifiable as one who seems to "change personality" dramatically when under the influence of psychoactive substances or cravings and urges associated with their abuse. This patient may seem quite compliant with the treatment regimen, and may relate in a friendly, cooperative manner with the therapist when he or she is clean and sober. The same patient may break appointments, drop out of sight, and avoid or otherwise disregard the therapist when he or she resumes drug use, and may engage in activities that seem to be completely "out of character."

For example, one of our patients demonstrated herself to be a conscientious, hard-working, likable person when she had been free of drugs for some time. Unfortunately, when she suffered a relapse, she resorted to thievery in order to obtain money for her habit. The crimes were not malicious but rather a matter of expediency—her values and priorities shifted dramatically when she used drugs (cf. Woody, Urschel, & Alterman, 1992). Family and friends (and the therapist) were shocked when these facts came to light.

Based on knowledge of her crimes of theft, and subsequent lies to cover up, this patient could be easily mistaken as having antisocial personality disorder. In actuality, she did not meet DSM-III-R criteria for any of the Axis II diagnoses. When she was abstinent from drugs, her most salient maladaptive beliefs were depressogenic, but not indicative of longstanding characterological issues. As an example, she believed "I'll never be able to find a job in which I will be trusted to be in a position of responsibility again," and "Something always seems to set me back just when I think I'm getting on my feet again."

On the other hand, while she was actively using, this patient's beliefs became even more problematic (i.e., more similar to those espoused by Axis II patients; see Beck et al., 1990), such as "I have to do what I have to do, no matter what anybody tells me" (similar to beliefs held by ASPD and passive–aggressive patients), and "I have to use drugs because I can't bear to face life in a straight frame of mind" (similar to beliefs put forth by avoidant personality disorder patients).

After successfully completing an inpatient detoxification program in a local hospital, this patient returned to cognitive therapy. She no longer gave credence to the beliefs that she had maintained during her relapse episode, and she once again became a very compliant and actively involved outpatient. The depressive beliefs persisted, however, and became ongoing issues, along with a focus on drug relapse prevention.

In other cases, it is not necessary for patients to be in a phase of active drug use for them to evince dysfunctional beliefs and behaviors that earmark them as personality-disordered patients. For example, when "Lee" was going through his initial intake assessment, he admitted to abusing amphetamines, and highlighted a myriad of life problems. When asked how the drug use had led to the various life dilemmas, he quickly corrected the intake therapist, saying, "Speed doesn't cause all my problems. I can get into all *kinds* of trouble, even if I'm *not* on the stuff, believe me!" In this case, the substance abuse coexisted with a number of personality disorders, which would complicate the drug abuse treatment and would need attention in their own right.

To identify the presence of a personality disorder in a substance-abusing patient requires a careful evaluation of the patient's drug-free beliefs and behavior patterns, and a comparison of these with beliefs and behaviors that are activated by psychoactive substances. A general rule of thumb holds that similarities between drug-free and drug-using beliefs and actions suggest a high probability of an Axis II component, while marked divergences give hope that the most noxious aspects of the patient's functioning will be extinguished if the drug-taking is brought under control. For example, a patient who maintains the belief that he must never follow anyone's rules but his own—and espouses this view whether or not he is drug free—is likely to demonstrate antisocial personality traits that will complicate treatment even if he is free from drugs. By contrast, a patient who typically believes that it is important to be an honest, responsible, cooperative person—that is, until she submits to her urges to use crack cocaine, whereupon she adopts an "I don't give a damn about anything" attitude—is more likely to make significant therapeutic strides in all aspects of her life if she overcomes her addiction.

Unfortunately, this assessment process is fraught with a number of difficulties. First, the optimal method of assessing drug-taking beliefs and actions is not readily apparent. We have noted earlier in this volume (Chapter 12) that the patient's "hot" cognitions are most salient to assessment and treatment, and that such affect-laden thoughts are highly accessible under conditions that closely simulate the target problems in question. In the case of the patient who suffers from a disorder such as panic, it is relatively safe and straightforward to contrive therapeutic situations that will elicit panic attacks in session, thus allowing the patient and therapist to have access to the hot cognitions.

In the case of the drug-abuser, however, it is neither wise nor ethical to encourage the patient to engage in substance-taking as a means of gaining access to key cognitions. Instead, we must use more indirect methods. One method involves having patients rely on free recall to remember what they believed and what they did while in the active phase of drug use. This technique is simple and safe, but may be subject to inaccuracies, owing to patients' memory distortions and deliberate confabulations.

Another method involves gaining data from more objective sources, such as the verbal reports of family members and the written reports of previous therapists and legal officers. Although these data help the therapist to ascertain the maladaptive actions of the drug-taking patient, they do not facilitate gaining an understanding of the subjective phenomenology of the patient who is under the influence of drugs.

We have found that the two approaches explained above are most informative when combined with clinical data that are obtained through provocative imagery exercises, such as patients' closing their eyes and imagining the houses where they use crack. These exercises, described earlier in this volume (Chapter 10), provide patients with the kinds of covert stimuli that will likely produce a reasonable experience of their hot cognitions. These techniques, free recall, third-party behavioral reports, and in-session imagery exercises, combine to help therapists to assess patients' drug-using beliefs and behaviors. As these data are obtained, it becomes more likely that therapists will be able to separate those aspects of patients' functioning that are part of a consistent personality characteristic from those aspects that are drug-related per se.

Still, there are further diagnostic problems. For example, when a 35-year-old drug-abusing patient notes that he has used hard-core drugs such as cocaine since the age of 15, the therapist is hard-pressed to view the patient's drug-related beliefs and actions as anything other than a major part of his personality characteristics. Here, there may not be a single person (the patient himself included) who could guess how the patient would function if he were not on drugs. In such cases, the line of distinction between Axis I and Axis II becomes quite clouded, and therapy may have to involve the teaching and nurturing of fundamental adaptive ways to view the self, the world, and the future practically from "scratch."

Yet another problem in distinguishing personality issues from substance-abuse issues involves the medical complications of long-term drug abuse. Specifically, it is likely that prolonged, heavy use of certain psychoactive substances causes progressive damage to the central nervous system (Karan et al., 1991; Nace & Isbell, 1991; O'Connor et al., 1992). As time goes on, rather permanent changes in personality may *result* from the abuse of drugs, such that even complete cessation of drug use may still leave behind the residual characterological dysfunction. As an example, one of our patients ended a 20-year habit of daily marijuana use after his wife threatened to leave him. Although he succeeded in stopping cold turkey, the patient then was dismayed that he began to feel perpetually depersonalized, to the point that he was "unable to focus my attention on anyone but myself and my own feelings." In a sense, the after-effects of the marijuana use seemed to be a narcissistic–schizoid personality style. This serious problem, along with his chronic anxiety, became the chief foci of therapy over the course of the next six months. Needless to say, there was a concomitant struggle to keep him from returning to regular marijuana use as well.

In sum, it is difficult to separate substance abuse symptoms from long-standing personality issues and disorders. Our experience has taught us that the majority of all substance-use cases will necessitate some sort of therapeutic focus on Axis II disorders, either as a contributory cause or as a consequence of the problematic taking of drugs. The best barometer for the concomitant presence of personality disorders is an assessment of the patient's beliefs—about drugs, and about the self, personal world, and future (the standard cognitive triad; cf. Beck, 1976), *when the patient is free of psychoactive substances.*

BELIEFS THAT FACILITATE
DRUG-TAKING ACROSS DIFFERENT
PERSONALITY DISORDERS

Beck et al. (1990) have outlined common beliefs that are held by patients who suffer from the various personality disorders as described by DSM-III-R. While it is beyond the scope of this text to describe fully each and every one of these disorders, along with their respective lists of beliefs, it is interesting to highlight some of the beliefs that feed into drug-taking. In each of the following examples, the treatment for drug addiction must attend to these concomitant maladaptive cognitive sets.

Many of our drug-using patients are chronically anxious and fearful, resorting to drugs as a way of feeling a greater degree of "safety" or "confidence." *Avoidant* personality patients, who experience chronic cross-situational, exaggerated feelings of threat to their physical and psychological well-being, fall into this category. They maintain beliefs that make the use of drugs seem quite enticing, certainly more attractive than facing up to (and solving) real problems. Such beliefs include "I cannot tolerate unpleasant feelings" and "If I feel or think something unpleasant, I should try to wipe it out with a drink or a drug."

Another type of anxious and fearful patient is the *dependent* personality. These patients do not believe that they can get by without "a little help from their friends" (e.g., drugs, and drug-using cohorts). Their drug-taking is facilitated by implicit assumptions such as "I can't cope as others can" and "I am needy and weak." This mind-set makes a patient easy prey for stimulants such as cocaine, crack, or amphetamines, which induce a temporary but powerful sense of confidence and control in the early stages of their abuse. In addition, peer pressure to engage in drug use is magnified greatly when dependent patients think that they must win the approval of their acquaintances at all costs.

Passive-aggressive patients are hesitant to act out their anger directly, instead choosing to ignore the rules set forth by authorities. They believe that it is safer simply to choose not to conform. For these patients, using drugs represents a way to rebel against disapproving members of their families and society, while maintaining erroneously that "It isn't hurting anybody, so what's the problem?" Meanwhile, these patients further neglect the obligations and responsibilities that they resent in the first place.

Drug use is also facilitated by *obsessive-compulsive* beliefs such as "My way of doing things is generally the best way," and "I need to be in complete control." Here, obsessive-compulsive drug-users maladaptively convince themselves that they know what is best; therefore the use of drugs "must not be a problem." Additionally, the false sense of omnipotence that cocaine can induce reinforces their mistaken notion that they are in complete control of themselves and their life situations.

Narcissistic patients believe that they are entitled to special treatment and privileges, and that they do not have to abide by the rules that most others must follow. They believe that they are special and powerful, and that they deserve to have all of their desires fulfilled. Obviously, these implicit points of view contribute to narcissistic patients' feeling free to engage in any behaviors that give them a sense of satisfaction (including the use of illicit drugs) without feeling that they have done anything wrong or unwise.

In the case of *histrionic* patients, drug use is facilitated by their beliefs that "I cannot tolerate boredom" and "If I feel like doing something, I should go ahead and do it." Furthermore, they want very much to be the center of attention, something that is more likely to occur if they are acting outrageously as a result of chemical intoxication.

Additionally, the beliefs of patients who suffer from *paranoid, schizoid,* and *schizotypal* personality disorders potentiate drug use in that these patients are looking for experiences that they can enjoy in solitude, and that help them to feel on their guard against intrusion or attack from others.

The Axis II disorders described present significant challenges to the therapist when patients also evidence substance abuse disorders. However, the most difficult and pernicious combinations involve, most notably, the borderline and antisocial personalities, which interact with chemical addictions to form a class of disorders that is substantially resistant to treatment of any kind.

Therapy for such noxious composite disorders must involve skilled application of (1) structured sessions, (2) between-session assignments and monitoring, (3) therapeutic relationship-building behaviors, and (4) sophisticated and flexible conceptualizations of patients' problems. In order to approach these objectives, we alert therapists to the following problems and complications that arise in the course of treatment with such patients.

BPD AND ASPD DRUG-ABUSING PATIENTS: CLINICAL MANIFESTATIONS AND IMPLICATIONS FOR COURSE OF COGNITIVE THERAPY

As separate entities, substance abuse disorders and personality disorders such as the borderline and antisocial syndromes are difficult to treat. In combination, the clinical picture becomes extremely challenging indeed. For example, one useful method of eliciting the active cooperation of a drug-taking patient is to help him or her to realize the long-term personal rewards of abstinence. For most patients, goals that appeal to self-interest are intrinsically attractive. However, imagine that such a patient has the following schema: "I'm bad, and I deserve to have my life fall apart." This schema, not uncommon for a borderline patient, may motivate the patient to deliberately steer clear of any strategy that might bring about personal success or recovery. As a result, the therapist's initial call to look at long-term benefits becomes meaningless to this patient. In such a case, the therapist must focus on modifying the extremely maladaptive beliefs that feed into self-hatred, fear of success, and compulsive self-sabotage.

As another example of the immense difficulties involved in treating the severely personality-disordered substance-abusing patient, consider the case of a man with antisocial personality disorder. In contrast to the borderline patient described above, self-interest is markedly *overdeveloped* in the antisocial patient. In turn, the capacity for feeling guilt is profoundly *underdeveloped*. As a result, the therapist's focusing on the harm that the patient is causing others as a result of the substance abuse loses practically all its motivational leverage. Furthermore, the antisocial patient's thirst for freedom and control, and his or her antipathy for authority (e.g., therapists), often leads such a patient to work extremely hard to fight against the work of therapy altogether.

The above examples offer but a glimpse at the dilemmas that face therapists who treat these most problematic of dual-diagnosis patients. We would like to note that although we present them as separate diagnostic categories, the borderline and antisocial personalities sometimes overlap. In fact, the co-occurrence of multiple Axis II diagnoses in the same patient is a common phenomenon (Gunderson & Zanarini, 1987). For the sake of clarity, however, we have chosen to discuss the special therapeutic issues of the borderline substance abuser and the antisocial substance abuser separately.

Antisocial

Antisocial patients rarely come into therapy of their own accord. They generally do not view themselves as having emotional problems of any sort. Instead, they view others around them as being the source of any problems that they may have ("They're hassling me, ripping me off, jerking me around, on my back all the time, setting me up," etc.). As a result, their appearance in therapy is likely to have been imposed on them against their will. In the case of substance-abusing antisocial patients, the source of this mandate usually is a legal authority. It is only natural then for such patients initially to view the therapist as part of the "system" that is trying to oppress them.

As a result, patients try to assert control in any manner possible, usually by passive resistance, sometimes by more radical means such as intimidation. It is especially important at times such as these that cognitive therapists remember to be collaborative, rather than acting controlling in their own right.

For example, when "Don" told one of us that he resented having to see a "shrink," the therapist avoided a response with paternal-sounding imperatives such as "Too bad, but you *have* to be here, buddy!" Instead, he surprised Don by stating, "I know that if it were up to you, you wouldn't be here in this office. You weren't given much of a choice, and that pisses you off. But you know something? We've got something in common. *I* didn't ask to see *you* either. You were assigned to me, and I didn't have much of a choice, just like you. So . . . since we seem to be stuck with each other, how are we going to make this a tolerable experience for both of us?"

This vignette underscores another principle of successfully engaging antisocial patients—keeping them entertained. As they are insatiable stimulus seekers, antisocial patients easily become bored and inattentive in session unless the therapists are willing to be energetic, innovative, and just a little bit confrontational (Doren, 1987). *To the extent that therapists can keep their antisocial patients stimulated, the patients will find the sessions engaging enough to want to return for further appointments.* These patients will be more likely to become actively involved in therapy if they feel that their relationships with their therapists pose interesting interpersonal challenges. As a caveat, therapists need to watch out that they do not fall into the trap of being so entertained *themselves* by the antisocial patient's tales of daring and horror that they are led completely astray—away from the agenda of drug abuse and other patient maladaptive behaviors.

Along these same lines, there is a great temptation on the part of therapists to fight to prevent their antisocial patients from gaining any degree of one-upmanship. These therapists believe that the only way to manage deceptive, manipulative patients is to browbeat them and to "show who's boss." This is a mistake. The therapist's job is not to impress the patient with his or her street smarts, nor to attempt to win every argument. The goal is to keep the patient interested in a therapeutic process that has the best chance of influencing behavioral change (Cummings, 1993; Doren, 1987). This may mean that the therapist has to allow the patient to "win a few." By being reasonably flexible, unpretentious, and willing to own up to mistakes or shortcomings in knowledge, therapists stand a fair chance of disabusing their antisocial patients of their commonly held beliefs that therapists are simply into head games and power trips.

To illustrate, one patient claimed that his barroom acquaintances, members of a local motorcycle gang, were responsible for his drug relapses. He reasoned that they challenged his manhood by daring him to get high with them. When the therapist suggested a few "middle-class, liberal" assertive comments for the patient to try out on these hoods, the patient just laughed and said "That intellectual shit might work in your neighborhood, but not in mine!" Rather than defend his position, the therapist admitted he had goofed on the matter, and said, "Yeh, you're right. I'd probably get my ass kicked if I said that to them." The therapist then proceeded to solicit suggestions for snappy retorts from the patient himself, a strategy that was much better received.

Another complicating factor in treating antisocial drug abusers is that their persistence in taking drugs throughout the course of therapy (and after treatment ends) seems to be worse than for the "average" substance abuser (Doren, 1987). While many addicted patients seem to decry their own drug use, and genuinely wish to kick the habit, antisocial patients often seem very much to *want* to continue their drug use. Rather than using therapy as a way to stop, they attempt to use their treatment to learn how to conceal it better. This may account, in part, for the generally poor outcome that has been reported in the literature for the ASPD drug-abusing patient (Alterman & Cacciola, 1991; Woody et al., 1990). Similarly, ASPD patients' self-report data are more likely to be falsified than are the average drug patients'. This would include information on their drug history, present-time drug self-monitoring, attendance at support group meetings, and adverse effects on their employment and relationships.

For therapists to be best equipped to catch such patients at baldfaced lying, they must take extensive notes. While this is true in treating all patients, it is especially so in treating these most difficult of patients, who weave elaborate webs of falsehoods around unsuspecting, well-meaning therapists. By writing complete notes, not only do therapists protect themselves from unnecessary legal risks, they will also be able to spot the inevitable inconsistencies in patients' reports that will serve as the basis for necessary therapeutic confrontations.

For example, a patient who missed an appointment with his therapist gave the alibi that, since his driver's license had been revoked, he was dependent on others to drive him to his sessions. He claimed that his "driver" failed to show up; therefore the missed session was not the patient's fault. The therapist documented this in great detail, including the "fact" that the license would not be restored for almost 6 months. One month later the same patient excused his lateness for a session by saying that he could not find a parking space. After determining that the patient had indeed driven himself to the therapist's office the therapist read aloud from his notes of the earlier session when the patient had bemoaned his lack of a driver's license. The patient, dumbfounded and annoyed at having been caught in a lie, admitted that he was driving on a suspended license. When pressed further, he was forced to admit that his lack of a license had been scarcely a deterrent to his driving, and that his absence from the previous session was due to something else—taking a "detour" to a bar, where he got drunk. The remainder of the session was spent discussing the patient's drinking, his illegal driving, and his avoidance of therapy sessions. Without the detailed therapy notes, this patient's important area of deceit might have gone unnoticed at the time.

When therapists challenge patients on the veracity of their statements, they may do so in a respectful, supportive way, but they must not shy away from expressing disbelief where it is called for. The following dialogue serves as an example:

TH: This is only the second time you've attended a therapy session in about two months, "Jackie." I'm wondering why it took so long for you to return my phone calls. Have you been in some sort of trouble?

PT: Oh, no! I've just been busy, you know. I'm working double shifts, you know, and I just didn't have time to get back to you, you know.
[Therapist noticed that Jackie was overly animated, and wondered if she was anxiously withholding important information. Her overuse of "you know" statements was a giveaway that Jackie was pretty wound up.]

TH: Jackie, I know that you work very hard at your job. You have always done so. But that never stopped you in the past from returning my calls, except for those times when you were actively using drugs.

PT: Oh, no, no, no! I haven't been using drugs.

TH: OK. I want to believe that. But I'm puzzled that you didn't call me for four weeks, even though I left numerous messages.

PT: I told you. I just didn't have time!

TH: Jackie, it's hard for me to accept what you're saying right now, because there have been many times in the past when you were very, very busy with your job, and with your family's problems, and you still managed to come to therapy sessions every week. You proved to me that you were capable of keeping your life organized and of not letting anything stand in the way of what you had to do. It's something I've always admired about you.

PT: (starts to cry)

TH: [Therapist wondered what Jackie was thinking as she started to cry, but did not want to get sidetracked just yet. He thought that the patient's tears might be real, but they might also be a manipulative ploy. Therefore, he decided to continue to press for the truth, albeit in a very supportive manner.] I'm on your side Jackie. I'm totally on your side, and I want to help you. What kind of trouble have you been in lately with drugs? I really want to help, but you have to be honest with me.

PT: (*Crying*) Everything's all messed up. [Jackie went on to say that she lost her job, and that she felt very ashamed. She and the therapist spent the rest of the session assessing her degree of drug abuse, hopelessness, and suicidality, and they arranged to have daily phone contacts for the next three days until the next face-to-face session. None of this would have come out had the therapist accepted everything that Jackie had said at face value.]

In this example, the therapist was very careful not to communicate an air of self-satisfaction because he had successfully caught the patient in a deception. The goal was to elicit information that could lead to the appropriate assessment and intervention, not to demonstrate that the therapist had superior savvy or to shame the patient. This underscores an important tenet of working with the antisocial drug abuser, namely, always treat the patient with respect, even as you are "winning" the struggle for control of the therapeutic agenda. By leaving the patient with a sense of dignity, collaboration is maintained and facilitated.

Antisocial patients are not altruists. They are not responsive to entreaties to "do the right thing"; they are turned off by the perception that others are moralizing, and they generally focus only on their own immediate wants and needs (e.g., a drug-based high). Therefore, *the therapist can make headway in treatment only to the extent that the patient becomes convinced that it is in his or her best interest to change.* Simply put, this involves helping patients to understand the relative costs and benefits of modifying the various aspects of their current functioning.

Unfortunately, antisocial patients are notoriously inept assessors of the consequences of their actions. Likewise, they are deficient in ascertaining the consequences of their thoughts, beliefs, and emotions as well. Walter is an excellent case in point. Each time he got a new job, he went out and "celebrated" by getting drunk and then using cocaine. This invariably led to tardiness, absenteeism, and the loss of the job. Walter once again would become depressed, and adopt the attitude "I don't give a shit anymore. Fuck it!" This would in turn lead to more drug use, and the downward cycle would continue.

A great deal of work (over a long time in therapy) was required in order for Walter to comprehend the amazingly simple fact that his own behaviors and thoughts were responsible for his downfall. A breakthrough of sorts was achieved when he was able to articulate the idea that his "celebrations" were at the root of his repeated firings. It took him considerably longer before he realized that the thoughts "I don't give a shit," and "Fuck it!" were also responsible for his continuing self-defeating behaviors.

One of the most effective methods of teaching patients to monitor the consequences of their responses is the advantages–disadvantages analysis (Chapter 9, this volume). For example, when a patient experiences a strong craving for drugs, he or she is instructed to examine the advantages and disadvantages for using, as well as the advantages and disadvantages of not using. Similarly, this same technique may be used for other maladaptive aspects of functioning, such as the pros and cons of (1) acting on an urge to seek revenge, (2) quitting a job, (3) engaging in high-risk sexual behavior, (4) dwelling on anger-producing thoughts, (5) discontinuing therapy, (6) contacting drug-using associates, and (7) adopting an "I don't give a damn" attitude, as well as many other "popular" modes of operation of the drug-taking antisocial patient.

As the patient begins to learn to use this technique with some degree of proficiency, he or she can be taught the next level on the hierarchy of difficulty, namely, distinguishing *short-term* pros and cons from *long-term* pros and cons. Typically, antisocial patients are driven by short-term rewards, and therefore often act out impulsively in a manner that is decidedly destructive in the long run. They seem to have a block in even thinking about or imagining long-term consequences.

It is a difficult task to help these patients to learn to envision the future and to delay gratification. One method is guided imagery exercises, where the therapist describes various outcomes for patients to picture in their mind's eye. Typically, the images depict aversive consequences for patients if they continue to use drugs, consequences such as loss of money, job, family, health, and freedom. It is important to make these images as graphic as possible, such as waking up in one's own urine in a roach-infested house, facing an accusatory tirade from the spouse or children, or having handcuffs slapped on in front of the neighbors. As this exercise is repeated, patients are asked to provide more and more of the description themselves. Along with the negatives mentioned above, *positive* images of the outcomes associated with *abstinence* from drugs should be generated in a detailed fashion as well. Therapists can teach their patients to practice these images every day, to help provide regular incentive to stay away from drugs.

Another technique encourages patients to "test their ability" (an appealing challenge to antisocial patients) to withstand urges to engage in impulsive behavior, such as drug use, violence, unsafe sex, and so on. When they get one such urge, they are instructed to monitor how long they can "bravely" fight off the temptation. While they are doing this, the second part of the skill involves thinking (and writing) of ways that it might be advantageous to "lay low, size up the situation real carefully, stay cool, and bide your time." An important goal here is to appeal to patients' intelligence by suggesting that they exercise their ability to think before they act (out). As a warning, therapists should emphasize to their patients that this technique works best when it is applied to cravings that arise spontaneously. It is inappropriate to use this technique by contriving high-risk and craving situations under the guise of "testing" oneself.

The methods described above are most effective when they are incorporated into regular therapeutic homework assignments. We cannot overemphasize the importance of between-session practice of the techniques and principles that are reviewed in the therapist's office (Newman, 1993; Newman & Haaga, in press). Without such regular application of therapy techniques, much of what goes on in session will go "in one ear and out the other." We advocate the taking of notes (by both the patient and the therapist) during the session. Further, *we suggest that patients keep a spiral notepad or folder where they can compile important therapeutic notes and homework assignments as they progress through treatment. In addition, we encourage patients to allow us to audiotape the goings-on in therapy, and for patients to take the tapes home to review the contents of the session again and again.* Sometimes, we have increased compliance by asking patients to listen to the tapes in order to remind us where we as therapists "goofed up," and where the patients made their most astute observations in the previous session.

In addition to their benefits as teaching devices and general interventions, homework assignments serve a useful assessment function as well. Patients with the higher levels of motivation will be the ones who are most likely to make earnest efforts to complete the assignments. The antisocial patients who are simply "playing the game" of therapy will find dozens of elaborate excuses for failing to do the homework as assigned (Doren, 1987). In this sense, a patient's willingness to collaborate in the therapeutic process can be gauged via his or her responses to homework assignments.

In any event, it is potentially useful to elicit the thoughts and beliefs that inhibited the patient from following through with the assignment. In the case of benign procrastination or lack of understanding, this is a rather straightforward task. On the other hand, the antisocial patient who is clandestinely trying to subvert the therapy process will be more difficult to pin down. Here, it may be more useful to ask the patient to express his or her *complaints* about the homework as an entry point into the assessment of thoughts that discouraged the patient from doing the assignment.

Sometimes the responses are quite surprising, such as one patient who resisted reading a book that we had recommended, even to the point of purchasing it and then throwing it out when he got home. After much careful probing by the therapist, the patient was finally able to explain that he noticed that the author of the book had been employed by the Center for Cognitive Therapy. He then reasoned, "You all just want to make more money by asking people like me to buy your books. You don't really care about helping *me!*" The fact that he was receiving free treatment in the first place did not seem to factor into his thinking, nor did the fact that the book was a very inexpensive paperback. He was simply primed to assume that "everyone will always try to get one over on me, if they get the chance." In his way of thinking, he certainly was not going to cooperate with anyone who was trying to take advantage of him, even if it meant wasting his money in the self-defeating act of throwing away a brand new book. This maladaptive mode of operation then became a focal point in therapy, along with his problematic substance abuse.

Although not commonly associated with the treatment of substance abuse or antisocial personality disorder, assertiveness training (Alberti & Emmons, 1974; Collner & Ross, 1978) is a useful part of treatment with this population. Most of these patients engage in dichotomous, all-or-none social behavior, acting either passively or aggressively. Assertiveness is not typically part of their repertoire. This leads to many obvious problems, such as an inability to say no to peers who want them to use drugs, and inappropriate ways of dealing with conflict situations with employers, significant others, parole officers, and therapists, among other people.

Although one may argue that teaching antisocial patients the skills of assertiveness is tantamount to instructing them in ways to be better manipulators of others, we have found that this is generally not the case. These patients wreak far more havoc by being passive aggressive (e.g., "forgetting" to pay child support) and aggressive (e.g, deliberate high-speed tailgating on the highway), rather than assertive (cf. Doren, 1987). Furthermore, the vicious cycles that are perpetuated by dysfunctional thoughts that lead to dysfunctional interpersonal behaviors that then lead to interpersonal consequences that further refuel maladaptive thoughts are slowed down when assertive behaviors prevail. An additional potential benefit of assertiveness training is that it may help patients to identify and articulate thoughts and feelings that previously were ignored or deliberately suppressed by the patients.

For example, a patient who believes that a therapist is trying to control and manipulate her may react in a hostile manner that results in greater attempts from the therapist to gain control over the patient's maladaptive behaviors, thus "confirming" the patient's suspicions. On the other hand, if a patient assertively and directly tells a therapist that she does not appreciate his heavy-handed therapeutic tactics and wishes that he would be a bit more lenient and understanding, the therapist is more likely to understand the patient's actions in a constructive light. Thus, a potentially destructive power struggle may be averted.

Borderline

Similar to the antisocial drug abuser, the borderline patient tends to act out impulsively, to experience extremely low frustration tolerance, to be deficient in learning from past mistakes, to use drugs in lieu of attempting to cope with stress, and to have difficulty in establishing stable, trusting relationships with caregivers.

In contrast to antisocial patients, borderline patients may use drugs more out of a sense of hopelessness than as thrill-seeking behavior. In addition, their behaviors are much more deliberately self-destructive than are the behaviors of antisocial patients or other personality-disordered patients. Owing to the borderline patients' tendency to maintain powerful negative beliefs about themselves, their hopelessness, and poor impulse control, the threat of suicide is far more prominent in the case of the borderline substance abuser. In contrast to antisocial patients, who often feel that they do not need to see a therapist, borderline patients more frequently are desperate for help. Nevertheless, they are apt to act in ways that sabotage the process of therapy, owing to their erratic emotionality, their difficulty in using thoughts (rather than raw emotions) to modulate their own behavior, and the extreme, conflicting demands that they make on their therapists.

Borderline patients pose a peculiar challenge to therapists in that they so readily avoid acting in their own best interests. It is one thing to motivate a patient to give up the use of drugs by appealing to an improved quality of life in the future. It is quite another thing to attempt this with a patient who states "I don't give a damn about what happens to me, now or ever, so I might as well do whatever it takes to kill the pain," or who maintains the belief "I hate myself and I deserve to have a messed up life."

On the other hand, borderline patients may be more likely than antisocial patients to profess concern and love for *others* in their lives, in spite of their lack of caring about themselves. For example, Dee experienced a life filled with sexual, physical, and emotional abuse, leading her to conclude that she was a "bad" person who was "dirty and used up." At the start of treatment, she professed not to care for herself, and she took a cavalier attitude about the possibility that she might wind up killing herself with a drug overdose. It was clear that she was not intent on doing the work of therapy in order to obtain the benefits for herself. Instead, Dee and her therapist focused on her baby daughter, whom she loved dearly. Therapeutic goals were set on the basis of the premise that the *baby* would become the ultimate beneficiary. This served as the "hook" that got Dee involved in the active process of trying to curtail her drug taking. She knew that she would take proper care of her beloved baby if she practiced abstinence from drugs. On the other hand, if she used drugs, Dee knew from experience that she would disregard everything in her life, even her own daughter. The prospect of this happening again frightened her and therefore served as an initial motivator for treatment.

Dee's case typifies the difficulties involved in treating this population. When she experienced a drug lapse, she would tend not to bring herself back into line by thinking about what was best for her daughter. Instead, she would look at her drug-using experience as "proof" that she was an evil person and a bad mother who deserved to die. She would think to herself that her baby would be better off if she had a different mother, and Dee would proceed to escalate her drug use into a full-blown relapse. As a result, Dee would get her "wish," in that her aunt would take custody of the baby. As she began the next cycle of recovery, Dee once again would yearn for her daughter, thus leading to more depressed affect, frustration, and rifts in the family. Such stressors precipitated significant drug-taking cravings and urges, which again would feed into Dee's extremely low self-esteem.

In dealing with cases such as Dee's, the therapist must be on the lookout for a number of emotional and cognitive dysfunctions typical of the borderline patient that exacerbate the patient's drug-taking habits. First, as mentioned above, *borderline patients are prone to self-sabotage, believing that they are undeserving and unable to change things for the better* (Layden, Newman, Freeman, & Byers-Morse, 1993). Such a mindset is wholly unconducive to acting in one's own best interest, in planning for the future, in collaborating with the therapist, and in resisting the temptation to abuse drugs. Therefore, the borderline patient's pathologically low self-image (i.e., beliefs about the self) must be assessed and addressed as part of the treatment for substance abuse.

Another factor is the borderline patient's propensity for feeling profoundly lonely and empty. Many of our patients have reported that the use of cocaine, crack, or heroin temporarily alleviates these feelings, causing them to feel no need for other people during the euphoric surge. It is therefore not surprising that borderline patients turn to drugs in response to interpersonal difficulties and the resultant dysphoria. Complicating matters is the fact that some of these patients view their drug-taking cohorts as their only source of "friends." The thought of losing these associates as a result of becoming abstinent is simply too threatening to entertain, and the drug use continues.

In order to deal with the problems associated with extreme loneliness, therapists must help their drug-using borderline patients to work at building new, drug-free relationships. In addition, it is often beneficial to assist these patients in trying to repair old relationships (e.g., with immediate family members) that were strained or severed due to their substance abuse. These are difficult tasks for the borderline patient, but they are necessary in order to provide an attractive alternative to the "loneliness-killing" qualities of drugs.

Yet another problem borderline patients pose is their hair-trigger hopelessness. As we discussed earlier in this volume (Chapter 12), patients are more likely to resort to the quick fix that drugs produce if they believe that the future holds no promise. The implication for therapy is that the patients' degree of hopelessness is a critical variable with which to contend if we are going to succeed in helping them become and remain drug-free.

Borderline patients, who are notorious for their extreme black-and-white thinking (cf. Beck et al., 1990; Layden et al., 1993), can change their outlook on life from optimistic to completely hopeless with relatively little provocation. We have seen such patients leave a productive therapy session in very high spirits, only to call the therapist the same evening in a state of deep dysphoria due to an objectively mild stressor. When drug abuse is part of the clinical picture, these patients are more likely to resort to getting high than they are to call their therapists for assistance. The upshot is that the borderline patient can flip very quickly from hopeful and abstinent to hopeless and using. Therefore, therapists need to remain vigilant in helping these patients to learn, practice, and, it is hoped, master the skills of decatastrophizing and problem-solving in the face of setbacks.

An offshoot of the borderline patient's problems with hopelessness is a pronounced risk for suicide (Linehan, 1987). Ideally, the patient's wish to live or die should be assessed at *every session*, and a verbal antisuicide contract should be made and renewed frequently. For example, Dee was periodically suicidal, and the therapist repeatedly stressed that she was to call him at work or at home in the event that she wanted to harm herself. She agreed to do so, but she was agonizingly inept in keeping ready access to the therapist's telephone numbers. Therefore, as a matter of ritual, the therapist assigned Dee the task of memorizing his telephone numbers, and quizzed her suddenly at various points during every therapy session.

As a population, substance-abusing borderline patients are more frequently in need of hospitalization than many other clinical patient groups. Even in an inpatient setting, such patients pose considerable management problems. If the patient is suicidal, the first order of business is to provide constant professional supervision. Although the acute risk for suicide may pass, this type of patient rarely is able to stay in the hospital long enough to deal adequately with the borderline disorder. When these patients reenter outpatient treatment, the therapist's tasks are daunting.

As with the antisocial drug-abusing patient, it is vitally important to carefully nurture and make clinical use of the therapeutic relationship (see Beck et al., 1990; Layden et al., 1993; Young, 1990; Chapter 4, this volume, for more detailed explications). The all-or-none thinking style of the borderline patient often shows itself in the way that the patient views the therapist, who may be seen as a savior one week (e.g., "Nobody else understands me the way you do. You're cool and I can trust you.") and a villain the next week ("You're just like all the rest! You don't care about me! You don't know what you're talking about! You're not helping me at all!"). Under such adverse interpersonal conditions, therapists must not allow themselves to buy into patients' extreme positive or negative feedback. Instead, they would do well simply to maintain their composure, to express an ongoing willingness to help, and to focus on the thoughts and beliefs that are behind the patients' polarized reactions.

Likewise, therapists must make every effort to teach these patients to think carefully before acting. This involves painstaking training in problem-solving (D'Zurilla & Goldfried, 1971; Nezu et al., 1989) and rational responding (Beck et al., 1979; Newman & Beck, 1990), skills that are most difficult (yet most necessary) to employ at times of extreme distress. Also similar to the treatment of the antisocial patient is the focus on helping the borderline patient acquire assertiveness skills, so as to reduce conflict in interpersonal situations.

All these interventions require numerous repetitions with both antisocial and borderline patients, as their psychological learning skills and levels of motivation to change are notoriously deficient.

SUMMARY

The existence of severe Axis II disorders in substance-abusing patients significantly complicates the treatment picture with these patients. In particular, antisocial and borderline patients pose tremendous challenges to therapists who are working diligently to help them to overcome addictions to drugs.

We have suggested ways that therapists may detect concomitant personality disorders in substance abusers, taking into account the fact that patients who are actively on drugs often seem to "change personality," thus confusing the diagnostic picture. Nevertheless, we posit that it is important to assess the presence or absence of personality disorders in substance-abusing patients, as the more extreme personality disorders will require awareness of special issues in clinical management, the likes of which we have reviewed.

Furthermore, assessing and understanding the substance abuser's characterological issues provides a window into the patient's beliefs or schemas about the self, world, and future, thus assisting the therapist in reaching a sound conceptualization of the case (Beck et al., 1990; Persons, 1989).

Finally, we would like to add that there is no tried-and-true starting point in the treatment of Axis II dual-diagnosis patients. The question whether to focus first on the substance abuse or on the personality disorder is a "chicken and egg" issue. Therapists must be prepared to attack these problems simultaneously, using their understanding of the patient's idiosyncratic dysfunctional beliefs to sympathetically earn increments of trust and cooperation in carrying out the treatment for drug abuse.

CHAPTER 17

Relapse Prevention in the Cognitive Therapy of Substance Abuse

$\mathbf{A}$fter the patient has quit using drugs, an even more formidable challenge begins. It is relatively easy for many people to change undesired behaviors temporarily; however, maintaining behavioral changes is much more difficult. In fact, it was Mark Twain who said, "To cease smoking is the easiest thing I ever did. I ought to know because I've done it a thousand times" (Prochnow, 1969).

Most people who quit using drugs have a lapse or a relapse (Saunders & Allsop, 1987; Vaillant, 1983), with the most likely time being within 90 days of the initiation of abstinence (Mackay, Donovan, & Marlatt, 1991). A lapse, or a "slip," is defined as the initial use of a substance after an individual has made a commitment to abstain from that substance. A relapse, on the other hand, is a full return to the maladaptive behaviors originally associated with use of the substance. In the cognitive therapy of substance abuse, a major goal is to have patients learn from whatever setbacks in long-term abstinence goals they may have (Moorey, 1989). It is hoped that the lessons learned from such experiences will ultimately improve an addict's planning skills, resolve, and self-confidence.

In this chapter we present cognitive therapy techniques for relapse prevention. Some of these techniques are an extension of methods used to help patients discontinue drug use in the first place (e.g., the development of a collaborative relationship, conceptualizing the patient's problems, guided discovery, structured sessions, advantages–

disadvantages analysis, and homework assignments.) Other techniques (e.g., identification of high-risk stimuli) are uniquely designed to assist patients in the relapse prevention process. Prior to presenting these techniques, the cognitive model of drug use and relapse is reviewed. This model provides a framework within which these techniques may be understood and applied.

THE COGNITIVE MODEL OF RELAPSE

The cognitive model of relapse (nearly identical to the model of *ongoing* use) is presented in Figure 17-1.

The cocaine addict is vulnerable to high-risk stimuli (HRS) (Marlatt & Gordon, 1985). These are internal and external "triggers" that stimulate the addict's appetite for drugs. Internal stimuli include emotional and physical factors such as depression, loneliness, boredom, anger, frustration, and physical pain (Mackay et al., 1991). External stimuli include people, places, and things that are related in some way to drug use (Shulman, 1989). HRS vary greatly from person to person. For example, possessing money may trigger some patients to use, while other patients may be more tempted to use when they feel upset about not having money. The difference lies in the personal meaning that the patient attaches to the stimulus.

The importance of HRS is that they may activate *basic drug-related beliefs* that have been overlearned by the patient. Examples of these beliefs are the following:

"Drugs are problems for some people, but they won't be for me."

"Drugs enhance my life by making it more fun."

"People who are against drugs don't really understand them."

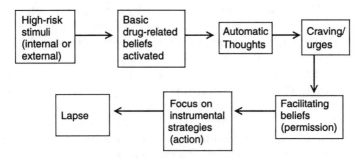

FIGURE 17.1. Cognitive model of relapse.

"As long as I am careful, drugs won't hurt me."

"Without drugs, life would be boring."

"When I have problems, drugs relieve the pain."

From these basic beliefs, *automatic thoughts* may be stimulated (e.g., "I need a hit!" "Time to party!" or "I've got to get high!"). Automatic thoughts are associated with *craving and urges*, and like other feelings, craving and urges themselves become internal HRS.

In response to craving and urges, the patient may engage in some *facilitating beliefs*. Facilitating beliefs are a subset of basic drug-related beliefs that give patients "permission" to use. Examples include the following:

"I can use just one more time."

"Nobody will find out."

"It will be OK to use again. I'll keep it limited."

Facilitating beliefs increase the likelihood that the addict will seek and eventually use drugs.

Instrumental strategies are the actual behaviors and activities involved in seeking, acquiring, and using drugs. These strategies, like basic drug-related beliefs, may vary from person to person and from time to time. For some, the craving for cocaine is so intense that the addict becomes obsessed with drug seeking, to the exclusion of all other considerations. Like a heat-seeking missile, the craving addict may focus on a target and let nothing get in the way of drug acquisition. As a result of this "drive" some addicts engage in violent or criminal behaviors to acquire cocaine.

If a patient has proceeded through the steps above, he or she is likely to have a slip. This slip, or *lapse*, then becomes a high-risk stimulus for the cycle to begin again. That is, on taking a hit, the addict may focus on his or her basic belief that "one hit means I'm out of control." This belief might be followed by a cascade of self-derogating automatic thoughts and negative feelings. The resulting urges may become stronger, and the use of drugs may escalate until the patient has a full-blown relapse.

To illustrate this process, we review the case of Mike, a 35-year-old salesman who had been abstinent from cocaine for six months. After two years of heavy use Mike chose to quit while hospitalized for cardiac problems (tachycardia and arrhythmias) associated with his cocaine use. Mike agreed to inpatient addiction treatment and, on completing a 28-day program, he entered outpatient psychotherapy and Narcotics Anonymous to deal further with his addiction. Prior to quitting, Mike had been having serious marital problems, as his wife "Judy" had recently given birth to their first child and had become increasingly frustrated with Mike's cocaine-related problems.

In spite of Mike's extended inpatient and outpatient drug treatment, he continued to crave cocaine. His internal (emotional) HRS included feelings of boredom, frustration, irritability, and anxiety. External high-risk stimuli included friends who used, parties, and arguments with Judy. After initial treatment Mike often "found himself" in high-risk situations. For example, he continued to spend time with his cocaine-using friends. Such behaviors made Judy quite angry and she eventually separated from him. In response to his separation, Mike felt depressed, anxious, bored, frustrated, and irritable; thus, he was at extremely high risk for relapse.

Mike's cocaine-using friend "Ryan," seeing Mike in "such bad shape," offered him a line of coke to "boost his spirits" (introducing another high-risk situation as well as a facilitating belief). Mike chose to accept Ryan's offer and in doing so he perceived himself as being "out of control." His automatic thoughts included "I can't resist" and "I can't handle life without drugs." He began to imagine and anticipate the extreme positive feelings he had previously associated with getting high: "I'll feel great!" and "It will relieve all of my pain." After very brief deliberation he took his first "hit," which led to a second, a third, and so forth (this episode became his initial lapse). As the effects of the drugs wore off, Mike began to feel dysphoric, agitated, and confused. He perceived this experience as proof that his substance abuse was an irreversible condition and he thought "once an addict, always an addict!" and "Now that I've started again I can't possibly stop using." As a result of this dichotomous thinking, Mike set the stage for a full relapse.

Relapses pose important challenges to both patient and therapist. They may trigger counterproductive thoughts in the therapist, such as "This patient's condition is hopeless!" and "I am wasting my time." Counterproductive thoughts in the patient might include, "I have failed and I always will fail," "I can't ever tell my therapist about my using," and "My therapist would surely reject me, or even hate me, if he knew I've been using!" The disadvantage of such all-or-none thinking processes is that they may result in a sense of hopelessness or apathy in the patient or therapist.

Ideally, the therapist helps the patient to construe lapses and relapses as opportunities to practice more adaptive ways of combatting drug use. For example, Mike's therapist could help him to understand that there were more adaptive ways to deal with his dysphoria over his marital separation than to use drugs. Rather than believing that his situation was hopeless, and that his only relief would be to accept his friend's offer of cocaine, he could focus on *productive* activities that would boost his mood and self-esteem. Further, even if he did *begin* to use cocaine, Mike did not have to believe that he was in an irreversible free fall. Instead, he could practice reciting some control beliefs that might help him to "pull out of the nose dive" (Shiffman, 1992) if confronted with similar situations in the future. Such control beliefs might be

"If I stop now, I can show myself that I am stronger than the drug."

"Walking *away* from drugs is the same as moving *toward* saving my marriage."

"I must seek *drug-free* friends when I feel this badly."

When the patient has maintained abstinence for an extended period of time and the therapist and patient are confident in the patient's ability to maintain abstinence, formal therapy may be terminated. At this time, "booster sessions" are arranged, which may include telephone calls, written correspondence, and face-to-face contacts. These sessions serve several purposes. First, they focus the patient's attention on the need for vigilance in combatting the relapse process. Second, the therapist's continued interest in the patient provides social support that motivates further abstinence. Third, the therapist can continue to provide expert guidance to a patient who may be at renewed risk for relapse.

Substantial gains may result from extended contact with the patient. Each booster visit or telephone call might decrease the likelihood that the patient will relapse, or at least will remind the addict that the therapist is a potential resource for coping with HRS. If the addict does relapse after therapy has been terminated, it is recommended that he or she be invited to return to therapy as soon as possible to work on improving coping skills. Again, careful analysis of each lapse and relapse provides the patient with an increased understanding and ultimately greater control over the relapse process.

At the same time, we must note the following two caveats. First, although we as therapists endeavor to provide ongoing help to patients who continue to be in need, we agree with Gawin and Kleber (1992) that, "The goal of relapse prevention is gradually to decrease the external controls placed on the abuser, by family and therapist, during initiation of abstinence, and gradually to facilitate development of the abuser's internal controls" (p. 47). Second, although it certainly is preferable for patients to learn from their lapses and relapses than merely to succumb to them, we must be careful not to convey the *wrong* message that we *encourage* lapses and relapses as growth-enhancing experiences. Therapists must make it clear to patients that the *best* learning occurs via ongoing drug-free coping with life's everyday and long-term demands.

TECHNIQUES FOR THE PREDICTION AND CONTROL OF RELAPSE

Identification of High-Risk Stimuli

People who suffer from drug and alcohol addictions inevitably encounter HRS. This is especially apparent when one considers the fact that all human beings experience some sadness, anxiety, nervousness, anger, or frustration (all internal HRS) at times. The identification of internal and external HRS is an extremely important component of the relapse prevention process, as it is not uncommon for the addict to lack an awareness of HRS.

By increasing awareness of HRS, the addict may reduce the likelihood of exposure and/or reflexive reaction to them. In sessions, patients are encouraged to carefully review recent and remote memories of relapses in order to discover the full range of HRS that might lead to future relapse. Here, a therapist–patient dialogue is presented to illustrate this "trouble-shooting" process:

TH: Mike, what types of situations are most likely to cause you to crave cocaine?

PT: I don't know.

TH: Well, let's try to think of some, so that you might learn to prepare and cope more effectively with them

PT: Yeah, I guess that makes sense. Now that you ask, when I am with certain friends I want to get high . . . but I can't think of anything else.

TH: OK, let's review your last binge. How did it begin?

PT: I had been clean for almost a month when I suddenly got the urge one night. The next thing I knew, I was with Bob and Ryan, smoking crack.

TH: Now think carefully, what actually happened that night? I would like to hear the details.

PT: Well, I was at home and my wife was in one of those moods where nothing I did was right.

TH: What happened next?

PT: I got pissed off at her and really let her have it. What I mean is, I really started to fight back.

TH: What happened next?

PT: She let me have it, even worse. She started screaming about how I'm a lazy, good for nothing so and so.

TH: And then?

PT: I stormed out of the house and went for a walk around the neighborhood. Sure enough, I saw Bob and Ryan sitting in front of the convenience store.

TH: What happened next?

PT: I walked over to them, and the next thing I knew we were all at Bob's house. The rest is history.

TH: So, there were actually several high-risk stimuli involved, weren't there? They included your wife's criticisms, your anger and frustration in response to her comments, your leaving home with the problem unresolved, walking around late at night, the convenience store where you guys typically meet, Bob and Ryan, and finally, being at Bob's house.

PT: Yeah, now that you mention it, I guess the situation was kind of complicated.

TH: How could you make this kind of situation "simpler" in the future?

PT: I don't know.

TH: Well, this is something we have to work on. For starters, you could make things simpler if you know how to *recognize* when you're upset and looking for an escape. Does that ring true for you?

PT: Yeah.

In this dialogue it became apparent that Mike had exposed himself to multiple HRS, thus dramatically increasing his likelihood of a lapse. Interestingly, Mike had difficulty seeing how he made decisions that led to a chain of events that led up to an ultimate lapse. Marlatt (1985) talks about such "accidental" exposures to HRS as resulting from "apparently irrelevant decisions." Carroll, Rounsaville, and Keller (1991) explain that such exposures may reflect underlying ambivalence about changing addictive behaviors. Thus, it is important that the therapist, under these circumstances, evaluate the status of the patient's decision to become abstinent from drugs and alcohol.

For example, Gorski and Miller (1982) highlight a number of telltale signs that signal a patient's starting along the road to relapse—

that is, being prone to exposure to high-risk situations, and ill-equipped to manage the thoughts, feelings, cravings, and actions that result. Such signs include, for example, (1) an increasingly noncha-lant attitude about remaining actively involved in ongoing self-help activities (e.g., attending therapy or support-group meetings, con-tinuing with homework derived from therapy), (2) regression into affective lability and hypersensitivity, (3) reduced willingness to talk about problems and concerns, (4) social withdrawal, (5) breakdown of healthy daily routines and structure, and (6) impulsive decision-making. A concrete example is a patient who begins to cancel therapy sessions for spurious reasons, and who denies *any* symptoms on the Beck inventories (BDI, BAI, BHS, etc.) in spite of obvious signs of stress. These early-warning indicators set the stage for the relapse process as depicted by the cognitive model flowchart, and must be given attention in their own right.

It is apparent that HRS are highly idiosyncratic for individual drug abusers (Carroll, Rounsaville, & Keller, 1991). It is recommended that the cognitive therapist carefully evaluate HRS for each individual patient. A useful method for doing so is self-monitoring homework. Specifically, the patient keeps a journal of hourly changes in cocaine (use and) craving in relation to internal and external events. This journal is reviewed in session to assess "previously unseen patterns in cocaine use" (Carroll, Rounsaville, & Keller, 1991). At the end of each session, the patient is asked to anticipate specific HRS that might occur between the present and the next session. Furthermore, the patient is asked to plan strategies for coping with such HRS.

Cognitive Strategies for Coping with HRS

The significance of HRS is that they trigger basic drug-related beliefs that increase vulnerability to lapses and relapses. Thus, a fundamental cognitive strategy for relapse prevention is the devel-opment of "control" beliefs that reduce vulnerability to lapses and relapses. The following are examples of control beliefs that reduce vulnerability to lapses and relapses:

"I don't need drugs to have fun."

"My life will improve without drugs."

"I can cope with unpleasant emotions without using drugs."

"I have control over my own behaviors, including my drug use."

"Even if I slip I don't have to continue using drugs."

"A lapse is not equivalent to failure."

The following patient–therapist encounter illustrates the process of guided discovery, used here to modify drug-related beliefs and to build control beliefs.

TH: I wonder how you make sense of your continued use of cocaine in spite of the destructive results?

PT: Well, for one thing, I feel like I have no control over my drug use when I am emotionally upset.

TH: What do you mean when you say "I have no control"?

PT: I just don't feel like I have any control.

TH: So you believe that you have "zero percent" control?

PT: I guess.

TH: Are you saying that each and every time you've ever had a craving for coke you've used?

PT: Well, no.

TH: How many times *have* you succeeded in not using in spite of having cravings and urges?

PT: Well, lots of times, actually. I guess most of the time now that I think of it.

TH: Does this mean that you've been able to demonstrate control?

PT: It never seems that way to me, but I guess I do have *some* control.

TH: And so you have just changed your belief from "I have no control" to "I have some control." As we have discussed, the first belief is an example of dichotomous, or "all-or-nothing" thinking, while the second thought is probably more objective, because it takes into account the "shades of grey."

PT: Yes, I know. So when I think that I have no control I am more likely to give in to the urges and use cocaine. But when I look carefully and I see that I have greater control, I'm likely to try to stay with my program.

TH: Yes, that's right.

In this example the patient is helped to see the advantages of changing his drug-related belief "I have no control" to "I have some control." Another cognitive strategy useful for dealing with HRS is distraction (Carroll, Rounsaville, & Keller, 1991). Specifically, the patient is encouraged to compile a list of distracting activities that might be used when HRS are encountered. Distracting activities may include any non–drug-related activity (e.g., exercise, singing, playing with children, and writing a letter). Although distraction techniques are only a short-term coping device, they serve the all-important function of providing a delay between the onset of cravings and the act of seeking and using drugs. Such a delay may provide patients with time to think of the full negative ramifications of using, as well as an opportunity to witness the diminishing of cravings if no drugs are taken (Carroll, Rounsaville, & Keller, 1991; Horvath, 1988).

Behavioral Strategies for Coping with HRS

After patients identify HRS and examine drug-related beliefs, they are helped to practice (i.e., rehearse) strategies for coping with certain HRS. For example, Mike might be assisted in developing and practicing methods for resolving conflicts with his wife. He might be encouraged to think about ways to give her and to ask her for more emotional support. He also might be encouraged to think about alternatives to going out alone, especially to areas where drug-using friends are located. Additionally, he would be helped to imagine ways of saying "no thanks" to his friends when they invite him to use drugs, in spite of his cravings and urges. As Mike's case illustrates, relapse prevention necessitates that patients learn to cope with both general life stressors (e.g., marital discord) and discomfort that specifically is related to *temptation to use drugs* (Wills & Shiffman, 1985).

A long-term goal for Mike, essential to most drug users' continued abstinence after termination from therapy, would be to establish and maintain meaningful relationships with people who are drug-free (Frances & Miller, 1991; Havassy et al., 1991). The phrase in 12-step groups that reflects this philosophy is "hugs, not drugs." Ultimately, the patient must learn to seek human contact, rather than drugs, in order to obtain gratification of dependency needs.

As an important part of this process, Mike would be taught to examine the beliefs that led to his high-risk behaviors. For example, the therapist might ask, "What were you thinking when you yelled at your wife?" The patient's automatic thoughts might have included: "I'll put a stop to this!" or "She can't talk to me that way." Underlying these thoughts are Mike's beliefs about his personal inadequacy and powerlessness, beliefs that trigger both drug urges and the accompanying belief that giving in to the urges is the only way to feel powerful.

Another behavioral relapse prevention strategy involves *planned, gradual* exposure to HRS (Mackay et al., 1991). Specifically, the patient and therapist construct a hierarchy of increasingly salient high-risk triggers and the patient is actually exposed to these in sessions (*in vitro*) and through homework (*in vivo*). The efficacy of this technique may be attributable to the cognitive changes in patients as they perceive themselves effectively dealing with these situations. In other words, patients gain an increased sense of self-efficacy as they successfully cope with increasingly high-risk situations.

Again, a word of caution is due. While we believe that exposure to high-risk situations is *inevitable* in life, and therefore gradually "inoculating" patients to these situations makes excellent clinical sense, this technique must be handled with care. Therapists must make sure that their patients have the requisite skills and motivation to manage their induced cravings in session before being asked to cope with cravings outside the office (Childress et al., 1990). Patients must be told that this type of assignment requires a detailed plan, as well as a safety valve contingency (e.g., calling the therapist) in case the cravings become hard to manage. Otherwise, patients may misuse this assignment by cavalierly "testing" themselves before they are ready to handle the resultant cravings (Carroll, Rounsaville, & Keller, 1991; Washton, 1988). An example is the patient who drives through the neighborhood where he used to buy heroin, "just to see if I can do it," *without preparing a plan of action* in advance, thus taking a huge gamble with his abstinence. By contrast, therapist-instructed graded-exposure assignments must be small, calculated risks that have excellent chances for success and backup plans in case things go wrong.

Keeping a Lapse from Becoming a Relapse

As mentioned earlier, lapses provide the addict with opportunities to apply cognitive skills and promote further understanding of the mechanisms involved in relapse. Thus, a lapse is not necessarily perceived as "bad"; instead it is "grist for the mill." An important theme of relapse prevention is helping the patient keep lapses from becoming relapses (Mackay & Marlatt, 1991).

There are many reasons why lapses occur. For example, addicts may choose to "slip" in order to test their ability to control their substance use. They might think, "I'll try it just this once. It will prove that I am in control of my addiction." As we've mentioned above, addicts may also "accidentally" or intentionally expose themselves to a high-risk stimulus without being prepared to respond cognitively or behaviorally to this stimulus. Another reason for a lapse may be that the addict once again believes that the advantages of using drugs outweigh the disadvantages.

Given the many reasons for lapses, an important component of relapse prevention involves the identification of *decision points* along the cognitive model of relapse. For example, did the lapse occur because the addict failed to avoid an external HRS? Or, did the lapse occur because the addict lacked appropriate control beliefs for resisting an inevitable HRS? Or, did the patient automatically engage in instrumental strategies for acquiring drugs in response to cravings, without waiting?

A lapse usually becomes a relapse as a result of underlying all-or-none beliefs; for example, "A lapse means I don't have any control," "Since I could not stay abstinent, the therapy isn't working," and "A lapse is a failure." Marlatt and Gordon (1985) call this thinking process and the resulting relapse the "abstinence violation effect." An important strategy for relapse prevention, then, is to challenge such dichotomous thoughts about lapses so that they do not become relapses.

When an addict has a lapse, imagery techniques are useful to reconstruct the sequence of stimuli, basic beliefs, automatic thoughts, and behaviors leading to the lapse. Additionally, it is important to use post-hoc rehearsal of techniques at each decision point to prepare the addict for similar future circumstances.

This strategy is illustrated in the following dialogue between Mike and his therapist. Prior to this interaction, the therapist learned that Mike had been walking near the areas where his drug-using friends, Ryan and Bob, get high together. In fact, Mike almost avoided his friends but he suddenly felt "obligated" to stop to talk to them. Bob asked Mike why he hadn't been around for awhile and he offered to drive Mike home. Mike accepted the offer and got into Bob's car. Once on the road, Bob explained that he had to make a quick stop at his house. While Bob was inside, Mike began to think that maybe he should join him in the house in order to be "sociable." Inside the house, Bob offered Mike "a quick hit." Although Mike felt that he did not really want any, he accepted the offer and took the hit.

There were several choices and decision points leading to this lapse. First, Mike decided to walk through a "high-risk zone" instead of choosing a "safe" route. Upon seeing his friends, he had the option of choosing to keep walking. When he was in the car outside of Bob's house he had the option of staying outside, rather than entering the house. And finally, when Bob offered him the hit, he had the opportunity to accept or refuse. The following dialogue is the therapist's and patient's "postmortem" evaluation of the sequence of events leading to the lapse. Mike had his eyes closed and was imagining the scene as if it were happening now.

TH: You were walking along and you happened to wander past the old hangout. What was the risk involved in taking that route?

PT: I guess that I might have seen Bob and Ryan. I knew it could have been a problem in the long run, but I like spending time with them. We really enjoy each other.

TH: What happened when you saw Bob?

PT: He called out to me and I thought "I ought to stop."

TH: Is there any problem with that thought?

PT: I couldn't turn my back on my friend.

TH: What do you risk by following the dictates of that thought? Do you give up your freedom of choice?

PT: I guess I could get into trouble that way.

TH: What happened next?

PT: I stopped and he offered to take me home.

TH: Did you have a choice?

PT: I felt that I should take him up on the offer.

TH: You often act instinctively but perhaps following those instincts may work against you . . . (*pause*) . . . Now, you're waiting in the car. What's going through your mind?

PT: I'm thinking that maybe I should go up there and be sociable.

TH: Are you feeling the urge to get high?

PT: Maybe in the back of my mind I may be thinking that it would feel good to take a hit.

TH: What are you thinking when Bob offers you some?

PT: I'm thinking that maybe I don't want to. But Bob offered it as a gesture of his friendship . . . I felt I should accept.

TH: Could you have asked yourself, "Am I being 'nice,' or am I just giving myself permission to use?"

PT: Yeh, I guess so.

TH: And what would the consequence have been of that thought?

PT: Maybe I would have realized how impulsive I was being. Maybe I wouldn't have taken the hit.

TH: After you took the hit, what were the thoughts that ran through your mind?

PT: I was thinking, "might as well finish the job I've started."

TH: And what was the meaning of that thought?

PT: It meant "one hit and I'm over the edge."

TH: That sounds like "all-or-nothing thinking."

PT: Yeh, you're right.

TH: And you proceeded to smoke crack at Bob's house all afternoon.

PT: Yes.

In this example, Mike was "guided" through the thoughts and images of his recent experiences so that he might review the decision points leading to his lapse. Upon arriving at his lapse, his therapist helped him to see that his dichotomous thinking led him to continue using after his initial hit. In the section that follows, Mike's therapist encouraged Mike to rehearse alternative methods for coping at each decision point.

TH: What could you have done instead of walking along the old route, past the old hangout?

PT: I guess there were lots of walks I could have taken which would have avoided those guys.

TH: And if you had still passed them, what could you have thought when they called out to you?

PT: I could have thought "Those guys put me at risk for relapse. Better keep walking."

TH: And what would your resulting behaviors have been?

PT: I would have waved in a friendly way and said "Hi guys! I'm in a hurry. Gotta run."

TH: And what if Bob had pulled up in his car and offered you a ride anyway?

PT: I could have continued to think "bad news. . . ."

TH: And the resulting behavior would have been what?

PT: I would have turned down the ride.

TH: And what if they convinced you to get in the car and you ended at Bob's house anyway?

PT: I still could have thought "Don't get out of the car. The house is a danger zone."

TH: And then what would have happened?

PT: Bob probably would have come back to the car and taken me home without using.

TH: And if that would have happened, how would you have felt?

PT: Probably relieved and proud of myself for exercising control over my life.

At this point, the therapist realized that Mike had other types of beliefs (relating to "loyalty" and "responsibility") that made him vulnerable to lapses and relapse. In the next segment, the therapist explored these beliefs.

TH: What were you thinking when you walked over to Bob's car?

PT: I thought, "I have really neglected my friends."

TH: What do you mean by that?

PT: I mean that I have to be friendly to these guys. After all, they are my friends.

TH: What do you mean when you use the phrase "have to"?

PT: I like to think of myself as a loyal friend.

TH: And what does "loyal" mean?

PT: It means that I should go along with what they want.

TH: Shoulds and musts.

PT: Yes.

TH: What do you know about shoulds and musts?

PT: I know that they aren't the best.

TH: And what are the results of shoulds and musts?

PT: Well, they can get me into trouble. Like in this case, they got me back into using.

Advantages–Disadvantages Analysis

Marlatt and Gordon (1985) explain that positive outcome expectancies contribute to relapse. Specifically, individuals who have been addicted to a substance perceive substantial positive advantages from using that substance. In fact, such people typically minimize or ignore the disadvantages of their drug use, especially when in high-risk situations.

The advantages–disadvantages analysis is a technique commonly used in cognitive therapy (see Chapter 9, this volume). This technique is particularly useful in relapse prevention, where addicts selectively perceive the advantages of drug use.

In the advantages–disadvantages analysis, the therapist constructs a four-cell matrix, with advantages–disadvantages on one axis, and use–nonuse on the other axis. Patients are asked to discuss the advantages and disadvantages of using and abstaining. The role of the therapist is to elicit objective data from patients, regarding such advantages and disadvantages. Additionally, patients are encouraged to understand that their exaggerated views about the advantages, along with their minimized views of disadvantages, contribute to their addiction.

The following dialogue is a continuation of the session with Mike. It illustrates the advantages–disadvantages analysis:

TH: Mike, when you were in the high-risk situation with your friends Bob and Ryan, what was going through your mind?

PT: I guess I thought, "Soon I'll get some relief from this bullshit."

TH: So you believed that an advantage of smoking crack was relief from your bad situation.

PT: I'd forget about my old lady for a few hours.

TH: What other advantages could you see?

PT: (*pauses*) Well, I can't think of any others.

TH: What were the disadvantages of using?

PT: Oh, the relief is only for a short time. I know that I am really making my marriage and my life worse.

TH: What other disadvantages are there to using?

PT: Well, I could lose my kid if my wife decides to split.

TH: What else?

PT: I can tell that my life is changing for the worse from this stuff. When I am really honest with myself I know that my health and self-confidence are going down the tubes.

TH: OK, What are the advantages of abstaining?

PT: Well, as I just said, I'm kinda wasting my life. Maybe my life would start to improve if I abstained.

TH: Can you think of any other advantages of abstaining?

PT: (*pause, tears in his eyes*) I guess I could start to be more of a father to my son; I never really had a father myself.

TH: Sounds like a very big advantage!

PT: Yeah, if I could only remember later how I feel right now!

In fact, Carroll, Rounsaville, & Keller (1991) suggest a method that facilitates remembering the advantages–disadvantages analysis. They suggest that the addict list the advantages of using cocaine on one side of an index card. The therapist then helps the patient to see the ultimate negative consequences of all advantages. For example, the "terrific high" is following by the "dreaded crash." On the flip side of the index card the patient lists the disadvantages of continued cocaine use. The card is then placed in the addict's wallet, near the money, so it will be accessible during periods of high vulnerability.

Development of Social Support Networks

Interpersonal conflict is a common high-risk stimulus for many addicts (Mackay et al., 1991). In fact, Cummings, Gordon, and Marlatt (1980) found that 44% of relapse experiences were linked to interpersonal conflicts. Loneliness is also a high-risk trigger, for two reasons. First, loneliness is an uncomfortable emotion (i.e., internal trigger) that may be anesthetized temporarily by cocaine. Second, heroin and cocaine use often take place in a social environment, which temporarily provides the addict with a sense of having "company" to relieve the loneliness. From these assumptions, we assume that relapse prevention efforts will be enhanced by the patient's acquisition of a drug-free social support network (cf. Frances & Miller, 1991).

It is important to understand that patients have numerous basic beliefs and automatic thoughts about relationships that influence their behaviors in relationships. For example, some addicts may believe "Only other users can understand me," "I will never be accepted by those who have never used drugs," "Nonusers are boring," and so forth. Obviously, such beliefs result in social discomfort, or anxiety, and a certain degree of social avoidance. Patients can be helped by the therapist's understanding of this process, as well as by modification of such beliefs.

Friends and family who do not use drugs may be excellent sources of support to the patient. Many addicts have avoided their nonusing family members and friends for fear of criticism and rejection. Twelve-step programs (e.g., Alcoholics Anonymous and Narcotics Anonymous) may also be sources of support for the addict. Therefore, patients should be encouraged to make use of these programs. By doing so they may experience multiple benefits, including social support, collaboration, an environment that is supportive of abstinence, and a way to spend time when suffering from boredom. Of course, cognitive therapists strive to be part of the patients' support network as well, but it is vital that drug-abusing patients have drug-free friends in their everyday lives "for the long haul."

SUMMARY

In this chapter, relapse prevention was presented as part of the cognitive therapy framework. This model emphasizes the role of beliefs as well as high-risk situations in the relapse process. Techniques were presented for predicting and controlling relapse, including identification of HRS, cognitive and behavioral strategies for coping with HRS, keeping a lapse from becoming a relapse, advantages–disadvantages analysis, and social support networks for relapse prevention.

We also alluded to the fact that long-term abstinence from drugs and alcohol entails broad-sweeping changes in attitudes and lifestyle. When therapists note that their patients are reverting back to former ways of viewing themselves, their world, and their future, it signals a need for the patients to reassess their self-efficacy and commitment to positive change.

In sum, the conceptual and technical skills that patients learn during the actual course of cognitive therapy must be practiced and "lived" in the months and years *after* formal treatment has terminated. Toward that end, we emphasize to our patients that they must learn to become their own cognitive therapists, and that the work of therapy needs to become a way of life.

POSTSCRIPT

The following is our version of the "Serenity Prayer," adapted for cognitive therapy substance abuse patients:

Cognitive Therapy Serenity Pledge

I pledge that I will strive to gain the strength to stay away from those drug triggers that I *can* avoid, the serenity and know-how to cope with those drug triggers that *can't* be avoided, and the wisdom to know the difference.

APPENDIX 1

BELIEFS ABOUT SUBSTANCE USE*

Name: _____ Date: _____

Listed below are some common beliefs about drug use. Please read each statement and rate how much you agree or disagree with each one.

1	2	3	4	5	6	7
Totally Disagree	Disagree Very Much	Disagree Slightly	Neutral	Agree Slightly	Agree Very Much	Totally Agree

_____ 1. Life without using is boring.

_____ 2. Using is the only way to increase my creativity and productivity.

_____ 3. I can't function without it.

_____ 4. This is the only way to cope with pain in my life.

_____ 5. I'm not ready to stop using.

_____ 6. The cravings/urges make me use.

_____ 7. My life won't get any better, even if I stop using.

_____ 8. The only way to deal with my anger is by using.

_____ 9. Life would be depressing if I stopped.

_____ 10. I don't deserve to recover from drug use.

_____ 11. I'm not a strong enough person to stop.

_____ 12. I could not be social without using.

_____ 13. Substance use is not a problem for me.

_____ 14. The cravings/urges won't go away unless I use drugs.

_____ 15. My substance use is caused by someone else (e.g., spouse, boyfriend/girlfriend, family member).

_____ 16. If someone has a problem with drugs, it's all genetic.

_____ 17. I can't relax without drugs.

_____ 18. Having this drug problem means I am fundamentally a bad person.

_____ 19. I can't control my anxiety without using drugs.

_____ 20. I can't make my life fun unless I use.

*This form was developed by Fred D. Wright, Ed.D.

CRAVING BELIEFS QUESTIONNAIRE (CBQ)*

Name: _____ **Date:** _____

Please read the statements below and rate how much you agree or disagree with each one.

1	2	3	4	5	6	7
Totally Disagree	Disagree Very Much	Disagree Slightly	Neutral	Agree Slightly	Agree Very Much	Totally Agree

_____ 1. The craving is a physical reaction, therefore, I can't do anything about it.

_____ 2. If I don't stop the cravings they will get worse.

_____ 3. Craving can drive you crazy.

_____ 4. The craving makes me use drugs.

_____ 5. I'll always have cravings for drugs.

_____ 6. I don't have any control over the craving.

_____ 7. Once the craving starts I have no control over my behavior.

_____ 8. I'll have cravings for drugs the rest of my life.

_____ 9. I can't stand the physical symptoms I have while craving drugs.

_____ 10. The craving is my punishment for using drugs.

_____ 11. If you have never used drugs then you have no idea what the craving is like (and you can't expect me to resist).

_____ 12. The images/thoughts I have while craving drugs are out of my control.

_____ 13. The craving makes me so nervous I can't stand it.

_____ 14. I'll never be prepared to handle the craving.

_____ 15. Since I'll have the craving the rest of my life I might as well go ahead and use drugs.

_____ 16. When I'm really craving drugs I can't function.

_____ 17. Either I'm craving drugs or I'm not; there is nothing in between.

_____ 18. If the craving gets too intense, using drugs is the only way to cope with the feeling.

_____ 19. When craving drugs it's OK to use alcohol to cope.

_____ 20. The craving is stronger than my will power.

*This form was developed by Fred D. Wright, Ed.D.

RELAPSE PREDICTION SCALE*

Name: _____ Date: _____

As you know, there are many situations that can trigger an urge to use cocaine or crack. This scale has *two parts*: (1) to determine *how strong you think* the urges will be in certain situations and (2) to determine the *likelihood that you will use* in these situations.

    Listed below are several situations that might trigger strong urges to use cocaine or crack. Read each item and imagine yourself in that situation. In the first column, "Strength of Urges," indicate how strong you think the urge will be. In the second column indicate the "Likelihood of Your Using" in these situations.

0	1	2	3	4
None	Weak	Moderate	Strong	Very Strong

	PREDICTION	
	Strength of Urges	Likelihood of Using
1. I am in a place where I used cocaine or crack before.	____	____
2. I am around people with whom I have previously used cocaine or crack.	____	____
3. I just got paid.	____	____
4. I see coworkers using.	____	____
5. I am leaving work.	____	____
6. It's Friday night.	____	____
7. I am at a party.	____	____
8. I am thinking of the last time I used.	____	____
9. I start talking with someone about using.	____	____
10. I feel bored.	____	____
11. I feel great!	____	____
12. I see a lover/ex-lover.	____	____
13. I am having a drink.	____	____
14. My friend is offering me some cocaine or crack.	____	____
15. I feel sad.	____	____

(OVER)

*This form was developed by Fred D. Wright, Ed.D.

	PREDICTION	
	Strength of Urges	Likelihood of Using
16. I see a prostitute.	____	____
17. I am out looking for sex.	____	____
18. I feel sexy.	____	____
19. I remember how good the high feels.	____	____
20. I feel angry.	____	____
21. I feel stressed out.	____	____
22. I feel guilty.	____	____
23. I just used drugs.	____	____
24. I just broke my abstinence.	____	____
25. I am getting ready for work.	____	____
26. I am tired.	____	____
27. I am frustrated.	____	____
28. I see an anti-drug use poster.	____	____
29. I see a pipe.	____	____
30. I am out gambling.	____	____
31. I just had a "coke dream."	____	____
32. I am watching sports.	____	____
33. I am getting dressed up.	____	____
34. I am under pressure at work.	____	____
35. I am thinking about having sex.	____	____
36. I am angry at my spouse/partner.	____	____
37. My spouse/partner is bugging me about my using.	____	____
38. My family is bugging me about my using.	____	____
39. I was just told I have a positive urine.	____	____
40. I didn't use, yet my urine was positive.	____	____
41. I am watching a drug-related movie.	____	____
42. I feel anxious.	____	____
43. Someone just criticized me.	____	____
44. I haven't used for a long time.	____	____
45. I feel tense.	____	____
46. Someone I care for is terminally ill.	____	____
47. I am in pain.	____	____
48. I feel a burden on my shoulders.	____	____
49. I am at a bar having a good time.	____	____
50. I had a fight with my family.	____	____

APPENDIX 2

CHECKLIST FOR DEALING
WITH AMBIVALENCE AND LAPSES*

____ 1. Set goals related to abstinence.
   "I want to keep job."
   "I'd like to get along better with family/girl friend/boyfriend."
   "I'd like to have more money to spend on things I want.

____ 2. Assess cocaine practices:
   a. Look for specific stimuli: money, cocaine paraphernalia (pipe, syringes, materials used in the preparation of freebase cocaine, etc.), exposure to cocaine itself or any white crystalline substance resembling cocaine, such as salt, sugar, snow, and even plaster dust; individuals and settings previously associated with cocaine use and cocaine paraphernalia. (Some intravenous users have reported intense subjective craving when their blood is drawn for determination of blood levels each week.)
   b. Determine whether other individuals in the patient's home, neighborhood, or workplace use cocaine; whether the patient is involved with selling cocaine and the nature of the patient's cocaine resources.
   c. Determine availability of money, use of other psychoactive substances, contact with cocaine using associates, and unstructured time spent without monitoring of the patient's activities.

____ 3. Begin therapy sessions with a review of all high-risk stimulus situations that were encountered by the patient during the past week and the coping strategies used by the patient, and *whether or not they were successful.*

____ 4. At end of interview, ask patient to anticipate any high-risk situations that may be encountered during the week ahead: Plan in advance how these might be avoided or successfully coped with.

____ 5. Address distress from abstinence.
   • Acknowledge patient's struggle
   • Acknowledge sense of deprivation

____ 6. Acknowledge patient's justifications for using.
   "There's nothing like a cocaine high."
   "Sex and coke go together."
   "I feel less anxious with people."
   "I get most of my money from dealing."

*Many of the items for this checklist were based on the text of Relapse Prevention Strategies for the Treatment of Cocaine Abuse by K. M. Carroll, B. J. Rounsaville, and D. S. Keller, 1991, *American Journal of Drug and Alcohol Abuse, 17*, pp. 249-265. Adapted by permission of Marcel Dekker Inc.

_____ 7. Identify patient's "compromise" with abstinence.
   • Spacing out use of cocaine (but not giving it up).
   • Continuing on high levels of alcohol or other psychoactive drugs
   • Staying in treatment only until "spouse or lover gets off my back"

_____ 8. Remind patient of the crash and dysphoria.

_____ 9. Assess whether patient has taken steps toward reducing cocaine avail-ability. Has the patient informed cocaine using associates of his/her intention to stop using?

_____ 10. Question: Has the individual resisted telling family and friends of his or her decision to stop using or reluctance to break ties with dealers?

_____ 11. If the patient has made no independent steps toward limiting cocaine availability, consider whether patient expects that mere exposure to treatment will "magically" produce abstinence with little or no participation or struggle on the part of the patient.

_____ 12. Determine whether the abusers, after an initial brief period of abstinence, expose themselves to a situation in which cocaine is available as a "test" of their ability to withstand temptation.

_____ 13. Encourage patient, at least at the beginning, to minimize deliber-ate exposure to cocaine-related cues and situations. Be ready to iden-tify unforeseeable "accidental" subintentional exposures ("appar-ently irrelevant decisions"). Example: A patient decided that since his problem was with cocaine, he would have a beer. After two beers, however, he ran into a friend who happened to have a gram of cocaine and a relapse occurred.

_____ 14. Teach the patient how to recognize and interpret such a decision chain leading to a lapse before it actually occurs.

_____ 15. Teach the patient how to detect the decisions that commonly occur during the beginning of the "accidental exposure" chain where risk, craving, and the availability of cocaine are relatively low. The patient should be able to regard certain feelings, such as boredom, as a "red flag." Part of the subintentional exposures (accidents) are manifested in the patient's "having" to do certain things that lead to high-risk activities or locations.

_____ 16. Elicit patient's relapse interpretation: "I blew it this time. I guess I'll never stop using cocaine, so I might as well keep using."

_____ 17. Check on psychological background to lapse: For example, some-times defiance or rebellion becomes a factor, as in the case of a person who had an argument with his wife and then had the thought that her efforts to monitor his actions made him her "pris-oner."

_____ 18. Look for "entitlement." For example, cocaine's initial euphorogenic properties may be sought to enhance positive feeling and then will be later used when the person feels "I am entitled to a reward."

_____ 19. Self-monitoring: Patient is asked to keep a log of hourly changes in cocaine craving and/or uses in relation to various external and internal events.

_____ 20. Increase abuser's ability to anticipate problems, prepare for them in advance, or avoid them entirely.

_____ 21. Maintain a balance between encouraging patient to avoid high-risk situations (at least initially) and utilizing behavioral and cognitive coping strategies when exposure/craving occurs.

_____ 22. Early in treatment, inquire about the intensity of craving. Patients often deny any craving at all. In later sessions, the patient might mention any of the following: "Seeing myself doing cocaine" or having a dream about cocaine or other experiences which may be indicative of some form of craving. Some descriptions are somatic ("a knot in my stomach . . . my blood racing . . . sweating . . . heart pounding," nervousness, excitement, smell or taste of cocaine).

_____ 23. Look for episodes of intense subjective craving for cocaine that are reported weeks or even months before the violation of abstinence.

_____ 24. Demystify the experience of craving by offering an explanation of conditioning experiments. Help the patient identify and tolerate conditioned craving when it occurs.

_____ 25. Explain the time-limited nature of cocaine craving. Craving usually peaks and dissipates in less than an hour *if not followed by cocaine use.* Distraction may be an effective strategy.

_____ 26. Lifestyle modification involves developing rewarding behavioral alternatives.

_____ 27. If the abuser is still working, the job in many cases has become only a means of acquiring money to buy cocaine and the fulfilling or challenging aspects of work have faded.

_____ 28. Anhedonic cocaine abusers may have difficulty seeing any activity or experience other than cocaine use as enjoyable. All other experiences are perceived as inferior to cocaine.

_____ 29. Encourage patient to look at slips as isolated incidents that can be conceived of as opportunities for learning.

APPENDIX 3

TYPICAL EXAMPLES OF DRUG USE ADVANTAGES AND DISADVANTAGES

ADVANTAGES OF USING

1. Feel like superman.

2. Took away shyness and insecurities.

3. Feel like king of the mountain.

4. Confident.

5. More sex.

6. It makes me feel good.

7. Fit in with the crowd.

8. I have more friends (until your money runs out).

9. Made me more social.

10. Reduces social anxiety.

11. Relaxes me.

12. It's fun.

13. A glass of wine is sometimes nice with dinner.

14. There are times when a single drink with a friend is a good thing—a little relaxation, sometimes mildly euphoric (nothing wrong with one drink, a lot of nice things about).

15. Reduced guilt (when leaving my daughter).

16. Ran away from loneliness.

17. Take mind off things.

18. Nothing bothered me when high.

DISADVANTAGES OF USING

1. Mental/physical beating your body is taking.
2. Relationships suffer.
3. Work suffers (don't show up for work because you are hurting so bad).
4. Big debt.
5. I lead a life that is a lie.
6. I'm in danger of legal consequences.
7. After using cocaine, feel bad about myself for picking up.
8. Hangover.
9. Sleep most of the day.
10. Stopped eating.
11. No motivation.
12. Didn't talk about anything meaningful.
13. Feel guilty in front of children.
14. Impotence.
15. Sterility.
16. Paranoia.
17. Laziness.
18. Loss of short-term memory.
19. Tensions in family.
20. Could get fired.
21. Injury to myself or others.
22. Less respect from others.
23. Self-esteem drops.
24. Not as comfortable meeting new people.
25. You don't achieve as much, you can't do constructive things after you've been drinking.
26. Interacts with medication.
27. Don't know if I'm helping myself when I go out and do in vivo exposures—whether it's me or the Xanax getting me through.
28. Hangovers.
29. Loss of control (e.g., saying something indiscreet during blackouts).
30. Drunk driving.
31. Discouragement for not being in control of a senseless urge.

32. I do and say things that I regret.
33. Have sex when I wouldn't normally.
34. Become too aggressive.
35. Impairing my reasoning.
36. Lack of control.
37. May lose house.
38. I could die.
39. Endanger self in bad areas of town.
40. Become isolated.

ADVANTAGES OF NOT USING

1. Keep your sanity.
2. Feel less paranoid.
3. Better relationship with spouse.
4. Feel great physically.
5. Save money.
6. Would not have to look over my shoulder.
7. Feel better about myself.
8. I can think clearly.
9. I feel like going to work.
10. Can pay my bills.
11. Not lazy.
12. Not flying off the handle.
13. Don't have to lie to family.
14. More time to practice hobbies.
15. It's a depressant and since I'm having problems in that area it's good to avoid.
16. Good for my weight (less calories).
17. You can accomplish more in the evening if you don't drink.
18. All around easier on my body not to drink.
19. Don't have to worry about making a fool of yourself at parties.
20. Don't wake up wondering what I did the night before (skinned hands, etc.).
21. No hangovers.
22. Self-confidence at having overcome a self-destructive urge.
23. Moral reward for overcoming unnecessary desire.
24. Wouldn't have bad reputation.
25. Wouldn't regret things—punching doors, being aggressive.
26. Health reasons.
27. Improved communication—not so snappy, talk better in *some* groups.
28. Sleep better.
29. Not so worried about others knowing.
30. Able to plan future.
31. Better relationship—better sex.
32. Less jealous.
33. More time (for self and family).

DISADVANTAGES OF NOT USING

1. I'm bashful around other people and it's hard to get over that.
2. Can't run away from the problems.
3. I'll be lonely.
4. I have to deal with urges.
5. Can't fall asleep at night.
6. Agitated.
7. Withdrawn—wouldn't talk to other people.
8. Feel hyper.
9. Social tension (being tempted).
10. Losing friends.
11. I wouldn't have the feelings that I get when I drink (the relaxed buzz).
12. It makes bars not quite as much fun.
13. It's awkward at cocktail parties or dinner having one drink or no drink and everyone else is having more.
14. I sometimes miss it (glass of good red wine with certain dinners).
15. Fear of intimacy while fully sober.
16. Uncomfortable in social situations.
17. Life wouldn't be as fun.
18. I'll have to deal with things.
19. Troubled by thoughts of future craving and relapse.

APPENDIX 4

DAILY RECORD OF CRAVINGS
(DTR ADAPTED FOR USE SPECIFICALLY WITH CRAVINGS)

Date	Situation	Thoughts or Feelings	Degree of craving (0–100)	Rational response and/or coping
6–12	Boss came down hard on me.	Felt stupid. Thought: I need a smoke.	50	I can try to work it out—waited it out for half an hour and craving went away.
6–25	Guys were going to the bar.	It's OK to be with them—I can handle craving now.	50	Went to bar and thought, "This is a mistake, and so I left."
7–4	I had to make a presentation.	Felt anxious, "I need a drink to do it."	40	"I don't need a drink. I can do it without it."
7–16	Had a fight with my wife.	Felt depressed and angry. Thought of taking a hit.	30	Decided to take a walk.
7–28	Got paid today.	Thought I should celebrate.	20	"I'll only feel worse later" so I went home. My wife will raise hell when she finds out.

APPENDIX 5

PATIENT'S REPORT OF THERAPY SESSION

Patient's Name: _____

Date of Session: _____ Time Session Began: _____ A.M. P.M.

Therapist's Name: _____

PART I. Please *circle* your response to each of the following:

1. Before you came in today, how much progress did you expect to make in dealing with your problems *in today's session*?

   MUCH PROGRESS   SOME PROGRESS   NO PROGRESS

2. *In today's session*, how much progress do you feel you actually made?

   MUCH   SOME   NO   THINGS GOT
   PROGRESS   PROGRESS   PROGRESS   WORSE

3. *In future sessions*, how much progress do you think you will be able to make in dealing with your problems

   MUCH PROGRESS   SOME PROGRESS   NO PROGRESS

4. How satisfied are you with *today's session*?

   VERY SATISFIED   SATISFIED   INDIFFERENT   DISSATISFIED

5. *In today's session*, how well do you think your therapist understood your problems?

   VERY WELL   FAIRLY WELL   POORLY

6. How well were you able to convey your concerns or problems *in this session*?

   VERY WELL   FAIRLY WELL   POORLY

7. *In today's session*, how much did you think you could trust (have confidence in) your therapist?

   VERY MUCH   SOME   NOT AT ALL

PART II. Please answer the following questions about *homework*.

1. Was homework assigned *last session*?   YES   NO

2. Did you discuss last week's homework *in today's session*?   YES   NO

3. How helpful was the homework and the discussion of it?

   VERY   SOMEWHAT   NOT AT ALL   NOT
   HELPFUL   HELPFUL   HELPFUL   APPLICABLE

324

4. How pleased are you with the homework that was assigned for *this coming week?*

| VERY PLEASED | SOMEWHAT PLEASED | NOT AT ALL PLEASED | NOT APPLICABLE |

PART III. Rate the extent to which you believe you gained the following skills *in this therapy session*. Please refer only to *this session*, realizing that not all of these skills can be gained in any one session.

	VERY MUCH	SOME	NONE
1. Better insight into and understanding of my psychological problems.	2	1	0
2. Methods or techniques for better ways of dealing with people (e.g., asserting myself).	2	1	0
3. Techniques in defining and solving my everyday problems (home, work, school).	2	1	0
4. Confidence in undertaking an activity to help myself.	2	1	0
5. Greater ability to cope with my moods.	2	1	0
6. Better control over my actions.	2	1	0
7. Greater ability to *recognize* my unreasonable *thoughts*.	2	1	0
8. Greater ability to *correct* my unreasonable *thoughts*.	2	1	0
9. Greater ability to *recognize* my self-defeating or erroneous *beliefs*.	2	1	0
10. Greater ability to *evaluate* my self-defeating or erroneous *beliefs*.	2	1	0

PART IV. Rate the extent to which your therapist was the following *in this session*.

	VERY MUCH	SOME	NOT AT ALL
1. Sympathetic and caring	2	1	0
2. Competent (knew what he/she was doing.)	2	1	0
3. Warm and friendly	2	1	0
4. Supportive and encouraging	2	1	0
5. Involved and interested	2	1	0

PART V. Please circle the response that applies to the way you perceived your therapist (or therapy) in this session.

1. My therapist talked down to me.	YES	NO
2. He/She was too quiet and passive.	YES	NO
3. He/She talked too much.	YES	NO
4. He/She was too bossy.	YES	NO
5. He/She seemed to miss the point.	YES	NO
6. This therapy (cognitive therapy) does not seem to be suited to me.	YES	NO

PART VI. In the remaining space, describe the most outstanding aspect of today's session and elaborate on any of the difficulties you experienced.

POSSIBLE REASONS FOR
NOT DOING SELF-HELP ASSIGNMENTS*
(to be completed by patient)

The following is a list of reasons that various clients have given for not doing their self-help assignments during the course of therapy. Because the speed of improvement depends primarily on the amount of self-help assignments that you are willing to do, it is of crucial importance to pinpoint any reasons that you may have for not doing this work. It is important to look for these reasons at the time that you feel a reluctance to do your assignment or a desire to put off doing it. Hence, it is best to fill out this questionnaire at that time. If you have difficulty filling out this form and returning it to the therapist, it might be best to do it together during a therapy session. [Rate each statement with a "T" (True) or "F" (False). "T" indicates that you agree with it; "F" means the statement does not apply at this time.]

1. It seems that nothing could help me so there is no point in trying. ____

2. I really can't see the point of what the therapist has asked me to do. ____

3. I feel that the particular method the therapist has suggested will not be helpful. It doesn't really make good sound sense to me. ____

4. "I am a procrastinator, therefore I can't do this." Then I end up not doing it. ____

5. I am willing to do some self-help assignments, but I keep forgetting. ____

6. I do not have enough time. I am too busy. ____

7. If I do something the therapist suggests it's not as good as if I come up with my own ideas. ____

8. I feel helpless, and I don't really believe that I *can* do anything that I choose to do. ____

9. I have the feeling that the therapist is trying to boss me around or control me. ____

10. I don't feel like cooperating with the therapist. ____

11. I fear the therapist's disapproval or criticism of my work. I believe that what I do just won't be good enough for him/her. ____

12. I have no desire or motivation to do self-help assignments or anything else. Since I don't feel like doing these assignments, it follows that I can't do them and I don't have to do them. ____

13. I feel too bad, sad, nervous, upset (underline appropriate word(s)) to do it now. ____

14. I am feeling good now and I don't want to spoil it by working on the assignment. ____

15. Other reasons (Please write them in)

_____

_____

_____

_____

APPENDIX 7

COGNITIVE THERAPY INTERVENTION
WITH HIV-POSITIVE DRUG ABUSERS*

Many chronic drug abusers engage in behavior that puts them at high risk for becoming HIV infected. The following is a brief outline for working with the HIV-positive population with regard to the emotional distress they will most likely experience when they become aware of, and try to cope with, their condition.

1. Educate patients about the physiological symptoms associated with psychological stress. Anxiety and depressive symptoms, such as hyperventilation and lightheadedness, or fatigue, anhedonia, lack of libido, irritability, and distractibility, are often misinterpreted as signs of a physical illness by distressed patients who have been informed that they are HIV positive. This common misinterpretation increases the sense of threat and loss, and intensifies the anxiety/depressive symptoms, which then reinforce the belief of a developing crisis ("I'm losing my mind," "I'm getting AIDS," etc.).

2. The therapist should encourage the drug abuser to remain free of drugs and alcohol in order to improve overall health in an effort to stay well long enough to see the day when more effective treatments are available for the disorder.

3. Review with patients cognitive coping techniques such as thought stopping, distraction, coping statements or flashcards, rational responding.

4. Help patients identify and modify dysfunctional thoughts and attitudes associated with being HIV positive. A typical thought might be, "This disease is my punishment for being a bad person." This dysfunctional thought is generated from unarticulated fundamental beliefs such as "I am bad" or "I am defective."

5. In addition to teaching patients to recognize distortions and the dysfunctional nature of specific automatic thoughts, therapists should train patients to label these distortions. Listed below are some common distortions associated with HIV-related emotional distress:

- *Catastrophizing.* "This is the end for me."
- *All-or-nothing thinking.* "If I'm not perfectly healthy, I can't enjoy anything."
- *Overgeneralization.* "This coughing means that my whole body is fall-

---

*From *Stress Prevention Training after HIV Antibody Testing: A Trainer's Manual* by B. Fishman, 1992, unpublished manuscript, Cornell University Medical College, New York. Copyright 1992 B. Fishman. Adapted by permission of the author.

ing apart."

- *Jumping to conclusions.* "My friend didn't want to go out this weekend; she must know I'm contagious and doesn't want to be around me."
- *Personalization.* "The grocer did not treat me well because he wants me to stay away from his store."

6. Teach patients to identify and modify dysfunctional behavioral habits. Throughout the treatment emphasize controlling high-risk sexual and IV drug use behaviors. Not only are unsafe IV drug use and sex dangerous in spreading HIV to uninfected individuals, but these behaviors also expose the HIV-infected patient to *reinfection, which may increase chances of the full AIDS syndrome.* Furthermore, the practice of high-risk behaviors is often experienced by patients themselves as impulsive and self-harming. Patients experience guilt, shame, loss of esteem, and an increased sense of vulnerability or "being out of control." Therefore, achieving effective control over these behaviors is extremely important.

Controlling high-risk behaviors requires three components:

- a. Reliable information and practical understanding about how HIV is transmitted, and how transmission can be avoided or prevented.
- b. Impulse control—habitual and automatic effort to perform the procedures necessary to avoid HIV transmission (using condoms, "bleaching" needles, etc.).
- c. Assertiveness—the ability to assert one's position under external social pressure without submission or aggression. Oftentimes difficulties in asserting wishes are based on distorted cognitions and dysfunctional assumptions such as "If I insist on using a condom, she will make fun of me," or "If I bleach my 'works,' they will think I'm not a real 'brother.'"

Summary

This outline has examined ways that therapists can help HIV-positive drug abusing patients cope with their disorder: (1) by educating them about the physiological symptoms associated with psychological stress and how these symptoms can be misinterpreted as signs of their illness, (2) by encouraging them to remain free of drugs and alcohol in order to improve overall health, (3) by reviewing with them the basic cognitive therapy techniques for coping with stress such as thought stopping, distraction, coping statements or flashcards, and rational responding, (4) by helping them identify and modify dysfunctional thoughts and attitudes associated with being HIV positive, (5) by teaching them to recognize and label distortions associated with HIV-related emotional distress (e.g., catastrophizing and all-or-nothing thinking), and (6) by teaching them to identify and modify dysfunctional behavioral habits such as not using condoms and not bleaching needles.

References

Abrams, D.B., & Niaura, R.S. (1987). Social learning theory. In H.T. Blane & K.E. Leonard (Eds.), *Psychological theories of drinking and alcoholism* (pp. 131–178). New York: Guilford.

Alberti, R.E., & Emmons, L. (1974). *Your perfect right* (2nd ed.). San Luis Obispo, CA: Impact.

Alterman, A.I., & Cacciola, J.S. (1991). The antisocial personality disorder diagnosis in substance abusers: Problems and issues. *Journal of Nervous and Mental Disease, 179*, 401–409.

Alterman, A.I., O'Brien, C.P., & McLellan, A.T. (1991). Differential therapeutics for substance abuse. In R.J. Frances & R.J. Miller (Eds.), *Clinical textbook of addictive disorders* (pp. 369–390). New York: Guilford.

Amaro, H., Fried, L.E., Cabral, H., & Zuckerman, B. (1990). Violence during pregnancy and substance abuse. *American Journal of Public Health, 80*, 575–579.

American Psychiatric Association. (1987). *Diagnostic and statistical manual of mental disorders* (3rd ed., rev.). Washington, DC: Author.

Ananth, J., Vandewater, S., Kamal, M., Brodsky, A., Gamal, R., & Miller, M. (1989). Missed diagnosis of substance abuse in psychiatric patients. *Hospital and Community Psychiatry, 40*(3), 297–299.

Annis, H.M. (1986). A relapse prevention model for treatment of alcoholics. In W.R. Miller & N. Heather (Eds.), *Treating addictive behaviors: Process of change* (pp. 407–421). New York: Plenum.

Babor, T.F., Korner, P., Wilber, C., & Good, S.P. (1987). Screening and early intervention strategies for harmful drinkers: Initial lessons from the amethyst project. *Australian Drug and Alcohol Review, 6*, 325–339.

Baker, T.B. (Ed.) (1988). Models of addiction [Special issue]. *Journal of Abnormal Psychology, 97*(2).

Bandura, A. (1969). *Principles of behavior modification.* New York: Holt, Rinehart & Winston.

Bandura, A. (1977). *Social learning theory.* Englewood Cliffs, NJ: Prentice-Hall.

Bandura, A. (1982). Self-efficacy mechanism in human agency. *American Psychologist, 97*, 122–147.

Beck, A.T. (1967). *Depression: Clinical, experimental, and theoretical aspects.* New York: Harper & Row.

Beck, A.T. (1976). *Cognitive therapy and the emotional disorders.* New York: International Universities Press.

Beck, A.T. (1986). Theoretical perspectives on clinical anxiety. In A.H. Tuma & J.D. Maser (Eds.), *Anxiety and the anxiety disorders* (pp. 183–196). Hillsdale, NJ: Erlbaum.

Beck, A.T. (1988). *Love is never enough.* New York: Harper & Row.

Beck, A.T. (1991). Cognitive therapy: A 30-year retrospective. *American Psychologist, 46*(4), 368–375.

Beck, A.T. (1993). Cognitive approaches to stress. In R. Woolfolk & P. Lehrer (Eds.), *Principles and practice of stress management* (2nd ed.) (pp. 333–372). New York: Guilford.

Beck, A.T., & Emery, G. (with Greenberg, R.L.). (1985). *Anxiety disorders and phobias: A cognitive perspective.* New York: Basic Books.

Beck, A.T., Epstein, N., Brown, G., & Steer, R.A. (1988). An inventory for measuring clinical anxiety: Psychometric properties. *Journal of Consulting and Clinical Psychology, 56*(6), 893–897.

Beck, A.T., Epstein, N., & Harrison, R. (1983). Cognitions, attitudes and personality dimensions in depression. *British Journal of Cognitive Psychotherapy, 1*(1), 1–16.

Beck, A.T., Freeman, A., & Associates. (1990). *Cognitive therapy of personality disorders.* New York: Guilford.

Beck, A.T., Rush, A.J., Shaw, B.F., & Emery, G. (1979). *Cognitive therapy of depression.* New York: Guilford.

Beck, A.T., & Steer, R.A. (1990). A reply to Tomasson: Hopelessness as a predictor of suicide [Letter to the editor]. *American Journal of Psychiatry, 147*(11), 1577–1578.

Beck, A.T., Steer, R.A., Kovacs, M., & Garrison, B. (1985). Hopelessness and eventual suicide: A 10-year prospective study of patients hospitalized with suicidal ideation. *American Journal of Psychiatry, 42*(5), 559–563.

Beck, A.T., Ward, C.H., Mendelson, M., Mock, J., & Erbaugh, J. (1961). An inventory for measuring depression. *Archives of General Psychiatry, 4,* 561–571.

Beck, A.T., Weissman, A., Lester, D., & Trexler, L. (1974). The measurement of pessimism: The hopelessness scale. *Journal of Consulting and Clinical Psychology, 42*(6), 861–865.

Beck, A.T., Wright, F.D., & Newman, C.F. (1992). Cocaine abuse. In A. Freeman & F. Dattilio (Eds.), *Comprehensive casebook of cognitive therapy* (pp. 185–192). New York: Plenum.

Beck, J. S. (in press). *Cognitive therapy: Basics and beyond.* New York: Guilford.

Beeder, A.B., & Millman, R.B. (1992). Treatment of patients with psychopathology and substance abuse. In J.H. Lowinson, P. Ruiz, R.B. Millman, & J.G. Langrod (Eds.), *Substance abuse: A comprehensive textbook* (2nd ed.) (pp. 675–690). Baltimore, MD: Williams & Wilkins.

Bernstein, D.A., & Borkovec, T.D. (1973). *Progressive relaxation training.* Champaign, IL: Research Press.

Blackburn, I.M., & Davidson, K.M. (1990). *Cognitive therapy for depression and anxiety: A practitioner's guide.* Oxford, England: Blackwell Scientific.

Blane, H.T., & Leonard, K.E. (1987). *Psychological theories of drinking and alcoholism.* New York: Guilford.

Brecher, E.M. (1972). *Licit and illicit drugs: The Consumers Union report on narcotics, stimulants, depressants, inhalants, hallucinogens, and marijuana—including caffeine, nicotine, and alcohol.* Boston: Little, Brown.

Brown, S.A., Goldman, M.S., Inn, A., & Anderson, L.R. (1980). Expectations of reinforcement from alcohol: Their domain and relation to drinking patterns. *Journal of Consulting and Clinical Psychology, 48,* 419–426.

Brown, V.B., Ridgely, M.S., Pepper, B., Levine, I.S., & Ryglewicz, H. (1989). The dual crisis: Mental illness and substance abuse. *American Psychologist, 44*(3), 565–569.

Brownell, K.D., Marlatt, G.A., Lichtenstein, E., & Wilson, G.T. (1986). Understanding and preventing relapse. *American Psychologist, 41*(7), 765–782.

Bunt, G., Galanter, M., Lifshutz, H., & Castaneda, R. (1990). Cocaine/"crack" dependence among psychiatric inpatients. *American Journal of Psychiatry, 147*(11), 1542–1546.

Burling, T.A., Reilly, P.M., Moltzen, J.O., & Ziff, D.C. (1989). Self-efficacy and relapse among inpatient drug and alcohol abusers: A predictor of outcome. *Journal of Studies on Alcohol, 50,* 354–360.

Burns, D.D. (1980). *Feeling good: The new mood therapy.* New York: William Morrow.

Burns, D.D., & Auerbach, A.H. (1992). Does homework compliance enhance recovery from depression? *Psychiatric Annals, 22,* 464–469.

Burns, D.D., & Nolen-Hoeksema, S. (1991). Coping styles, homework compliance, and the effectiveness of cognitive-behavioral therapy. *Journal of Consulting and Clinical Psychology, 59,* 305–311.

Cameron, D.C. (1968). Youth and drugs. *Journal of the American Medical Association, 206*(6), 1267–1271.

Carey, K.B. (1991). Research with dual diagnosis patients: Challenges and recommendations. *Behavior Therapist, 14,* 5–8.

Carroll, K.M. (1992). Psychotherapy for cocaine abuse: Approaches, evidence, and conceptual models. In T.R. Kosten & H.D. Kleber (Eds.), *Clinician's guide to cocaine addiction: Theory, research, and treatment* (pp. 290–313). New York: Guilford.

Carroll, K.M., Rounsaville, B.J., & Gawin, F.H. (1991). A comparative trial of psychotherapies for ambulatory cocaine abusers: Relapse prevention and interpersonal psychotherapy. *American Journal of Drug and Alcohol Abuse, 17,* 229–247.

Carroll, K.M., Rounsaville, B.J., & Keller, D.S. (1991). Relapse prevention strategies for the treatment of cocaine abuse. *American Journal of Drug and Alcohol Abuse, 17,* 249–265.

Castaneda, R., Galanter, M., & Franco, H. (1989). Self-medication among addicts with primary psychiatric disorders. *Comprehensive Psychiatry, 30,* 80–83.

Centers for Disease Control. (1991a). Smoking-attributable mortality and years of potential life lost: United States, 1988. *Morbidity and Mortality Weekly Report, 40,* 62–71.

Centers for Disease Control. (1991b). Cigarette smoking among adults: United States, 1988. *Morbidity and Mortality Weekly Report, 40,* 757–765.

Chiasson, R.E., Bacchetti, P., Osmond, D., Moss, A., Onishi, R., & Carlson, J. (1989). Cocaine use and HIV infection in intravenous drug users in the United States. *Journal of the American Medical Association, 261,* 2677–2684.

Chiauzzi, E.J. (1991). *Preventing relapse in the addictions.* New York: Pergamon.

Childress, A.R., Hole, A.V., & DePhilippis, D. (1990). *The coping with craving program: Active tools for reducing the craving/arousal to drug-related cues.* Unpublished treatment manual. Philadelphia, PA: Addiction Research Center, University of Pennsylvania.

Clark, D.M., Salkovskis, P.M., & Chalkley, A.J. (1985). Respiratory control as a treatment for panic attacks. *Journal of Behavioral Therapy and Experimental Psychiatry, 16,* 23–30.

Clayton, R.R. (1992). Transitions in drug use: Risk and protective factors. In M.D. Glantz & R.W. Pickens (Eds.), *Vulnerability to drug abuse* (pp. 15–52). Washington, DC: American Psychological Association.

Closser, M.H. (1992). Cocaine epidemiology. In T.R. Kosten & H.D. Kleber (Eds.), *Clinician's guide to cocaine addiction: Theory, research, and treatment* (pp. 225–240). New York: Guilford.

Cohen, S. (1991). Causes of the cocaine outbreak. In A.M. Washton & M.S. Gold (Eds.), *Cocaine: A clinician's handbook* (pp. 3–9). New York: Guilford.

Collner, D., & Ross, S. (1978). The assessment and training of assertiveness skills with drug addicts: A preliminary study. *International Journal of the Addictions, 13,* 227–239.

Covi, L., Baker, C.D., & Hess, J.M. (1990). *An integrated interpersonal/cognitive-behavioral counseling approach to cocaine abuse.* Unpublished treatment manual. Baltimore, MD: National Institute on Drug Abuse, Addiction Research Center.

Cummings, C., Gordon, J.R., & Marlatt, G.A. (1980). Relapse: Prevention and prediction. In W.R. Miller (Ed.), *The addictive behaviors: Treatment of alcoholism, drug abuse, smoking, and obesity* (pp. 291–321). New York: Pergamon.

Cummings, N.A. (1993). Psychotherapy with substance abusers. In G. Stricker & J. R. Gold (Eds.), *Comprehensive handbook of psychotherapy integration* (pp. 337–352). New York: Plenum.

Current disease model of addiction is overstated, expert suggests. (1992, March 6). *Psychiatric News,* pp. 13–21.

Davis, D.I. (1984). Differences in the use of substances of abuse by psychiatric patients compared with medical and surgical patients. *Journal of Nervous and Mental Disease, 172*(11), 654–657.

Doren, D.M. (1987). *Understanding and treating the psychopath.* New York: Wiley.

Drake, R.E., & Vaillant, G.E. (1985). A validity study of Axis II of DSM-III. *American Journal of Psychiatry, 142*(5), 553–558.

D'Zurilla, T.J., & Goldfried, M.R. (1971). Problem-solving and behavior modification. *Journal of Abnormal Psychology, 78*, 107–126.

Ellis, A. (1962). *Reason and emotion in psychotherapy.* New York: Lyle Stuart.

Ellis, A., McInerney, J.F., DiGiuseppe, R., & Yeager, R.J. (1988). *Rational-emotive therapy with alcoholics and substance abusers.* New York: Pergamon.

Estroff, T.W. (1987). Medical and biological consequences of cocaine abuse. In A.M. Washton & M.S. Gold (Eds.), *Cocaine: A clinician's handbook* (pp. 23–32). New York: Guilford.

Evans, K., & Sullivan, J.M. (1990). *Dual diagnosis: Counseling the mentally ill substance abuser.* New York: Guilford.

Fingarette, H. (1988). *Heavy drinking.* Berkeley: University of California Press.

Fishman, B. (1992). *Stress prevention training after HIV antibody testing: A trainer's manual.* Unpublished manuscript, Cornell University Medical College, New School for Social Research and Testing and Counseling Center, New York.

Frances, R.J., & Miller, S.I. (1991). Addiction treatment: The widening scope. In R.J. Frances & S.I. Miller (Eds.), *Clinical textbook of addictive disorders* (pp. 3–22). New York: Guilford.

Frances, R.J., & Miller, S.I. (Eds.). (1991). *Clinical textbook of addictive disorders.* New York: Guilford.

Fullilove, R.E., Fullilove, M.T., Bowser, B.F., & Gross, S.A. (1990). Risk of sexually transmitted disease among black adolescent crack users in Oakland and San Francisco, California. *Journal of the American Medical Association, 263*, 851–857.

Galanter, M. (1993, January). Psychotherapy for substance abuse; interestingly, it's at the cutting edge. *Newsletter, the American Academy of Psychiatrists in Alcoholism and Addictions*, pp. 1–2.

Gawin, F.G., & Ellinwood, E.H. (1988). Cocaine and other stimulants: Actions, abuse, and treatment. *New England Journal of Medicine, 318*(18), 1173–1182.

Gawin, F.H., & Kleber, H.D. (1986). Abstinence symptomatology and psychiatric diagnosis in cocaine abusers. *Archives of General Psychiatry, 43*, 107–113.

Gawin, F.H., & Kleber, H.D. (1988). Evolving conceptualizations of cocaine dependence. *Yale Journal of Biology and Medicine, 61*, 123–136.

Gawin, F.H., & Kleber, H.D. (1992). Evolving conceptualizations of cocaine dependence. In T.R. Kosten & H.D. Kleber (Eds.), *Clinician's guide to cocaine addiction* (pp. 33–52). New York: Guilford.

Glantz, M., & Pickens, R. (Eds.) (1992). *Vulnerability to drug abuse.* Washington, DC: American Psychological Association.

Goldsmith, M.F. (1988). Sex tied to drugs = STD spread. *Journal of the American Medical Association, 260*, 2009.

Gomberg, E.S.L., & Nirenberg, T.D. (1991). Women and substance abuse. *Journal of Substance Abuse, 3*, 255–267.

Goodwin, D.W. (1981). *Alcoholism: The facts*. New York: Oxford University Press.

Gorski, T.T., & Miller, M. (1982). *Counseling for relapse prevention*. Independence, MO: Herald House/Independence Press.

Gorski, T.T., & Miller, M. (1986). *Staying sober: A guide for relapse prevention*. Independence, MO: Herald House/Independence Press.

Grabowski, J., Stitzer, M.L., & Henningfield, J.E. (Eds.). (1984). *Behavioral techniques in drug abuse treatment*. (Research Monograph No. 46). Rockville, MD: National Institute on Drug Abuse.

Grande, T.P., Wolf, A.W., Schubert, D.S.P., Patterson, M.B., & Brocco, K. (1984). Associations among alcoholism, drug abuse, and antisocial personality: A review of the literature. *Psychological Reports, 55*, 455–474.

Grant, M. (1986). From contemplation to action: The role of the World Health Organization. In W.R. Miller & N. Heather (Eds.), *Treating addictive behaviors: Processes of change* (pp. 51–57). New York: Plenum.

Grossman, J., & Schottenfeld, R. (1992). Pregnancy and women's issues. In T.R. Kosten & H.D. Kleber (Eds.), *Clinician's guide to cocaine addiction: Theory, research, and treatment* (pp. 374–388). New York: Guilford.

Gunderson, J.G., & Zanarini, M.C. (1987). Current overview of the borderline diagnosis. *Journal of Clinical Psychiatry, 48*, 5–11.

Hall, S.M., Havassy, B.E., & Wasserman, D.A. (1991). Effects of commitment to abstinence, positive moods, stress, and coping on relapse to cocaine use. *Journal of Consulting and Clinical Psychology, 59*, 526–532.

Harstone, E., & Hansen, K.V. (1984). The violent juvenile offender. In R. Mathias, P. DeMuro, & R.S. Allinson (Eds.), *An anthology on violent juvenile offenders* (pp. 83–112). Newark, NJ: National Council on Crime and Delinquency.

Hatsukami, D., & Pickens, R.W. (1982). Posttreatment depression in an alcohol and drug abuse population. *American Journal of Psychiatry, 139*, 1563–1566.

Havassy, B.E., Hall, S.M., & Wasserman, D.A. (1991). Social support and relapse: Commonalities among alcoholics, opiate users, and cigarette smokers. *Addictive Behaviors, 16*, 235–246.

Heath, A.W., & Stanton, M.D. (1991). Family therapy. In R.J. Frances & S.I. Miller (Eds.), *Clinical textbook of addictive disorders* (pp. 406–430). New York: Guilford.

Heatherton, T.F., & Baumeister, R.F. (1991). Binge eating as an escape from self-awareness. *Psychological Bulletin, 110*, 86–108.

Helzer, J.E., & Pryzbeck, T.R. (1988). The co-occurrence of alcoholism with other psychiatric disorders in the general population and its impact on treatment. *Journal of Studies on Alcohol, 49*(3), 219–224.

Henningfield, J.E., Clayton, R., & Pollin, W. (1990). Involvement of tobacco in alcoholism and illicit drug use. *British Journal of Addiction, 85*, 279–291.

Hesselbrock, M.N., Meyer, R.E., & Kenner, J.J. (1985). Psychopathology in hospitalized alcoholics. *Archives of General Psychiatry, 42*, 1050–1055.

Hesselbrock, V.M., Hesselbrock, M.N., & Stabenau, J.R. (1985). Alcoholism in men patients subtyped by family history and antisocial personality. *Journal of Studies on Alcohol, 46*(1), 59–64.

Hollon, S.D., & Beck, A.T. (in press). Cognitive and cognitive-behavioral therapies. In A.E. Bergin & S.L. Garfield (Eds.), *Handbook of psychotherapy and behavior change: An empirical analysis* (4th ed.). New York: Wiley.

Horney, K. (1950). *Neurosis and human growth.* New York: W. W. Norton.

Horvath, A.T. (1988). Cognitive therapy and the addictions. *International Cognitive Therapy Newsletter, 4,* 6–7.

Horvath, A.T. (in press). Enhancing motivation for treatment of addictive behavior: Guidelines for the psychotherapist. *Psychotherapy: Theory, Research and Practice.*

Hudson, C.J. (1990). Anxiety disorders and substance abuse. In D.F. O'Connell (Ed.), *Managing the dually diagnosed patient: Current issues and clinical approaches* (pp. 119–316). New York: Haworth.

Hunt, W.A., Barnett, L.W., & Branch, L.G. (1971). Relapse rates in addiction programs. *Journal of Clinical Psychology, 27,* 455–456.

Institute of Medicine. (1987). *Causes and consequences of alcohol problems.* Washington, DC: National Academy Press.

Institute of Medicine. (1990a). *Broadening the base of treatment for alcohol problems.* Washington, DC: National Academy Press.

Institute of Medicine. (1990b). *Treating drug problems* (Vol. 1). Washington, DC: National Academy Press.

Jellinek, E.M. (1960). *The disease concept of alcoholism.* Highland Park, NJ: Hillhouse Press.

Jennings, P.S. (1991). To surrender drugs: A grief process in its own right. *Journal of Substance Abuse Treatment, 8,* 221–226.

Jones, R.T. (1987). Psychopharmacology of cocaine. In A.M. Washton & M.S. Gold (Eds.), *Cocaine: A clinician's handbook* (pp. 55–72). New York: Guilford.

Karan, L.D., Haller, D.L., & Schnoll, S.H. (1991). Cocaine. In R.J. Frances & S.J. Miller (Eds.), *Clinical textbook of addictive disorders* (pp. 121–145). New York: Guilford.

Khantzian, E.J. (1985). The self-medication hypothesis of addictive disorders: Focus on heroin and cocaine dependence. *American Journal of Psychiatry, 143,* 1259–1264.

Khantzian, E.J. (1988). The primary care therapist and patient needs in substance abuse treatment. *American Journal of Drug and Alcohol Abuse, 14,* 159–167.

Khantzian, E.J., & Treece, C. (1985). DSM-III psychiatric diagnosis of narcotic addicts: Recent findings. *Archives of General Psychiatry, 42,* 1067–1071.

Koenigsberg, H.W., Kaplan, R.D., Gilmore, M.M., & Cooper, A.M. (1985). The relationship between syndrome and personality disorder in DSM-III: Experience with 2,462 patients. *American Journal of Psychiatry, 142*(2), 207–212.

Kosten, T.R., & Kleber, H.D. (Eds.). (1992). *Clinician's guide to cocaine addiction.* New York: Guilford.

Kosten, T.R., Rounsaville, B.J., & Kleber, H.D. (1986). A 2.5 year follow-up of depression, life events, and treatment effects on abstinence among opioid addicts. *Archives of General Psychiatry, 43,* 733-738.

Kranzler, H.R., & Liebowitz, N.R. (1988). Anxiety and depression in substance abuse: Clinical implications. *Medical Clinics of North America, 72*(4), 867-886.

Kushner, M.G., Sher, K.J., & Beitman, B.D. (1990). The relation between alcohol problems and the anxiety disorders. *American Journal of Psychiatry, 147*(6), 685-695.

LaBounty, L.P., Hatsukami, D., Morgan, S.F., & Nelson, L. (1992). Relapse among alcoholics with phobic and panic symptoms. *Addictive Behaviors, 17,* 9-15.

Lang, A.R. (1992). Parental drinking and child behavior problems: A case of bidirectional influences? *The Behavior Therapist, 15,* 15-17.

Layden, M.A., Newman, C.F., Freeman, A., & Morse, S.B. (1993). *Cognitive therapy of borderline personality disorder.* Needham Heights, MA: Allyn & Bacon.

Levin, J.D. (1990). *Alcoholism: A bio-psycho-social approach.* New York: Hemisphere.

Lewis, C.E., Robins, L., & Rice, J. (1985). Association of alcoholism with antisocial personality in urban men. *Journal of Nervous and Mental Disease, 173,* 166-174.

Linehan, M.M. (1987). Dialectical behavior therapy for borderline personality disorder. *Bulletin of the Menninger Clinic, 5,* 261-276.

Lingswiler, V.M., Crowther, J.H., & Stephens, M.A.P. (1989). Affective and cognitive antecedents to eating episodes in bulimia and binge eating. *International Journal of Eating Disorders, 5,* 533-539.

Linnoila, M.I. (1989). Anxiety and alcoholism. *Journal of Clinical Psychiatry, 50*(Suppl. 11), 26-29.

Lyon, D., & Greenberg, J. (1991). Evidence of codependency in women with an alcoholic parent: Helping Mr. Wrong. *Journal of Personality and Social Psychology, 61,* 435-439.

Mackay, P.W., Donovan, D.M., & Marlatt, G.A. (1991). Cognitive and behavioral approaches to alcohol abuse. In R.J. Frances & S.I. Miller (Eds.), *Clinical textbook of addictive disorders* (pp. 452-481). New York: Guilford.

Mackay, P.W., & Marlatt, G.A. (1991). Maintaining sobriety: Stopping is starting. *International Journal of Addictions, 25,* 1257-1276.

Marlatt, G.A. (1978). Craving for alcohol, loss of control, and relapse: A cognitive-behavioral analysis. In P.E. Nathan, G.A. Marlatt, & T. Loberg (Eds.), *Alcoholism: New directions in behavioral research and treatment* (pp. 271-314). New York: Plenum.

Marlatt, G.A. (1982). Relapse prevention: A self-control program for the treatment of addictive behaviors. In R.B. Stuart (Ed.), *Adherence, compliance, and generalization in behavioral medicine* (pp. 329-378). New York: Brunner/Mazel.

Marlatt, G.A. (1983). The controlled-drinking controversy: A commentary. *American Psychologist, 38,* 1097-1110.

Marlatt, G.A. (1985). Cognitive factors in the relapse process. In G.A. Marlatt & J.R. Gordon (Eds.), *Relapse prevention: Maintenance strategies in the treatment of addictive behaviors* (pp. 128–200). New York: Guilford.

Marlatt, G.A., & Gordon, J.R. (1985). *Relapse prevention: Maintenance strategies in the treatment of addictive behaviors.* New York: Guilford Press.

Marzuk, P.M., Tardiff, K., Leon, A.C., Stagis, M., Morgan, E.R., & Mann, J.J. (1992). Prevalence of cocaine use among residents of New York City who committed suicide during a one-year period. *American Journal of Psychiatry, 149,* 371–375.

McCord, J. (1992). Another time, another drug. In M.D. Glantz & R.W. Pickens (Eds.), *Vulnerability to drug abuse* (pp. 473–490). Washington, DC: American Psychological Association.

McDermut, W., Haaga, D.A.F., & Shayne, V.T. (1991). Schemata and smoking relapse. *Behavior Therapy, 22,* 423–434.

McLellan, A.T., O'Brien, C.P., Metzger, D., Alterman, A.I., Cornish, J., & Urschel, H. (1991). How effective is substance abuse treatment—compared to what? In C.P. O'Brien & J.H. Jaffe (Eds.), *Understanding the addictive states* (pp. 231–252). New York: Raven Press.

Medical Letter on Drugs and Therapeutics. (1993). *35,* p. 5.

Mental Health Report. (1992, January 2). *Study shows cocaine use increased in 1991,* p. 5.

Metzger, D., Woody, G., DePhilippis, D., McLellan, A.T., O'Brien, C.P., & Platt, J.J. (1991). Risk factors for needle sharing among methadone-treated patients. *American Journal of Psychiatry, 148,* 101–105.

Miller, N.S. (1991). Special problems of the alcohol and multiple-drug dependent: Clinical interactions and detoxification. In R.J. Frances & S.I. Miller (Eds.), *Clinical textbook of addictive disorders* (pp. 194–218). New York: Guilford.

Miller, R.L. (1991). *The case for legalizing drugs.* New York: Praeger.

Miller, W.R., & Hester, R.K. (1980). Treating the problem drinker: Modern approaches. In W.R. Miller (Ed.), *The addictive behaviors: Treatment of alcoholism, drug abuse, smoking, and obesity* (pp. 11–141). Oxford, England: Pergamon.

Miller, W.R., & Hester, R.K. (1986). The effectiveness of alcoholism treatment: What research reveals. In W.R. Miller & N. Heather (Eds.), *Treating addictive behaviors: Process of change* (pp. 121–174). New York: Plenum.

Miller, W.R., & Munoz, R.F. (1976). *How to control your drinking.* Englewood Cliffs, NJ: Prentice-Hall.

Miller, W.R., & Rollnick, S. (1991). *Motivational interviewing.* New York: Guilford.

Mirin, S.M., & Weiss, R.D. (1991). Substance abuse and mental illness. In R.J. Frances & S.I. Miller (Eds.), *Clinical textbook of addictive disorders* (pp. 271–298). New York: Guilford.

Moorey, S. (1989). Drug abusers. In J. Scott, J.M.G. Williams, & A.T. Beck (Eds.), *Cognitive therapy in clinical practice: An illustrative casebook.* London: Routledge.

Mullaney, J.A., & Trippett, C.J. (1979). Alcohol dependence and phobias: Clinical description and relevance. *British Journal of Psychiatry, 135,* 565–573.

Musto, D.F. (1991). Opium, cocaine and marijuana in American history. *Scientific American, 265*(1), 40–47.

Nace, E.P., Davis, C.W., & Gaspari, J.P. (1991). Axis-II comorbidity in substance abusers. *American Journal of Psychiatry, 148,* 118–120.

Nace, E.P., & Isbell, P.G. (1991). Alcohol. In R.J. Frances & S.I. Miller (Eds.), *Clinical textbook of addictive disorders* (pp. 43–68). New York: Guilford.

Nace, E.P., Saxon, J.J., & Shore, N. (1983). A comparison of borderline and non-borderline alcoholic patients. *Archives of General Psychiatry, 40,* 54–56.

Nace, E.P., Saxon, J.J., & Shore, N. (1986). Borderline personality disorder and alcoholism treatment: A one-year follow-up study. *Journal of Studies on Alcohol, 47*(3), 196–200.

Nathan, P.E. (1988). The addictive personality is the behavior of the addict. *Journal of Consulting and Clinical Psychology, 56*(2), 183–188.

National Institute of Alcohol Abuse and Alcoholism (1990). *Seventh special report to the U.S. Congress on alcohol and health.* Rockville, MD: Author.

Newman, C.F. (1988). Confrontation and collaboration: Congruent components in cognitive therapy. *Cognitive Behaviorist, 10,* 27–30.

Newman, C.F. (1990). Therapy-threatening behaviors on the part of the cognitive-behavior therapist in the treatment of the borderline patient. *Behavior Therapist, 13,* 215–216.

Newman, C.F. (1993). The importance of between-sessions homework assignments in the cognitive therapy of depression. *Verhaltenstherapie und Psychosoziale Praxis, 25*(2), 205–224.

Newman, C.F., & Beck, A.T. (1990). Cognitive therapy of the affective disorders. In B.B. Wolman & G. Stricker (Eds.), *Handbook of affective disorders: Facts, theories, and treatment approaches* (pp. 343–367). New York: Wiley.

Newman, C.F., & Haaga, D.A.F. (in press). Cognitive skills training. In W. O'Donohue & L. Krasner (Eds.), *Handbook of psychological skills training.* Needham Heights, MA: Allyn & Bacon.

Newman, C.F., & Wright, F.D. (in press). Crisis intervention with substance abusing patients. In F. Dattilio & A. Freeman (Eds.), *Cognitive-behavior therapy and crisis intervention.* New York: Plenum.

Nezu, A.M., Nezu, C.M., & Perri, M.G. (1989). *Problem-solving therapy for depression: Theory, research, and clinical guidelines.* New York: Wiley.

O'Brien, C.P. (1992). Conditioned responses, craving, relapse, and addiction. *Facts About Drugs and Alcohol, 1,* 1–3.

O'Brien, C.P., McLellan, A.T., Alterman, A., & Childress, A.R. (1992). *Psychotherapy for cocaine dependence. Cocaine: Scientific and social dimensions* (Ciba Foundation Symposium 166). Chichester, England: Wiley.

O'Connell, D.F. (Ed.) (1990). *Managing the dually diagnosed patient: Current issues and clinical approaches.* Cambridge, MA: Haworth.

O'Connor, P.G., Chang, G., & Shi, J. (1992). Medical complications of cocaine use. In T.R. Kosten & H.D. Kleber (Eds.), *Clinician's guide to cocaine addiction: Theory, research, and treatment* (pp. 241–272). New York: Guilford.

Ola, P., & D'Aulaire, E. (1991). Cocaine: The devil within. *Reader's Digest*, *138*, 51–58.

Overholser, J.C. (1987). Facilitating autonomy in passive-dependent persons: An integrative model. *Journal of Contemporary Psychotherapy*, *17*(4), 250–269.

Overholser, J.C. (1988). Clinical utility of the Socratic method. In C. Stout (Ed.), *Annals of clinical research* (pp. 1–7). Des Plaines, IL: Forest Institute.

Peele, S. (1985). *The meaning of addiction: Compulsive experience and its interpretation*. Lexington, MA: Lexington Books.

Peele, S. (1989). *Diseasing of America: Addiction treatment out of control*. Lexington, MA: Heath.

Peele, S., Brodsky, A., with Arnold, M. (1991). *The truth about addiction and recovery: The life process program for outgrowing destructive habits*. New York: Simon & Schuster.

Penick, E.C., Powell, B.J., Othmer, E., Bingham, S.F., Rice, A.S., & Liese, B.S. (1984). Subtyping alcoholics by coexisting psychiatric syndromes: Course, family history, outcome. In D.W. Goodwin, K.T. VanDusen, & S.A. Mednick (Eds.), *Longitudinal research in alcoholism* (pp. 167–196). Boston: Kluwer-Nijhoff.

Perez, J.F. (1992). *Alcoholism: Causes, effects, and treatment*. Muncie, IN: Accelerated Development.

Persons, J.B. (1989). *Cognitive therapy in practice: A case formulation approach*. New York: W. W. Norton.

Persons, J.B., Burns, D.D., & Perloff, J.M. (1988). Predictors of drop-out and outcome in cognitive therapy for depression in a private practice setting. *Cognitive Therapy and Research*, *12*, 557–575.

Pierce, J.P., Fiore, M.C., & Novotny, T.E. (1989). Trends in cigarette smoking in the United States: Projections to the year 2000. *Journal of the American Medical Association*, *261*, 61–65.

Platt, J.J., & Hermalin, J. (1989). Social skill deficit interventions for substance absuers. *Psychology of Addictive Behaviors*, *3*, 114–133.

Prochaska, J.O., & DiClemente, C.C. (1986). Toward a comprehensive model of change. In W.R. Miller & N. Heather (Eds.), *Treating addictive behaviors: Processes of change* (pp. 3–27). New York: Plenum.

Prochaska, J.O., DiClemente, C.C., & Norcross, J.C. (1992). In search of how people change: Applications to addictive behaviors. *American Psychologist*, *47*, 1102–1114.

Prochnow, H.Z. (1969). *Treasury of humorous quotations*. New York: Harper & Row.

Quitkin, F.M., Rifkin, A., Kaplan, J., & Klein, D.F. (1972). Phobic anxiety syndrome complicated by drug dependence and addiction: A treatable form of drug abuse. *Archives of General Psychiatry*, *27*, 159–162.

Rawson, R.A., Obert, J.L., McCann, M.J., Smith, D.P., & Ling, W. (1990). Neurobehavioral treatment for cocaine dependency. *Journal of Psychoactive Drugs*, *22*, 159–171.

Regier, D.A., Boyd, J.H., Burke, J.D., Rae, D.S., Myers, J.K., Kramer, M., Robins, L.M., George, L.K., Karno, M., & Locke, B.Z. (1988). One-month prevalence of mental disorders in the United States. *Archives of General Psychiatry, 45*, 977–986.

Regier, D.A., Farmer, M.E., Rae, D.S., Locke, B.Z., Keith, S.J., Judd, L.L., & Goodwin, F.K. (1990). Comorbidity of mental disorders with alcohol and other drug abuse: Results from the Epidemiological Catchment Area (ECA) study. *Journal of the American Medical Association, 264*(19), 2511–2518.

Robins, L.N., Davis, D.H., & Goodwin, D.W. (1974). Drug use by U.S. army enlisted men in Vietnam: A follow-up on their return home. *American Journal of Epidemiology, 99*, 235–249.

Ross, H.E., Glaser, F.B., & Germanson, T. (1988). The prevalence of psychiatric disorders in patients with alcohol and other drug problems. *Archives of General Psychiatry, 45*, 1023–1031.

Rounsaville, B.J., Anton, S.F., Carroll, K., Budde, D., Prusoff, B.A., & Gawin, F. (1991). Psychiatric diagnoses of treatment-seeking cocaine abusers. *Archives of General Psychiatry, 48*, 43–51.

Rounsaville, B.J., & Kleber, H.D. (1986). Psychiatric disorders in opiate addicts: Preliminary findings on the course and interaction with program type. In R.E. Meyer (Ed.), *Psychopathology and addictive disorders* (pp. 140–168). New York: Guilford.

Rush, B. (1790). *An inquiry into the effects of spirituous liquors on the human body*. Boston: Thomas & Andrews.

Saunders, B., & Allsop, S. (1987). Relapse: A psychological perspective. *British Journal of Addiction, 82*, 417–429.

Schneier, F.R., & Siris, S.G. (1987). A review of psychoactive substance use and abuse in schizophrenia: Patterns of drug choice. *Journal of Nervous and Mental Disease, 175*(11), 641–652.

Schuckit, M.A. (1985). The clinical implications of primary diagnostic groups among alcoholics. *Archives of General Psychiatry, 42*, 1043–1049.

Schwartz, J.L. (1987). *Review and evaluation of smoking cessation methods: The United States and Canada, 1978–1985* (NIH Publication No. 87-2940). Washington, DC: U.S. Government Printing Office.

Shiffman, S. (1992). Relapse process and relapse prevention in addictive behaviors. *Behavior Therapist, 15*, 9–11.

Shulman, G.D. (1989). Experience with the cocaine trigger inventory. *Advances in Alcohol and Substance Abuse, 8*, 71–85.

Smart, R.G. (1991). Crack cocaine use: A review of prevalence and adverse effects. *American Journal of Drug and Alcohol Abuse, 17*, 13–26.

Smart, R.G., & Adlaf, E.M. (1990). Trends in treatment admissions for cocaine and other drug abusers. *Canadian Journal of Psychiatry, 35*(7), 621–623.

Smart, R.G., Murray, G.F., & Arif, A. (1988). Drug abuse and prevention programs in 29 countries. *International Journal of the Addictions, 23*(1), 1–17.

Sobell, L.C., Sobell, M.B., & Nirenberg, T.D. (1988). Behavioral assessment and treatment planning with alcohol and drug abusers: A review with an emphasis on clinical application. *Clinical Psychology Review, 8,* 19–54.

Sobell, M.B., Sobell, L.C., Bogardis, J., Leo, G.I., & Skinner, W. (1992). Problem drinkers' perceptions of whether treatment goals should be self-selected or therapist selected. *Behavior Therapy, 23,* 43–52.

Spitzer, R.L., Williams, J.B.W., & Gibbon, M. (1987). *Instruction manual for the Structured Clinical Interview for the DSM-III-R (SCID).* New York: New York State Psychiatric Institute.

Stabenau, J.R. (1984). Implications of family history of alcoholism, antisocial personality, and sex differences in alcohol dependence. *American Journal of Psychiatry, 141*(10), 1178–1182.

Stacy, A.W., Newcomb, M.D., & Bentler, P.M. (1991). Cognitive motivation and drug use: A 9-year longitudinal study. *Journal of Abnormal Psychology, 100*(4), 501–515.

Stimmel, B. (1991). *The facts about drug use: Coping with drugs and alcohol in your family, at work, in your community.* New York: Consumer Reports Books.

Stine, S.M. (1992). Cocaine abuse within methadone maintenance programs. In T.R. Kosten & H.D. Kleber (Eds.), *Clinician's guide to cocaine addiction: Theory, research, and treatment* (pp. 359–373). New York: Guilford.

Stitzer, M.L., Grabowski, J., & Henningfield, J.E. (1984). Behavioral interventions in drug abuse treatment. In J. Grabowski, M.L. Stitzer, & J.E. Henningfield (Eds.), *Behavioral techniques in drug abuse treatment* (Research Monograph No. 46). Rockville, MD: National Institute on Drug Abuse.

Tarter, R.E., Ott, P.J., & Mezzich, A.C. (1991). Psychometric assessment. In R.J. Frances & S.I. Miller (Eds.), *Clinical textbook of addictive disorders* (pp. 237–267). New York: Guilford.

Thomason, H.H., & Dilts, S.L. (1991). Opioids. In R.J. Frances & S.I. Miller (Eds.), *Clinical textbook of addictive disorders* (pp. 103–120). New York: Guilford.

Tiffany, S.T. (1990). A cognitive model of drug urges and drug-use behavior: Role of automatic and non-automatic processes. *Psychological Review, 97,* 147–168.

Tucker, J.A., & Sobell, L.C. (1992). Influences on help-seeking for drinking problems and on natural recovery without treatment. *Behavior Therapist, 15,* 12–14.

Vaillant, G.E. (1983). *The natural history of alcoholism: Causes, patterns, and paths to recovery.* Cambridge, MA: Harvard University Press.

Velten, E. (1986). Withdrawal from heroin and methadone with rational-emotive therapy: Practice and theory. *British Journal of Cognitive Psychotherapy, 4,* 19–24.

Walfish, S., Massey, R., & Krone, A. (1990). Anxiety and anger among abusers of different substances. *Drug and Alcohol Dependence, 25,* 253–256.

Washton, A.M. (1988). Preventing relapse to cocaine. *Journal of Clinical Psychiatry, 49,* 34–38.

Watkins, K., Metzger, D., Woody, G., & McLellan, A.T. (1991, April). *The sexual behaviors of intravenous drug users: Implications for the spread of HIV infection.* Paper presented at the University of Pennsylvania Department of Psychiatry Research Retreat, Philadelphia, PA.

Weiner, H., & Fox, S. (1982). Cognitive-behavioral therapy with substance abusers. *Social Casework, 63,* 564–567.

Weinstein, S.P., Gottheil, E., & Sterling, R.C. (1992). Cocaine users in medical practice: A five-year follow-up. *American Journal of Drug and Alcohol Abuse, 18,* 157–166.

Weiss, C.J., & Millman, R.B. (1991). Hallucinogens, phencyclidine, marijuana, inhalants. In R.J. Frances & S.I. Miller (Eds.), *Clinical textbook of addictive disorders* (pp. 146–170). New York: Guilford.

Weiss, R.D. (1992). The role of psychopathology in the transition from drug use to abuse and dependence. In M.D. Glantz & R.W. Pickens (Eds.), *Vulnerability to drug abuse* (pp. 137–148). Washington, DC: American Psychological Association.

Weissman, A.N., & Beck, A.T. (1978). *Development and validation of the Dysfunctional Attitudes Scale: A preliminary investigation.* Paper presented at the Annual Meeting of the American Educational Research Association, Toronto, Canada.

Westermeyer, J. (1991). Historical and social context of psychoactive substance disorders. In R.J. Frances & S.I. Miller (Eds.), *Clinical textbook of addictive disorders* (pp. 23–40). New York: Guilford.

Wills, T.A., & Shiffman, S. (1985). Coping and substance use: Conceptual framework. In S. Shiffman & T.A. Wills, (Eds.), *Coping and substance use* (pp. 3–24). New York: Academic Press.

Wilson, G.T. (1987a). Cognitive studies in alcoholism. *Journal of Consulting and Clinical Psychology, 55*(3), 325–331.

Wilson, G.T. (1987b). Cognitive processes in addiction. *British Journal of Addiction, 82,* 343–353.

Wilson, G.T. (1988). Alcohol and anxiety. *Behavioral Research and Therapy, 26*(5), 369–381.

Wolf, A.W., Schubert, D.S.P., Patterson, M.B., Grande, T.P., Brocco, K.J., & Pendleton, L. (1988). Associations among major psychiatric diagnoses. *Journal of Consulting and Clinical Psychology, 56*(2), 292–294.

Woody, G.E., Luborsky. L., McLellan, A.T., O'Brien, C.P., Beck, A.T., Blaine, J., Herman, I., & Hole, A. (1983). Psychotherapy for opiate addicts: Does it help? *Archives of General Psychiatry, 40,* 1081–1086.

Woody, G.E., McLellan, A.T., & O'Brien, C.P. (1990). Research on psychopathology and addiction: Treatment implications. *Drug and Alcohol Dependence, 25,* 121–123.

Woody, G.E., Urschel, H.C. III, & Alterman, A. (1992). The many paths to drug dependence. In M.D. Glantz & R.W. Pickens (Eds.), *Vulnerability to drug abuse* (pp. 491–507). Washington DC: American Psychological Association.

Young, J.E. (1990). *Cognitive therapy for personality disorders: A schema-focused approach.* Sarasota FL: Professional Resource Exchange.

Zanarini, M.C., Gunderson, J.G., & Frankenburg, F.R. (1989). Axis I phenomenology of borderline personality disorder. *Comprehensive Psychiatry*, *30*(2), 149–156.

Ziedonis, D.M. (1992). Comorbid psychopathology and cocaine addiction. In T.R. Kosten & H.D. Kleber (Eds.), *Clinician's guide to cocaine addiction: Theory, research, and treatment* (pp. 335–358). New York: Guilford.

Zotter, D.L., & Crowther, J.H. (1991). The role of cognitions in bulimia nervosa. *Cognitive Therapy and Research*, *15*, 413–426.

Zung, W.W.K. (1986). Prevalence of clinically significant anxiety in a family practice setting. *American Journal of Psychiatry*, *143*(11), 1471–1472.

Author Index

Abrams, D.B., 13
Adlaf, E.M., 7
Alberti, R.E., 254, 264, 286
Allsop, S., 292
Alterman, A.I., 7, 51, 236, 273, 281
Amaro, H., 196, 220, 252
Ananth, J., 10
Anderson, L.R., 33
Annis, H.M., 157
Arif, A., 3
Arnold, M., 4
Auerbach, A.H., 109, 136, 185

Babor, T.F., 3
Baker, C.D., 7
Baker, T.B., 12
Bandura, A., 13, 33
Barnett, L.W., 10, 11
Baumeister, R.F., 38
Beck, A.T., 10, 14, 27, 35, 42, 48, 49, 50,
    51, 52, 69, 82, 93, 94, 95, 100, 135,
    140, 143, 169, 173, 226, 227, 230,
    234, 244, 252, 258, 269, 273, 276,
    289, 290, 291, 327
Beck, J.S., 86
Beeder, A.B., 257
Beitman, B.D., 257
Bentler, P.M., 13
Bernstein, D.A., 168, 264
Blackburn, I.M., 108
Blane, H.T., 12
Bogardis, J., 16
Borkovec, T.D., 168, 264
Bowser, B.F., 209
Branch, L.G., 10, 11
Brecher, E.M., 3, 5, 6
Brocco, K.J., 268
Brodsky, A., 4

Brown, G., 94
Brown, S.A., 33
Brown, V.B., 10, 268
Brownell, K.D., 11
Bunt, G., 10
Burling, T.A., 228
Burns, D.D., 109, 117, 136, 143, 185, 327

Cabral, H., 196
Cacciola, J.S., 236, 281
Cameron, D.C., 3
Carey, K.B., 187, 270, 272
Carroll, K.M., 30, 32, 57, 124, 152, 154,
    157, 298, 299, 300, 301, 302, 307,
    315
Castaneda, R., 10, 27, 59, 152, 158
Chalkley, A.J., 264
Chang, G., 206
Chiasson, R.E., 209
Chiauzzi, E.J., 11
Childress, A.R., 50, 51, 52, 157, 159, 302
Clark, D.M., 264
Clayton, R.R., 5, 9
Closser, M.H., 197, 208
Cohen, S., 7
Collner, D., 254, 264, 286
Cooper, A.M., 269
Covi, L., 7, 55, 124, 157
Crowther, J.H., 38
Cummings, C., 308
Cummings, N.A., 216, 271, 280

D'Aulaire, E., 7
Davidson, K.M., 108
Davis, C.W., 27
Davis, D.H., 24
Davis, D.I., 10
DePhilippis, D., 50

346

Subject Index